Practical
Gastroenterology

Practical Gastroenterology

Editor

V Balakrishnan
MD, DM, FACG, FAMS
Professor of Gastroenterology
Amrita Institute of Medical Sciences and
Research Centre, Cochin, Kerala
India

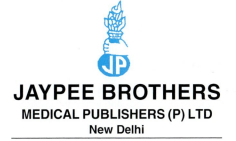

JAYPEE BROTHERS
MEDICAL PUBLISHERS (P) LTD
New Delhi

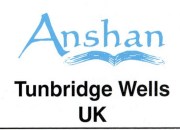

Tunbridge Wells
UK

First published in the UK by

Anshan Ltd
in 2007
6 Newlands Road
Tunbridge Wells
Kent TN4 9AT, UK

Tel: +44 (0)1892 557767
Fax: +44 (0)1892 530358
E-mail: info@anshan.co.uk
www.anshan.co.uk

ISBN 10 1-905740-58-1
ISBN 13 978-1-905740-58-1

British Library Cataloguing in Publication Data
A catalogue record for this book is available from the British Library

Printed in India by Ajanta Offset & Packagings Ltd., New Delhi

Contributors

Anil John, MD, DM (Gastro), DNB (Gastro)
Associate Professor of Gastroenterology
Amrita Institute of Medical Sciences,
Cochin, Kerala, India

Balakrishnan V, MD, DM, FACG, FAMS
Professor of Gastroenterology
Amrita Institute of Medical Sciences,
Cochin, Kerala, India

Deepak Suvarna, MD
DNB Trainee in Gastroenterology
Amrita Institute of Medical Sciences,
Cochin, Kerala, India

Elango EM, MSc, PhD
HOD, Department of Molecular Biology
Amrita Institute of Medical Sciences,
Cochin, Kerala, India

George Thomas, MD, DM
Consultant Gastroenterologist
Pushpagiri Medical College & Hospital
Thiruvalla, Kerala, India

Jose V Francis, MD, DM
Consultant Gastroenterologist
Lakeshore Hospital, Cochin, Kerala
India

Madhu S Menon, MBBS
Resident in Gastroenterology
Amrita Institute of Medical Sciences,
Cochin, Kerala, India

Mathew Philip, MD, DM (Gastro), DNB
(Med), DNB (Gastro)
Senior Consultant Gastroenterologist
Lakeshore Hospital, Cochin, Kerala,
India

Musthafa CP, MD, MRCP
Assistant Professor in Gastroenterology
Amrita Institute of Medical Sciences,
Cochin, Kerala, India

Nandakumar R, MD, DM (Gastro),
DNB (Med), DNB (Gastro)
Assistant Professor in Gastroenterology
Amrita Institute of Medical Sciences,
Cochin, Kerala, India

Narayanan VA, MD, DM
Professor and HOD of Gastroenterology
Amrita Institute of Medical Sciences,
Cochin, Kerala, India

Narendranathan M, MD, DM, MPH
Senior Consultant Gastroenterologist
KIMS and Cosmopolitan Hospitals
Thiruvananthapuram, Kerala, India

Padmanabhan TK, MD
Professor and HOD of Radiation Oncology
Amrita Institute of Medical Sciences,
Cochin, Kerala, India

Padma S Sundaram, MBBS, DRM
Consultant, Dept of Nuclear Medicine
Amrita Institute of Medical Sciences,
Cochin, Kerala, India

Pavithran K, MD, DM (Med Oncology)
Consultant, Department of Medical
Oncology, Amrita Institute of Medical
Sciences, Cochin, Kerala, India

Philip Augustine, MD, DM
HOD of Gastroenterology and Medical
Director
Lakeshore Hospital, Cochin, Kerala,
India

Prakash Zacharias, MD, DM
HOD of Gastroenterology
Malabar Institute of Medical Sciences,
Calicut, Kerala, India

Prem Nair
       MD, Dip AB (Med), Dip AB (Gastro)
Gastroenterologist and Medical Director
Amrita Institute of Medical Sciences,
Cochin, Kerala, India

Raj VV, MD, DM
Consultant Gastroenterologist
Manipal Hospital, Bangalore
Karnataka, India

Rajeendranath T, MD, DM
Senior Consultant Gastroenterologist
Baby Memorial Hospital, Calicut,
Kerala, India

Rajesh G, MD
DNB Trainee in Gastroenterology
Amrita Institute of Medical Sciences,
Cochin, Kerala, India

Rajiv Mehta, MD, DNB (Gastro)
Assistant Professor in Gastroenterology
Amrita Institute of Medical Sciences,
Cochin, Kerala, India

Ramachandran TM, MD, DM
Assistant Professor in Gastroenterology
Medical College Hospital, Calicut,
Kerala, India

Ramesh GN, MD, DM
Senior Consultant in Gastroenterology
Lakeshore Hospital, Cochin, Kerala,
India

Ramesh H, MS, MCh, FACS
HOD, Surgical Gastroenterology
Lakeshore Hospital, Cochin, Kerala,
India

Saju Xavier, MD, DM
Consultant Gastroenterologist
Al-Shifa Hospital, Perinthalmanna,
Kerala, India

Shanmuga Sundaram P,
 MBBS, DRM, DNB (Nuclear Med) MNAMS
HOD, Department of Nuclear Medicine
Amrita Institute of Medical Sciences
Cochin, Kerala, India

Shine Sadasivan, MD, DNB (Gastro)
Assistant Professor in Gastroenterology
Amrita Institute of Medical Sciences,
Cochin, Kerala, India

Sobhana Devi R, MD, DM
Professor and HOD of Gastroenterology
Medical College Hospital, Kottayam,
Kerala, India

Srikanth Moorthy, MD, PDDC
HOD, Department of Radiology and
Imaging Services
Amrita Institute of Medical Sciences,
Cochin, Kerala, India

Sreekumar KP, MD
Consultant, Department of Radiology
and Imaging Services
Amrita Institute of Medical Sciences,
Cochin, Kerala, India

Subhalal N, MS, MCh, FACS
Professor of Surgical Gastroenterology
Medical College Hospital
Thiruvananthapuram, Kerala, India

Sudhindran S, MS, FRCS,
HOD, Department of Gastrointestinal
Surgery
Amrita Institute of Medical Sciences,
Cochin, Kerala, India

Sudheer K, MD
Professor of Radiology
Pushpagiri Medical College & Hospital,
Thiruvalla, Kerala, India

Sudheer OV, MS, MCh
Consultant GI Surgeon
Amrita Institute of Medical Sciences,
Cochin, Kerala, India

Sunil Mathai, MD, DM
Senior Consultant Gastroenterologist
Medical Trust Hospital, Cochin, Kerala,
India

Thankappan KR, MD, DM,
(Presently Consultant
Gastroenterologist, Kingdom of
Saudi Arabia)
Professor of Gastroenterology (Retd)
Medical College Hospital,
Thiruvananthapuram, Kerala, India

Thomas Alexander
MD, DM, DNB (Gastro)
HOD, Department of Gastroenterology
VSM Hospital, Mavelikkara, Kerala,
India

Varghese Thomas, MD, DM
HOD, Department of Gastroenterology
Medical College Hospital, Calicut,
Kerala, India

Vinayakumar KR, MD, DM
Professor of Gastroenterology
Medical College Hospital,
Thiruvananthapuram, Kerala, India

Vinod Kumar V, MD, DM
HOD, Department of Gastroenterology
Ernakulam Medial Centre, Cochin,
Kerala, India

Viswanath N, MD, DM
HOD, Department of Gastroenterology
Mother Hospital, Thrissur, Kerala, India

Preface

Long before, we were conducting continuing medical education programmes for practitioners regularly in the Gastroenterology Department at Medical College, Trivandrum. After a few years, we compiled the entire course material prepared by the faculty of our department and M/s Jaypee Brothers Medical Publishers (P) Ltd. New Delhi published this as a book *Common Problems in Gastroenterology*. This book was warmly welcomed by doctors and it soon went into a second edition. There must have been a continuing demand for such a book as evidenced by an enquiry recently made by the publishers whether I could bring out a revised edition of this book.

Gastroenterology, like the rest of medicine, has made phenomenal advances in the past few years in theory and practice. Keeping in tune with this, the book has been totally re-written by an entirely new panel of authors, and several newer chapters included. Reflecting the emphasis the book lays on a practical approach to day-to-day gastroenterology care, so the book is entitled *Practical Gastroenterology*. This is a collective effort where an array of eminent gastroenterologists including a few from allied specialties from across the state, have contributed their valuable time and effort. I am deeply indebted to all of them. It is hoped this book will be a handy, comparatively inexpensive, ready reference in gastroenterology for practitioners and doctors in training all over India. My special thanks are due to Mr N Sudhakaran who has rendered invaluable help to me with secretarial assistance in the preparation of the manuscript. I should express my sincere gratitude to M/s Jaypee Brothers Medical Publishers (P) Ltd. New Delhi and Anshan in the UK for the excellent support they have extended in publishing this book.

V Balakrishnan

Contents

1

George Thomas

Managing Dysphagia

INTRODUCTION

'Dysphagia' is the sensation of difficult passage of food from the mouth into the stomach. (Greek—Dys: difficulty, Phagia: eat). This common clinical problem almost always denotes malfunction of the esophagus.

MECHANISMS

Functionally, the esophagus has been divided into upper esophageal sphincter (UES), body and lower esophageal sphincter (LES). The UES, upper esophagus and the muscles involved in oropharyngeal phase of swallowing are striated. Lower 2/3 of esophagus and LES are smooth muscles. Swallowing is facilitated by voluntary and involuntary control mechanisms located in the CNS, the peripheral nerves and muscles of the esophagus.

The act of deglutition initiates integrated esophageal motor activity leading to aboral peristaltic waves. Exaggeration of normal physiologic activity or its abnormalities can result in motor disorders. The accumulated food bolus distends the esophageal lumen, producing discomfort, which is perceived as dysphagia. It can also occur with luminal obstruction.

CLASSIFICATION

1. Oropharyngeal dysphagia: Caused by abnormalities of pharynx and the neuromuscular mechanisms of UES.
2. Esophageal dysphagia: Due to disorders that affect the esophageal body.

COMMON CAUSES OF DYSPHAGIA

Oropharyngeal
1. **Neuromuscular**
   Cerebrovascular accident
   Parkinson's disease
   Brainstem tumors
   Multiple sclerosis
   Amyotrophic lateral sclerosis
2. **Mechanical obstruction**
   Retropharyngeal abscess
   Zenker's diverticulum
   Thyromegaly
   Cervical osteophyte

Esophageal
1. **Mechanical obstruction**
   Benign strictures
   Webs and rings
   Diverticuli

2. **Motility disorders**
   Achalasia
   Spastic motility disorders
   Scleroderma
   Chaga's disease

3. **Skeletal muscle disorders**
   Polymyositis
   Muscular dystrophies
   Myasthenia gravis
   Metabolic myopathies
4. **Miscellaneous**
   Decreased saliva (medication, Sjögren's syndrome)
   Alzheimer's disease
   Depression

3. **Miscellaneous**
   Diabetes mellitus
   Chronic alcoholism
   Gastroesophageal reflux disease
   (GERD)

OROPHARYNGEAL DYSPHAGIA (TRANSFER DYSPHAGIA)

Patients are unable to initiate swallowing and have difficulty in propelling food from mouth into esophagus. This is perceived as food not having left the oropharynx, and discomfort is felt at the cervical esophagus. Food impaction and regurgitation of liquids into trachea can occur, leading to recurrent pulmonary infection. Hoarseness of voice occurs due to recurrent laryngeal nerve dysfunction or intrinsic muscular disease. Weakness of soft palate and pharyngeal constrictors produces dysarthria and pharyngonasal regurgitation. These can lead to reluctance to eat and weight loss. Myasthenia gravis, polymyositis, Alzheimer's disease and depressive illness can also be associated with oropharyngeal dysphagia.

ESOPHAGEAL DYSPHAGIA (TRANSIT DYSPHAGIA)

Mechanical obstructions and motility disorders produce difficulty in transporting food bolus down the esophagus after initiation of swallowing. Symptoms are often localised to restrosternal area. Dysphagia for solids as well as liquids, waxing and waning severity over long periods of time and episodic chest pain are characteristic of motility disorders. Provocation of symptoms by liquids at extremes of temperature, relief by physical maneuvres like elevation of arms, systemic symptoms like chronic cough, recurrent aspiration pneumonia are often associated.

Dysphagia only to solids and never with liquids alone is indicative of mechanical obstruction, unless the obstruction is high grade. Progressive symptoms indicate peptic stricture or carcinoma. Nonprogressive dysphagia without weight loss can occur with esophageal webs and rings. Esophagitis due to corrosives, drugs or viruses have dysphagia along with odynophagia.

INVESTIGATIONS

Radiology

Esophagogram and video fluroscopy can detect many of UES lesions. Double contrast mucosal detail techniques are useful to study diseases of esophageal body. Special techniques like iced barium suspension and solid bolus methods can detect motility disorders.

Radionuclide Studies

Scintigraphy is used to study bolus transit through the esophagus and can be quantified.

Video Endoscopy

Primarily used to diagnose structural lesions of esophagus, endoscopy can detect tracheobronchial aspiration and secondary changes in neurogenic dysphagia (Fig. 1.1)

Manometry

Muscle contraction patterns of body and LES are measured indirectly, by placing recording probes comprising of fused small calibre catheters in the lumen, that

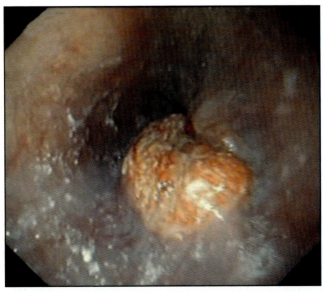

Fig. 1.1: Upper GI endoscopy showing proliferative mass in the lower esophagus suggested esophageal counter

are sensitive to pressures generated by circular muscle layer. Based on peristaltic wave patterns, contraction wave configuration, LES basal pressure and LES relaxation, various motor disorders can be identified.

Classification of Esophageal Motility Disorders

- Inadequate LES relaxation
  Achalasia
  Atypical disorders of LES relaxation
- Uncoordinated contractions
  Diffuse esophageal spasm
- Hyper contraction
  Nut cracker esophagus
  Isolated hypertensive LES
- Hypocontraction
  Ineffective esophageal motility.

Disorders of UES and Cervical Esophagus

Primary CNS disease like cerebrovascular accidents (damage to swallowing centre or the motor nuclei controlling striated muscles of swallowing), Parkinsonism, multiple sclerosis, focal cranial neuropathies, diabetic autonomic neuropathy or diffuse skeletal muscle disorders result in dysphagia. These should be differentiated from 'globus sensation' where there is a sensation of cervical fullness (but no true dysphagia), and a visceral sensory abnormality has been postulated.

Treatment

The diseases producing motor dysfunction of UES and upper esophagus are progressive and supportive measures alone are feasible.
a. Maintenance of nutrition
b. Prevention of tracheobronchial aspiration by improving swallowing function (adjustments of head and body posture; modifying consistency, volume and rate of delivery of food)
c. Indirect therapy to improve neuromuscular controls
d. Medical therapy of primary disorder, cricopharnygeal myotomy, maxillofacial prostheses.

Specific Motor Disorders

Achalasia (failure to relax)

Pathophysiology: There is increased resting basal pressure of LES due to reduction in number of inhibitory ganglion cells in the intramural plexus, degeneration in vagal motor nucleus, and denervation of smooth muscle segment.

Clinical features: Onset is in 3rd to 5th decades, with equal gender distribution. Slowly progressive dysphagia with fluctuating severity is typical. Chest pain, bronchopulmonary aspiration and weight loss can occur.

Diagnosis

1. Compatible clinical history.
2. *Barium swallow:* Failure of peristalsis to clear barium from esophagus, dilatation of distal body, air fluid level and bird's beak appearance are characteristic.
3. Endoscopy is done to evaluate the mucosa and to exclude other causes.
4. Manometry: Incomplete relaxation of LES along with aperistalsis in body is confirmatory. LES pressure is elevated.

Differential Diagnosis (pseudo achalasia)

Carcinoma of lower esophagus or cardia, sarcoidosis, amylodosis, post vagotomy states.

Treatment

1. *Pharmacotherapy:* Nitrites and calcium channel blockers relax LES. Long-term efficacy is poor.
2. *Botulinum toxin:* When injected circumferentially at the level of LES, toxin binds to cholinergic receptors irreversibly inhibiting acetyl choline release. This decreases LES tone. Recurrence rate is high.
3. *Dilatation:* Forceful dilation of LES, producing tearing of circular muscles leads to long lasting reduction in LES tone. Pneumatic dilators are commonly used with 60-80% response. Complication—perforation in 5%.
4. *Myotomy:* Modified Heller's anterior myotomy or minimally invasive surgery, (transthoracic or laparoscopic) has 80-90% response. Complication: Gastroesophageal reflux.

Complications of achalasia include esophagitis, aspiration and 20% incidence of carcinoma.

Other Hypermotility Disorders

Spectrum of diseases exemplified by diffuse esophageal spasm and nutcracker esophagus present usually in 4th decade, commoner in females. Up to 60% have intermittent nonprogressive dysphagia of varying severity [with no weight loss], often associated with chest pain, heartburn and psychological dysfunction.

Diagnosis

Barium swallow: Shows non-propulsive contractions and indentation of barium column—'cork screw' appearance.

Manometry: Diffuse esophageal spasm shows repetitive, nonperistaltic, simultaneous contractions of long duration after initiation of swallow. Nutcracker esophagus is characterized by high amplitude peristaltic waves in distal esophagus.

Treatment: Essentially symptomatic. Exclude coronary artery disease, GERD by appropriate investigations. Low dose anti depressants, nitrites, calcium channel blockers are useful.

Esophageal Hypomotility

Connective tissue disorders, scleroderma, CREST syndrome and polymyositis show muscle atrophy and fibrosis. Heartburn, dysphagia due to associated esophagitis, and strictures are common. Manometry shows aperistalsis in body and hypotensive LES. Treatment involves antireflux therapy.

Diabetes mellitus, hypothyroidism and ageing also show failed contractions in the body leading to hypomotility symptoms.

Obstructive Lesions

Tumors

Both squamous cell carcinoma and adenocarcinoma produce significant rapidly progressive dysphagia, associated with weight loss.

Diagnosis is made by barium studies and endoscopy and histological examination, which is confirmatory. CT and endoscopic ultrasonography help in evaluating operability.

Treatment: Primary modes of treatment are surgery, radiotherapy and chemotherapy. Since most patients present with advanced stages of tumor, endoscopic palliation is the commonly used option to either displace (dilatation, stenting) or ablate tumor tissue (thermal methods, lasers, debulking agents and photodynamic therapy).

Dilatation: Lateral shearing force is used to stretch and tear stenotic tissue using polyvinyl dilators (Savary Guilliard) or hydrostatic 'through the scope' (TTS) balloons.

Debulking agents injection therapy: Alcohol, polidocanol, etc. can be injected for debulking.

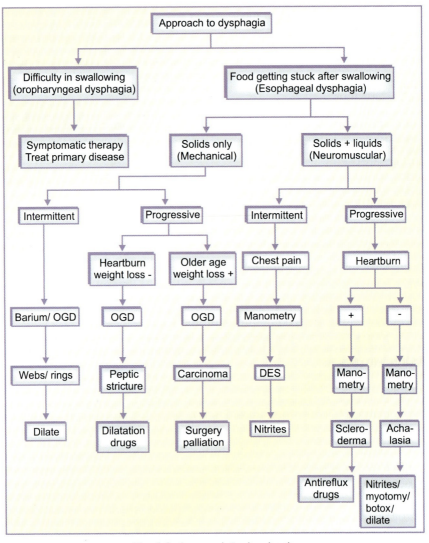

Fig. 1.2: Approach to dysphagia

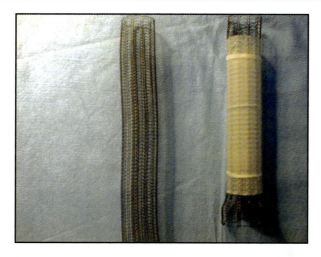

Fig. 1.3: Self-expanding metallic stents used for dysphagia palliation in patients with inoperable esophageal cancer.

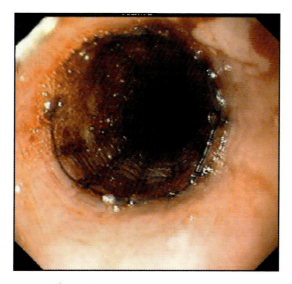

Fig. 1.4: Upper GI endoscopy showing self-expanding metallic stent following deployment.

Contact-thermal methods: Application of electrosurgical BICAP probe to ablate tissue.

Endoscopic laser therapy: Delivery of Nd-YAG, Argon laser energy burns tumor tissue to produce adequate lumen. Argon plasma coagulation is less useful, since only superficial necrosis occurs.

Esophageal stents: Self-expandable metallic stents (SEMS) offer excellent relief of dysphagia and have replaced the older plastic rigid ones. Newer innovations include Ultraflex stent, Z stent (expensive). Tumor ingrowth, stent migration and chest pain are complications.

Photodynamic therapy: Photosensitizing agents, when administered, are retained in tumor cells. These are activated by delivering low dose laser energy, resulting in local cytotoxicity and tissue necrosis (Figs 1.3 and 1.4)

Benign tumors such as leiomyoma, hemangioma, hamartoma and lipoma produce luminal obstruction, which are all amenable to surgery. Lymphoma and metastases from melanoma and breast cancers can also produce dysphagia.

SUGGESTED READING

1. Castell DO, Kartz PO. Approach to the patient with dysphagia. Yamada T,Textbook of Gastroenterology. 3rd Edn, 1999.
2. AGA medical position statement on management of Oropharyngeal dysphagia. Gastroenterology 1999;116.
3. Spechler SJ. American gastroenterological association medical position statement on treatment of patients with dysphagia caused by benign disorders of the distal esophagus. Gastroenterology 1999; 117:229-33.
4. Lind CD. Dysphagia evaluation and treatment—Gastroenterol Clin North Am 2003; 32: 553-75.
5. Saud B. A diagnostic approach to dysphagia—Clin Fam Pract—2004; 6: 525.
6. Cook IJ, Kahrilas PJ. AGA technical review on the management of oropharyngeal dysphagia. Gastroenterology 1999; 116:455-78.

2

Saju Xavier

Treating Gastroesophageal Reflux Disease

INTRODUCTION

Gastroesophageal reflux disease (GERD) is a common but fascinating problem in GI practice. Once thought to be entirely the domain of gastroenterologist, now the spectrum of presentation extends to the otolaryngologist, the pulmonologist and even the cardiologist.

DEFINITION

The term GERD describes any symptomatic condition or histopathologic alteration resulting from episodes of gastroesophageal reflux. Reflux esophagitis is a condition experienced by a subset of GERD patients with endoscopically evident lesions in the esophageal mucosa.

EPIDEMIOLOGY

Seven percent of western population experience reflux daily, 14% at least once weekly and 48-79% of pregnant women experience reflux. Asians seem less symptomatic, compared to western population, and less prone to complications, of GERD.

PATHOPHYSIOLOGY

The classical teaching is that GERD is a progressive disease spectrum from non-erosive disease to complicated disease. This may not be the case and the spectrum may in fact be three distinct groups, nonerosive reflux disease, erosive disease and Barrett's disease, which do not switch from one to another. The different responses of the mucosa to acid reflux is probably the reflection of differing immune responses in various individuals to acid exposure; interleukin 1β, interleukin 8 and interferon- v consistent with T-helper cell 1 activation in nonerosive and erosive GERD and IL-4 suggestive of T-helper cell 2 activation in Barrett's esophagus. Reactive epithelial changes occur even without endoscopically evident esophagitis. There is hyperplasia of the basal zone and elongation of the papillae such that they extend more than two thirds of the way to the surface. In addition, there may be increased mitotic figures, vascularization of the epithelium with dilated vessels at the apices of the papillae, increased papillae, loss of longitudinal orientation of the surface epithelium, and balloon cells. When there is epithelial damage, ulceration of the mucosa with inflammatory infiltrate of neutrophils and eosinophils are seen.

MECHANISMS OF REFLUX

Transient lower esophageal sphincter relaxation (TLESR): This is a vagally mediated reflex, provoked by distension of fundus. In GERD, TLESR occurs independent of food, lasts longer than 10 seconds, not accompanied by peristalsis and accompanied by diaphragmatic inhibition. Mild disease is most often due to TLESR.

Hypotensive lower esophageal sphincter (LES): The normal LES pressure ranges from 10-30 mmHg. Low LES pressure predisposes to strain induced reflux and when LES pressure is below 4 mmHg, free reflux results.

Hiatus hernia: Abolishes the pinch-cock effect of crural diaphragm, decreases basal LES pressure and also increases TLESR.

Delayed gastric emptying of diverse: Etiology also predisposes to reflux.

CLINICAL FEATURES

Typical

- Heartburn (pyrosis)—discomfort and burning sensation from epigastrium to neck usually within 60 minutes of eating, during exercise and recumbency
- Regurgitation—Effortless return of gastric contents without retching
- Dysphagia (30%)—Possibly due to abnormal sensitivity to bolus movement. Schatsky's ring and peptic stricture are other important causes.

Atypical

- Posterior laryngitis—chronic hoarseness, posterior laryngeal edema, contact ulcer of vocal cords and vocal cord granuloma
- Asthma—77% of asthmatics have heartburn and 55% have regurgitation
- Chronic cough—GERD accounts for 10-40% of chronic cough. Of these 50-75% do not have any reflux related symptoms. It is a vagally mediated esophagobronchial reflux.

  Nocturnal symptoms, post prandial symptoms and symptoms provoked by recumbency are clues to suggest underlying GERD. Patients may be prone to get "sleep apnoea".

Non-cardiac Chest Pain

Thirty percent of patients with chest pain have normal coronaries on angiography. Most such cases are due to GERD and esophageal motility disorders.

Natural History

Eighty percent of patients with severe GERD relapse in six months of cessation of therapy. The non-erosive group fare better and as many as 56% remain in remission at six months

Differential Diagnosis

Infectious esophagitis, pill esophagitis: Odynophagia and characteristic endoscopic findings are useful differentiating points.

- Peptic ulcer
- Nonulcer dyspepsia
- Biliary colic
- Motility disorders
- Coronary artery disease (particularly inferior wall Ischemia): Diaphoresis, dyspnea and fatigue are useful cues to ischemic heart disease.

Investigations and Management

GERD is diagnosed most often on the basis of history. American College of Gastroenterology and ASGE recommend lifestyle alteration and empirical drug therapy for patients with typical history and uncomplicated GERD. Investigations are required only in the atypical and refractory cases.

Upper gastrointestinal endoscopy is the first investigation of choice. Presence of erosive esophagitis is 90-95% specific for the diagnosis of GERD but is only 30-40% sensitive. Endoscopy is indicated in:

1. Alarm symptoms: Dysphagia, odynophagia, gastrointestinal bleed and weight loss
2. Persistent and progressive symptoms while on treatment
3. Extra-esophageal symptoms
4. Esophageal symptoms in immunocompromised patients
5. Presence of mass or stricture on esophagogram
6. Iron deficiency anemia

   Various grading systems are available for grading the severity of esophagitis. The Los Angeles grading scheme is one of the more accepted and objective grading systems.

Los Angeles endoscopic grading scheme for esophagitis severity

Grade A	One or more mucosal breaks not longer than 5 mm in length and do not extend between the tops of adjoining folds
Grade B	One or more mucosal breaks longer than 5 mm in length and do not extend between the tops of adjoining folds
Grade C	One or more mucosal breaks that are continuous between the tops of two or more folds but involve less than 75% of the circumference
Grade D	Mucosal breaks that involve at least 75% of the circumference

The presence of Barrett's esophagus and stricture is not considered in the grading and is mentioned separately.

Bernstein test: This test is useful to confirm if a patient's symptoms are due to reflux disease and consists of perfusing the patient's esophagus with 0.1 N Hcl. If patient's symptoms are reproduced with Hcl but not with normal saline, the test is considered positive. Though it is a very specific test, its sensitivity in the evaluation of patients with atypical symptoms is too low for routine practice

Esophageal pH metry: Ambulatory 24 hour pH monitoring is done with a pH probe placed 5 cm above the LES as determined by manometry. The patient keeps a symptom diary during the period. Esophageal pH remaining below four for more than 3.5% of time is considered significant.

Guidelines for the Clinical use of Esophageal pH Recording

Indications

- To document abnormal esophageal acid exposure in an endoscopy-negative patient being considered for surgical anti-reflux repair (pH study done after withholding anti-secretory drug regimen for $\geq$ one week)
- To evaluate patients after antireflux surgery who are suspected to have ongoing abnormal reflux (pH study done after withholding anti-secretory drug regimen for ≥ 1 week).
- To evaluate patients with either normal or equivocal endoscopic findings and reflux symptoms that are refractory to proton pump inhibitor therapy (pH study done after withholding anti-secretory drug regimen for $>$ one week)
- To detect refractory reflux in patients with chest pain after cardiac evaluation using a symptom reflux association scheme, preferably the symptom association probability calculation (pH study done after a trial of proton pump inhibitor therapy for at least four weeks)
- To evaluate a patient with suspected otolaryngologic manifestations (laryngitis, pharyngitis, chronic cough) of gastroesophageal reflux disease after symptoms have failed to respond to at least four weeks of proton pump inhibitor therapy (pH study done while the patient continues taking their anti-secretory drug regimen to document the adequacy of therapy)
- To document concomitant gastroesophageal reflux disease in an adult onset, non-allergic asthmatic suspected of having reflux-induced asthma (pH study done after withholding anti-secretory drugs for $\geq$ one week). Note: a positive test does not prove causality

- To detect or verify reflux esophagitis (this is an endoscopic diagnosis)
- To evaluate for "alkaline reflux".

Therapeutic Trial with Proton Pump Inhibitors

One to two week trial of proton pump inhibitors will identify most patients who are likely to respond to PPI and is useful to detect patients who are negative on pH studies.

Treatment

Nonprescription Therapy

- Head of the bed elevation with 6-8 inch blocks
- Avoidance of tight fitting garments
- Weight loss
- Dietary modification –   avoidance of fat, chocolate
                                avoid eating within three hours of bedtime
                                decreasing the quantity of food
- Restriction of alcohol use and elimination of smoking
- Antacids as needed.

Drug Therapy

Proton Pump Inhibitors

They are the most effective drugs available to control symptoms of reflux and promote healing of erosions. Omeprazole, lansoprazole, pantoprazole, rabeprazole and esomeprazole are available in the Indian market.

Caveats in Usage of PPI

- Ideally given before breakfast
- Twice daily dosing is more effective at prolonged acid suppression and symptom control
- Pantoprazole has least interaction with cytochrome p450 and is safe for coprescription
- Rabeprazole has the fastest onset of action
- Esomeprazole has the longest duration of action.

H_2 **receptor antagonist:** They are effective in controlling nocturnal and fasting acid secretion but are not effective against postprandial acid secretion.

Famotidine and ranitidine are available in the Indian market and famotidine remains the most economical acid reducing agent available. Though not the most potent agent, it is effective in many patients with mild disease.

Prokinetic agents: Metaclopramide, domperidone, mozapride, cizapride and itopride are the prokinetic agents available in the Indian market. Cizapride has been found to be equivalent to ranitidine in efficacy; but QT prolongation and the possibilities of cardiac arrhythmias have decreased its use.

Modulators of TLESR

Cholecystokinin A (CCK_A) antagonist loxiglumide, a nitric oxide (NO) synthase inhibitor and *l*-Baclofen, are agents shown to decrease TLESR. Their role in clinical practice is yet to be clarified.

Maintenance Therapy

Severe GERD relapses in 80% patients upon cessation of therapy. Proton pump inhibitors have been shown to be most effective in prevention of relapse and majority of patients require the initial dose for maintenance of remission. For many patients with mild disease and NERD the strategy of SOS usage of PPI is sufficient and patients have been shown to remain off drugs for up to six months or more.

Endoscopic Treatment Modalities

These methods are likely to rewrite the management algorithms in the days to come. There are three such systems available, which require a lot more finetuning before getting worldwide acceptance.

Radiofrequency ablation (Stretta procedure): Involves delivering radio frequency energy to the GE junction and gastric cardia. PPI requirement has been shown to decrease from 88 to 30%.

Endoscopic suturing devices: Four systems are available. The endocinch and full thickness plicator have been approved by FDA. The syntheon antireflux device and endoscopic sewing system (Wilson Cook) are the others available. These have been shown to decrease GERD related quality of life and usage of PPI. However, the experience and expertise is not well established to recommend its routine use.

Injection of inert materials into the GE junction is another strategy on trial. Enteryx (ethylene vinyl alcohol polymer), the gatekeeper (expandable hydrogel prosthesis placed into the submucosa) and artecol (gelatinous implant composed of plexiglass beads) are the agents undergoing evaluation. Sham trials are underway and these are yet to reach the practicing clinician.

Surgery

Surgical therapy should be considered in those individuals with documented GERD who:
1. Have failed medical management
2. Opt for surgery despite successful medical management (due to lifestyle considerations including age, time or expense of medications, etc.)
3. Have complications of GERD (e.g., Barrett's esophagus; grade III or IV esophagitis)
4. Have medical complications attributable to a large hiatus hernia. (e.g., bleeding, dysphagia)
5. Have "atypical" symptoms (asthma, hoarseness, cough, chest pain, aspiration) and reflux documented on 24 hour pH monitoring.

Surgical Techniques

The 360° or Nissen-type fundoplication has emerged as the most widely accepted procedure for patients with normal esophageal motility. For patients with compromised esophageal motility, one of the various partial fundoplications should be considered to decrease the possibility of postoperative dysphagia.

Laparoscopic antireflux surgery: In expert hands it is as good as open fundoplication with much less morbidity. It should only be offered by surgeons skilled in the equivalent open antireflux procedure.

Complications of GERD

Peptic stricture: Strictures respond well to endoscopic dilatation. Long term acid suppression is essential to prevent further recurrence. Malignancy needs to be excluded with multiple biopsies. (Fig. 2.1)

Barrett's esophagus: Defined as columnar lined esophagus with specialized intestinal metaplasia.
a. This alteration is associated with an increased propensity for malignant transformation and warrants aggressive approach. It is divided into two types.

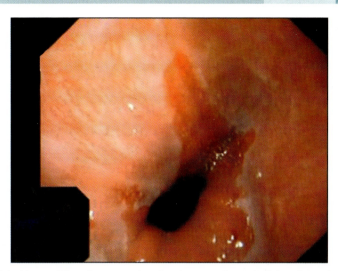

Fig. 2.1: Upper GI endoscopy showing tongue shaped pink color columnar mucosa above the squamocolumnar junction (Z-line) indicates presence of Barrett's esophagus

b. Long segment–columnar epithelium extends beyond 3 cm of the gastroesophageal junction and associated with greater risk of dysplasia.

c. Short segment. Columnar epithelium limited to 3 cm from the GE junction.

Management: Symptoms of GERD are managed with proton pump inhibitors or surgery as the case may be. Ablative therapies have been tried for dysplastic and nondysplastic Barrett's esophagus.

Endoscopic mucosal resection: Endoscopic ultrasound guided EMR of focal lesions is very successful in determining the depth of invasion and deciding which patients need esophagectomy. It is therapeutic in a large number of patients with early carcinoma (T1m and T1sm)

Photodynamic therapy: The dysplastic epithelium concentrates porphyrins and makes them susceptible to light energy. 5-aminolevulinic acid is given orally followed by laser treatment of dysplastic mucosa. A very promising technique, still not recommended outside study protocols.

Other techniques are argon plasma coagulation (APC), multipolar electrocoagulation and laser.

Surveillance

Barrett's without dysplasia	2-3 yearly follow up is advised
Low grade dysplasia	Review by an expert pathologist, treat for 12 weeks and repeat biopsy; if positive, repeat 6 monthly for 1 year and then yearly if there is no progression.

If high-grade dysplasia is confirmed, surgery or ablation therapy, as an alternate therapy (e.g., APC) is needed.

Conclusion

GERD is a common condition with intestinal and extraintestinal manifestations. Lifestyle modifications and PPI remain the backbone of therapy. Minimally invasive surgery is an attractive maintenance option. Endoscopic techniques of sphincter augmentation are exciting evolving prospects.

SUGGESTED READING

1. Current opin in Gastroenterol. 2003; 19:373 – 8,
2. Proceedings of the DDW – Medscape—Gastroenterology 2004. url-www.medscape.com
3. AGA guidelines for the use of Esophageal pH measurement
4. Gastroesophageal Reflux. Curr Opin Gastroenterol 2004; 20(4):369-74.
5. Richter J.E. Gastroesophageal reflux disease during pregnancy. Gastroenterol Clin North Am 2003: 32: 235-61.
6. Fass R., Bautista J., Janarthanan S Treatment of gastroesophageal reflux disease. Clin Cornerstone 2003; 5: 18-31.
7. Waring J.P., Surgical and endoscopic treatment of gastroesophageal reflux disease. Gastroenterol Clin North Am 2002; 31: S89-S109.
8. Cappell Mitchell S. Clinical presentation, diagnosis, and management of gastroesophageal reflux disease Med Clin North Am—2005; 892: 243-29.
9. Ramirez B, Richter JE. Review article: promotility drugs in the treatment of gastroesophageal reflux disease. Aliment Pharmacol Ther 1993; 7:5-20.

3

Ramachandran TM

Nausea and Vomiting: A Common Clinical Problem

INTRODUCTION

Nausea and vomiting is one of the most common symptoms in clinical practice. Vomiting can be a manifestation of disease affecting any system in the human body including psychiatric illness. The cause of vomiting can vary from a simple one to a very serious and life threatening condition. Hence a meticulous approach to proper diagnosis is of paramount importance.

Nausea is an unpleasant sensation of impending vomiting.

Vomiting refers to forceful expulsion of the gastric contents through the mouth. Vomiting may be preceded by nausea but not invariably so. In other words, nausea is a feeling and vomiting is an act.

Retching is vigorous, spasmodic respiratory and abdominal movements where the inspiratory movement of chest and diaphragm is opposed by expiratory movements of abdominal muscles.

Related Terms

Regurgitation is effortless passive expulsion of gastric and esophageal contents into the mouth in small quantities.

Rumination is chewing and swallowing of the regurgitated material.

Pathophysiology of Vomiting

Vomiting is a complex viscero-somatic process controlled by the central nervous system. Vomiting centre is located in the dorsal portion of the medulla closely associated with respiratory, vasomotor and salivatory centers. Recent studies indicate that this is more of a pharmacological than anatomical entity. Closely related to the vomiting centre, but a distinct entity is chemoreceptor trigger zone (CTZ) located in the floor of fourth ventricle, which is outside the blood brain barrier. CTZ cannot function independently but acts as relaying centre of noxious chemical stimuli to the vomiting centre. The main receptors for the vomiting centre are dopamine(D2) receptor, 5-hydroxytryptamine(5HT3) receptor, histamine (H1) receptor and muscarinic (M1) receptor.

The main afferent inputs are:
1. Stimuli from gastrointestinal tract, peritoneum, bile duct, mesentery and vasculature, pharynx, heart and pericardium, mediated by vagus
2. Stimuli from vestibular and cochlear structure

3. Supra medullary (corticobulbar) stimuli for smell, taste, sight, emotional disturbances and also impulse from thalamus and hypothalamus.
4. Noxious chemicals, drugs, toxins, etc. detected and transmitted to vomiting center through CTZ.

Act of Vomiting

The efferent pathway for vomiting includes vagus, phrenic and spinal nerves. The sequence of events is contraction of the proximal small intestine and duodenum followed by that of antrum of stomach. The body and fundus of stomach get relaxed. Retrograde peristalsis pushes the gastric contents into the esophagus through the relaxed lower esophageal sphincter. Just before the expulsion the cricopharyngeus muscle relaxes and upper esophageal sphincter opens. Simultaneously the abdominal muscle and diaphragm contract, respiration is suspended and glottis closed, thus forcefully ejecting the contents out.

Because of the proximity of other medullary centers, there is salivation, cardiac arrhythmia, vasomotor instability, etc. associated with nausea and vomiting.

Approach to a Patient with Vomiting

The main objectives are:
1. To define the cause of vomiting
2. To assess the effect of vomiting on the body in terms of fluid and electrolyte imbalance, malnutrition, etc.
3. To plan the treatment – pharmacological or interventional, depending upon the cause

From the gastroenterological aspect, it is important to differentiate between the obstructive cause and non-obstructive cause. The important causes for vomiting and features suggestive of luminal obstruction are given in Table 3.1.

Clinical Features of Luminal Obstruction

Gastric outlet obstruction
- Stale food vomiting
- Non-bilious vomiting
- Pain relieved by vomiting
- Rolling sensation in upper abdomen
- Visible peristalsis

Table 3.1: Common causes of vomiting (*indicates recurrent or chronic causes)

1. **Intra-abdominal inflammation**
   a. Appendicitis
   b. Cholecystitis
   c. Pancreatitis
   d. Peritonitis
   e. Acute gastroenteritis
2. **Luminal obstruction**
   a. Chronic duodenal ulcer*
   b. Neoplasm* – gastric antrum, colon, small intestine, pancreatic and intestinal lymphoma.
   c. Intestinal tuberculosis*
   d. Crohn's disease*
   e. Ischemic strictures*
   f. Adhesions
   g. Volvulus
   h. Internal hernias
   i. Intussusceptions
   j. Foreign body impaction
3. **Metabolic and endocrine causes**
   a. Diabetic ketoacidosis
   b. Endocrine disorders* – Addison's disease, hyper-and hypothyroidism, hypercalcemia.
   c. Chronic renal failure*
4. **Nervous system disorders**
   a. Meningitis
   b. Encephalitis
   c. CNS tumors*
   d. Raised intracranial tension of any origin
   e. Migraine*
   f. Labyrinthitis*
   g. Menier's disease*
5. **Medications and toxins**
   a. Anti-arrhythmic drugs
   b. Chemotherapeutic agents
   c. NSAIDs
   d. Antibiotics
   e. Digoxin
   f. Phenytoin
   g. Excess alcohol
6. **Motility disorders***
   a. Achalasia cardia
   b. Gastroparesis
      i. Diabetes mellitus
      ii. Post-surgical (vagotomy)
      iii. Visceral neuromyopathies
      iv. Amyloidosis
      v. Medications
      vi. Idiopathic
7. **Other conditions**
   a. Myocardial infarction
   b. Acute hepatitis
   c. Pregnancy
   d. Radiation induced vomiting
   e. Psychogenic vomiting*

- Succusion splash
- Fasting gastric aspiration more than 200 ml
- Saline load test: more than 400 ml residual gastric aspiration 30 min after nasogastric instillation of 750 ml normal saline.

Intestinal obstruction
- Colicky pain relieved by vomiting.
- Bilious, stale food vomiting.
- Intestinal type of visible peristalsis (step-ladder pattern).
- Feculent odour may be present in lower GI obstruction.
- Alteration in bowel habits.

In the clinical evaluation the following points are to be noted:

Duration of vomiting is important in terms of differential diagnosis (Table 3.1). Timing in relation to food intake, content of the vomitus and associated symptoms are important points to be elicited. Early morning vomiting can occur in pregnancy and also in chronic alcoholic patients. Chronic vomiting soon after food intake without much constitutional disturbances could indicate psychogenic cause. Gastroparesis or luminal obstruction has to be considered in cases of delayed vomiting many hours after food intake (Table 3.1).

The content of vomitus as regard to presence of stale food (food taken many hours earlier), bilious or non-bilious, and the presence of blood in the vomitus should be noted. Blood in the vomitus may be due to peptic ulcer or variceal bleed, or it could be the effect of vomiting as in Mallory–Weiss tear. In lower gut obstruction there may be feculent odour for the vomitus. Feculent vomiting can also occur in ileus, gastro-colic fistula, or bacterial overgrowth.

The associated symptoms like abdominal pain, jaundice, diarrhea and fever should be evaluated. Pain relieved by vomiting may be due to peptic ulcer disease or small intestinal obstruction. Severe pain not relieved by vomiting could indicate pancreatitis or cholecystitis. Fever and localized tenderness could point to intra abdominal sepsis-appendicitis, cholecystitis and diverticulitis.

Special care should be given to elicit non-gastrointestinal symptoms like chest pain, headache, vertigo, fits or neurological deficits. Projectile vomiting, i.e. vomitus ejected forcefully from mouth, is usually associated with raised intracranial tension even though not specific for the condition. It may also occur in pyloric obstruction with gastric stasis. Weight loss and features of malnutrition are important. History of drug intake, alcohol habits and menstrual history could give a clue regarding the aetiolgy of vomiting. Also features suggestive of chronic renal failure, diabetes mellitus and its complications should get due attention. History of abdominal surgery in the past and the nature of surgery should be evaluated.

Detailed physical examination with special attention to dehydration, pallor and malnutrition, jaundice, lymphadenopathy and abdominal examination should include presence of surgical scar, hernia, abdominal distension and visible peristalsis. On palpation, presence of guarding, tenderness, organomegaly, masses, succussion splash and presence of bruit should be noted. Per rectal and per vaginal examination should also be done.

Detailed neurological, cardiovascular examination and in suspected cases, psychiatric evaluation also need to be done.

Complications of Vomiting

1. Metabolic derangements
   Hypokalemia, hyponatremia, metabolic alkalosis
2. Volume depletion
3. Prerenal azotemia
4. Pulmonary complication: aspiration
5. Bleeding due to mucosal tear at GE junction: Mallory-Weiss tear
6. Rupture of Esophagus: Boerhaave's syndrome
7. Malnutrition in chronic vomiting
8. Dental erosions in chronic vomiting.

Investigations

The following are the battery of investigations to evaluate cause for vomiting. The selection of investigations should be *individualized* based on clinical findings.

Laboratory Investigations

- Hemoglobin, total and differential blood count, sedimentation rate
- Blood sugar and urine ketone bodies
- Renal function tests, liver function tests
- Serum electrolytes
- Endocrinological workup: TSH, fasting cortisol, serum calcium
- Urine pregnancy test.

Imaging Studies

- Plain X-ray abdomen for distended bowel loops, radio-opaque shadows (renal stones, pancreatic calculi, gall-stones), free intra-peritoneal air
- Ultrasound scan abdomen for evidence of cholecystitis, parenchymal liver disease, evidence of biliary obstruction, bowel wall thickening, pelvic masses and lymph nodes, ascites
- CT scan abdomen
- Barium studies: barium meal follow through/enteroclysis(small bowel enema) for small intestinal diseases and tumors. Barium enema for evaluation of colon.

Endoscopic Studies

- Upper GI endoscopy to detect peptic ulcer disease and its complications, Esophageal / gastric neoplasms.
- Colonoscopy

Table 3.2: Antiemetics

Drug	Dose	Indications/side effects
I. Dopamine (D2) receptor antagonists		
1. Metaclopramide	Dose: 10-20 mg 6-8 hourly i.v: 0.5-2 mg 8 hourly	Dystonia, dyskinesia, Galactorrhoea
2. Domperidone	Oral: 10-20 mg 8 hourly	
3. Promethazine	Oral: 25-50 mg 8 hourly i.m: 25 mg 8 hourly	Sedation, hypotension
4. Prochlorperazine	Oral: 10-20 mg 6 hourly im/iv: 10-20 mg 6 hourly	Sedation, hypotension
II. Serotonin 5-HT3 antagonists		
1. Ondansetron	Oral: 4-8 mg 8 hourly i.v: 4-8 mg slow i.v. [higher dose for chemotherapy induced vomiting (upto 32 mg)]	These drugs are usually used for chemotherapy induced vomiting.
2. Granisetron	Oral: 1 mg twice daily i.v.: 1-2 mg s.o.s.	Side effects are minimal and include headache,
3. Tropisetron	Oral: 5 mg 6-8 hourly i.v.: 5-10 mg slow iv 30 min before chemotherapy.	constipation/diarrhea, transient elevation in LFT.
III. Anticholinergics (M1 receptor antagonists)		
1. Hyoscine	Transdermal application 1.5 mg s.o.s.	Mainly used for motion sickness.
2. Scopolamine		May cause drowsiness.
IV. Antihistamines (H1 receptor antagonists)		
1. Dimenhydrinate	Oral: 50 mg 6-8 hourly	Used for motion sickness
2. Cyclizine	Oral: 50 mg 6-8 hourly	and pregnancy induced
3. Meclizine	Oral: 50 mg 6-8 hourly	vomiting.
4. Promethazine	Oral: 25-50 mg 8 hourly i.m: 25 mg	May cause drowsiness.
V. Other drugs		
1. Dexamethasone	10-20 mg i.v	Mainly used for
2. Dronabinal (cannabinoid receptor agonist)	Oral:10 mg iv.: 5 mg/m^2 one hour before chemotherapy.	chemotherapy induced vomiting.

Special Investigations

- GI manometry
- Scintigraphy
- Radionuclide gastric emptying study
- Electrogastrography

Treatment

The principles involved are general measures, pharmacological measures and specific treatment for the cause.

General measures: Proper hydration, restoration of electrolyte imbalance, correction of metabolic derangements like hyperglycemia, ketosis and hypercalcemia should get immediate attention. In suspected gastric stasis and luminal obstruction, nasogastric suction with parenteral fluid administration should be done.

In chronic vomiting, nutritional therapy, either enteral or parenteral, depending on the severity of the condition, is to be instituted.

Pharmacological treatment: The list of drugs available are given in Tables 3.2 and 3.3. It has to be noted that in severe vomiting like that of chemotherapy-induced and radiation-induced vomiting, a combination of drugs may be required.

Specific treatment depends upon the underlying cause.

Table 3.3: Prokinetic agents		
Generally, this group has weak antiemetic action, but they are useful in gastroparesis and other dysmotility conditions.		
1. **Cisapride** (cholinomimetic and 5-HT4 agonist)	Oral: 10 mg t.i.d.	QT prolongation, diarrhea, crampy abdominal pain.
2. **Mosapride** (5-HT4 agonist)	Oral: 5 mg t.i.d.	Minimal side effects
3. **Itopride** (dopamine antagonist and cholinomimetic)	Oral: 5 mg t.i.d.	Prolactinemia in higher doses, headache, diarrhea.
4. **Erythromycin** (motilin agonist)	Oral: 250 mg t.i.d.	Gastritis, vomiting, liver dysfunction.

Non-pharmacological Approach

Surgery may be indicated in case of acute inflammatory conditions, luminal obstruction and malignancy.

Luminisation by dilatation, laser therapy and stenting options are available in malignant obstruction not amenable to surgery.

SUGGESTED READING

1. Goodman, Gilman. The pharmacological basis of therapeutics, 10th edition, 2002.
2. Quigley EM, Hasler WL, Parkman HP. AGA technical review on nausea and vomiting. Gastroenterology 2001; 120:263–86.
3. Quigley EMM. Gastric and small intestinal motility in health and disease. Gastroenterol Clin North Am 1996; 25:113-45.
4. Tramer MR, Moore RA, Reynolds DJ, McQuay HJ. A quantitative systemic review of ondansetron in treatment of established post-operative nausea and vomiting. BMJ 1997; 314:1088-92.
5. Osoba D, Warr D, Fitch MI, Nakashima L, Warren B. Guidelines for the optimal management of chemotherapy-induced nausea and vomiting: a consensus. Can J Oncol 1995; 5:381-400.

4

Rajesh G

Managing Recurrent Hiccups

INTRODUCTION

Hiccups (hiccoughs) or singultus are involuntary spasmodic and coordinated contractions of inspiratory muscles associated with delayed and sudden closure of the glottis, which is responsible for the characteristic noise.

Occasional hiccup is a ubiquitous human experience, rarely warranting designation as a symptom. Adults are less prone to hiccups than children. Most cases of occasional hiccups are never reported to a doctor. They either remit spontaneously or respond to one of several 'grandmother's remedies'. Chronic hiccups or those recurring as repetitive attacks are the ones usually needing medical attention. Hiccups continuing even during sleep are definitely pathological.

The **reflex arc** for hiccup comprises:
1. *Afferent limb:* vagus nerve, phrenic nerve, or thoracic sympathetic fibres.
2. *Central connections:* located between C3-C5 segments of spinal cord with additional probable complex supraspinal connections between the respiratory center, phrenic nerve nuclei, reticular formation, and hypothalamus.
3. *Efferent limb:* primarily the phrenic nerve.

Classification

Hiccups can be classified by duration as:
1. **Acute:** lasting upto 48 hours
2. **Persistent:** longer than 48 hours
3. **Intractable (diabolic):** more than 2 months

There are close to a hundred causes for hiccups, the most common of which are gastrointestinal.

Selected Causes of Hiccups

Irritation of vagus nerve
Abdominal branches
    Gastric distension
    Gastritis
    Hepatomegaly
    Gallbladder distension
    Pancreatitis
    Bowel obstruction
    Peritonitis

Irritation of phrenic nerve
Diaphragmatic
    Subphrenic abscess
    Tumor
Mediastinal tumor
Cervical tumor

Central nervous system
    Intracranial tumors

Intra-abdominal hemorrhage   Brainstem lesions
Tumor   Basilar arterial insufficiency
Thoracic branches   Head injury
  Esophageal reflux   Encephalitis
  Esophageal obstruction   Meningitis
  Pneumonia
  Coronary occlusion   **Toxic**
Laryngeal branches   Alcohol
Pharyngeal branches   Renal failure
Auricular branches   **Drugs**
Meningeal branches   **Psychogenic**

Drugs Inducing Hiccups

The diagnosis of drug-induced hiccup is difficult and often achieved only by a process of elimination; the mechanisms of these adverse drug reactions are also unclear. Hiccups secondary to high dose corticosteroids are a well-recognized problem in neurosurgery. Other drugs include anti-depressants, dopaminergic anti-Parkinsonian drugs, antibiotics (beta-lactams, macrolides, fluoro-quinolones), digitalis, opioids, and NSAIDs. The same agents that are used to treat hiccups may also induce them.

Hiccups during General Anesthesia or Sedation

Acute hiccup can be a minor complication in this setting and can disturb the surgical field, interfere with lung ventilation, or hamper diagnostic procedures.

Hiccups during Stroke Rehabilitation

Significant complications in this setting include aspiration pneumonia, respiratory arrest, and nutritional depletion with increased need for gastrostomy feedings and prolonged rehabilitation stay. Sedation can be an unwanted side effect of many treatment measures, including chlorpromazine administration.

Hiccups in Terminally ill Patients

In terminal cancer, gastric distension is the commonest cause. Other relatively common causes include diaphragmatic irritation, and toxicity (uremia or infection). Less common causes include phrenic nerve irritation and CNS tumor. Rarely hiccups can be a major cause of distress, interrupting talking, eating, and sleeping; and resulting in weight loss, exhaustion, and depression. Hiccup is occasionally the presenting symptom of neoplasms of the brainstem and esophagus.

TREATMENT

Non-pharmacological Treatment

Stimulation of the pharynx or palate using a rubber catheter or cotton swab is effective in most hiccups, and suggests a pharyngeal 'gate-control' mechanism. Most of the 'grandmother's remedies' for hiccup involve pharyngeal stimulation either directly or indirectly:

1. Rapid ingestion of two heaped teaspoons of granulated sugar;
2. Rapid ingestion of two glasses of liquid;
3. Swallowing dry bread;
4. Swallowing crushed ice;
5. Drinking from the wrong side of a cup;
6. A cold key dropped down the collar of ones' shirt or blouse;
7. Having someone shout 'Boo!' loudly in order to produce a startle response;
8. Forceful tongue retraction sufficient to induce a gag reflex.

Breath holding and rebreathing into a bag are also physiological; the resultant hypercapnia has a central depressant effect and blocks the central component of the reflex. Deep breathing and chest physiotherapy may also disrupt the repetitive diaphragmatic spasms. Valsalva manoeuvre, carotid sinus massage, digital rectal massage, and even sexual intercourse have been reported to terminate hiccups.

It is preferable to direct treatment at the cause of hiccup, if identifiable. However, in many instances, a cause cannot be identified; hence general measures should be instituted.

Hiccups: Causes and Treatments

Causes	Treatments
Gastric distension	Reduce tube feeding
	Defoaming antiflatulent (simethicone)
	Prokinetic (metaclopromide)
Esophageal reflux	H_2 blocker (ranitidine) or proton pump inhibitor (lansoprazole)
Anxiety	Calm environment
Drug induced (benzodiazepines corticosteroids, barbiturates)	Stop, wean, or decrease the drug
Electrolyte imbalances	Supplement deficiency

Pharmacological Treatments

Most treatments are based on anecdotal experience or case reports, as the infrequent occurrence of hiccups precludes large controlled clinical trials.

Baclofen has emerged now as a safe and acceptable first-line drug in most situations. It is effective in doses as small as 5-10 mg/day, although occasionally 20 mg TDS is necessary.

Metaclopramide 10-20 mg QID orally

Nifedipine 10-20 mg TDS orally

Gabapentin can be used as add-on therapy with baclofen.

Haloperidol 1-4 mg TDS orally

Anticonvulsants like **phenytoin** 300 mg/day, **carbamazepine** 800 mg/day or **sodium valproate** 800 mg/day are more appropriately used with hiccups of central origin.

Lignocaine 1 mg/kg IV bolus followed by 2-4 mg/min IV infusion.

Chlorpromazine widely used previously, almost always works (probably by a diffuse depressant effect on the reticular formation), but does not correct gastric distension. Adverse drug reactions are common (e.g. sedation, dry mouth, postural hypotension) particularly in elderly debilitated patients. If used, chlorpromazine should be given in a test dose of 10-25 mg orally, and repeated BD/TDS either as needed or prophylactically, according to circumstances. If still intractable, chlorpromazine 25 mg IV can be given slowly over 2-3 minutes. The patient should lie down for 30-60 minutes, and be warned about drowsiness, light-headedness, and palpitations.

Midazolam 5-10 mg IV can be used to control hiccups in terminally ill patients. Maintenance treatment is by subcutaneous infusion of 30-120 mg/24 hours. Sedation is a concomitant side effect.

Glucagon which has a relaxant effect on the sphincter of Oddi is said to help if hiccup is caused by distension of the gallbladder secondary to opioid-induced constriction of the sphincter and minimal food.

Other measures for resistant cases include:
- Endoscopic maneuvers involving gentle massage over the cardia
- Crushing one or both phrenic nerves
- Phrenic nerve stimulation

- Hypnosis
- Acupuncture

Leg traction used by osteopaths, relaxes the ipsilateral psoas muscle and terminates spasm of the diaphragm.

Breathing pacemaker devices control excursions of the diaphragm by electric stimulation of the phrenic nerve.

SUGGESTED READING

1. Howard RS. Persistent hiccups. British Medical Journal, 1992; 305:1237-8.
2. Kranke P, Eberhart LH, Morin AM, Cracknell J, Greim CA, Roewer N. Treatment of hiccups during general anesthesia or sedation: a qualitative systemic review. Eur J Anaesthesiol 2003; 20: 239-44.
3. Levine JS. Hiccups. In: Levine JS(ed) Decision making in Gastroenterology. 2nd ed. St. Louis, CV Mosby 1992;92.
4. Lewis J. Hiccups: causes and cures. J Clin Gastroenterol. 1985; 7: 539-52
5. Smith HS, Busracamwongs A. Management of hiccups in the palliative care population. Am J Hosp Palliative Care 2003; 20: 149-54.
6. M.J. Pollack Intractable hiccups serious sign of underlying systemic disease. J Clin Gastroenterol 2003; 37 272-3.
7. Hernández JL. Gabapentin for intractable hiccup. Am J Med 2004; 117: 279-81.
8. Rousseau P. Hiccups. South Med J. 1995; 88:175-81.

5

Nandakumar R

The Differential Diagnosis of Abdominal Pain

INTRODUCTION

Abdominal pain is the most common gastrointestinal symptom encountered by gastroenterologists and primary care physicians alike.

PAIN TYPES

Pathophysiologically, there are three types of pain. They are:

Visceral pain: This is experienced when noxious stimuli trigger visceral nociceptors. Pain is usually dull and poorly localized in the abdomen; e.g. acute pancreatitis.

Parietal pain: This results from noxious stimulation of the parietal peritoneum and is generally more intense and more precisely localized than visceral pain. e.g. McBurney's point tenderness in acute appendicitis.

Referred pain: This is felt in areas remote to the diseased organ. It is a result of convergence of visceral afferent neurons with somatic afferent neurons from different anatomic regions on second order neurons in the spinal cord in the same spinal segment. e.g., shoulder pain in acute cholecystitis.

Clinical Pain Syndromes

1. Acute abdominal pain
2. Chronic abdominal pain   Intermittent
                                        Constant

Acute Abdominal Pain

The goal of the evaluation is to make an early, efficient and accurate diagnosis. A good clinical history, physical examination and selective use of appropriate lab and radiographic examinations are necessary for this.

Important Elements in Patient History

Onset of pain: Abrupt onset suggests a vascular cause e.g., mesenteric infarction, ruptured abdominal aortic aneurysm or perforation or volvulus of an abdominal organ e.g., perforated duodenal ulcer, sigmoid volvulus.

Extra abdominal causes of sudden pain that are referred to abdomen include inferior wall myocardial infarction, spontaneous pneumothorax, etc.

Pain onset is acute in conditions like appendicitis, cholecystitis and pancreatitis.

Site: This may give a clue to the underlying pathology

Right upper quadrant	Cholecystitis, liver abscess
Central	Peptic ulcer disease, pancreatitis, small intestinal colic
Left upper quadrant	Splenic infarct, splenic flexure ischemia
Right lower quadrant	Appendicitis, mesenteric adenitis
Left lower quadrant	Diverticulitis

Certain diseases specific to women can cause pain in both lower quadrants-salpingitis, ruptured ectopic, tubo-ovarian disorders.

Radiation: Cholecystitis-pain radiating to right shoulder/inferior angle of scapula, pancreatitis-pain radiasing to back and ureteric colic to loin.

Character: Peptic ulcer patient may present with a burning upper abdominal pain. Colic is a sharp intermittent griping pain that comes on suddenly and has a waxing and waning quality lasting a few minutes i.e., intestinal colic and ureteric colic.

Aggravating and relieving factors: Vomiting may give a transient relief of pain in intestinal colic, sitting up and leaning forward gives pain relief in pancreatitis. Ingestion of food can worsen the pain in bowel obstruction, fatty foods can aggravate cholecystitis and any body movement worsens the pain of peritonitis.

Associated intestinal symptoms: Hematemesis can occur in peptic ulcer disease. Diarrhea associated with crampy abdominal pain is present in gastroenteritis. Jaundice and abdominal pain suggest liver disease or biliary tract obstruction.

Associated extraintestinal symptoms: Significant fatigue and weight loss may indicate inflammatory bowel disease or malignancy as the underlying cause of abdominal pain. Inflammatory bowel disease (IBD) can have extra intestinal manifestations like iritis, arthritis, apthous ulcers, erythema nodosum and pyoderma gangrenosum. A history of skin rash that resolved over 7-10 days suggests neuropathic pain of herpes zoster. In female patients of child bearing age a missed period may be a clue to diagnosis of ectopic pregnancy. Referred pain from a cardiac or pulmonary origin should be considered if patient complains of shortness of breath, cough or chest pain.

Pastmedical and surgical history: Patients with known gallstones or diverticular disease may be experiencing a recurrence. A history of hypertension/vascular disease is a risk factor for a vascular cause. Ketoacidosis can present with abdominal pain and should be considered in a diabetic patient. Patients with a previous history of abdominal surgery are at risk for bowel obstruction caused by adhesions.

Drug history: NSAIDS can cause H.pylori-negative peptic ulcer disease. Azathioprine, didanosine and thiazide diuretics can cause pancreatitis.

Medical causes of acute abdominal pain—inferior wall myocardial infarction, diabetic ketosis, acute intermittent porphyria, sickle cell crises and lead colic.

Physical Examination

Patience in the examination of the patient and occasionally repeated examinations are required to make a diagnosis. Examination begins with the assessment of vital signs. This helps in grading the severity and choosing the probable surgical candidates.

Posture: Patients with peritonitis prefer to be still whereas patients with renal or intestinal colic will be restless. Patients with pancreatitis tend to sit up and lean forward. A proper and thorough inspection can give valuable clues. Sluggish movement of abdominal wall indicates peritonitis, a "step ladder" pattern of visible peristalsis indicates small bowel obstruction. Inspection of hernial orifice may reveal femoral hernia as the cause of the intestinal obstruction. Scars of previous surgery should be noted.

Palpation

Start palpating lightly in areas away from the abdominal pain. A positive Murphy's sign is supportive of a diagnosis of cholecystitis and rebound tenderness at McBurney's point suggests appendicitis. Generalized severe abdominal tenderness is indicative of diffuse peritoneal inflammation. A note should be made of hernias and abdominal lumps. Significant abdominal pain in the absence of physical examination findings in an elderly person may be a clue to mesenteric ischemia. A rectal examination should be performed in all cases. In male patients external genitalia should be examined as pain from testicular torsion or epididymitis may be referred to abdomen. In women, a pelvic examination should be performed to check for pelvic masses, cervical motion tenderness and discharge.

Auscultation: Hyperactive bowel sounds occur with partial bowel obstruction whereas a silent abdomen indicates generalized peritonitis. An abdominal bruit suggests potential vascular pathology.

A careful examination of respiratory system for basal lung or pleural involvement and spine should be done.

Investigations

Lab studies should include complete blood count (CBC), urine analysis and in women of childbearing age, a pregnancy test. Other tests commonly obtained include liver function test (LFT), renal function test (RFT), blood sugar, amylase and lipase.

Test	Clinical state
CBC	Infection, anemia, hemorrhage
Urine analysis	Urinary tract infection, stones, diabetes
LFT	Cholecystitis, liver abscess, hepatitis
Amylase, lipase	Pancreatitis
RFT, blood sugar, electrolytes	Renal impairment, diabetes, assess hydration

Plain X-ray Abdomen

Should include two views viz; supine and upright. If the patient is unable to sit upright, lateral decubitus view should be obtained. Plain films are useful in evaluating for intestinal obstruction and for free air, which signifies a perforated viscus. Even though yield is low for a diagnostic abdominal abnormality this should be done because it is readily available and inexpensive. Additional information is limited but include evidences of kidney stones, gallstones (if radio opaque) and pancreatic calcification.

Ultrasound Abdomen

This is a very useful investigation in suspected gallstones, renal stones, pancreatitis, appendicitis and gynecologic causes.

CT Abdomen

CT abdomen has an important role in evaluating undifferentiated acute abdominal pain with a diagnostic yield of more than 90%. Contrast enhanced CT (CECT) has made important advances in deciding the management of conditions like acute pancreatitis where the severity can be graded (Balthazar's grading).

Laparoscopy

The role for laparoscopy is in situations where diagnostic uncertainty exists and the patient's condition demands intervention.

Guidelines for Management

Initial stabilization: This includes administration of colloids/crystalloids/blood products, e.g., in a case of peritonitis while making a diagnosis.

Treatment of Cause

Broad-spectrum antibiotics should be started in cholecystitis, pancreatitis, diverticulitis and salpingitis. Surgery may be indicated in appendicitis, perforated duodenal ulcer and ruptured ectopic pregnancy.

Chronic Abdominal Pain

Common Causes

Chronic intermittent pain

Inflammatory
- Inflammatory bowel disease
- Endometriosis
- Recurrent pancreatitis.

Mechanical
- Intermittent intestinal obstruction

Metabolic/Neurologic
- Porphyria
- Uremia
- Diabetic radiculopathy
- Abdominal epilepsy

Miscellaneous
- Irritable bowel syndrome
- Peptic ulcer
- Nonulcer dyspepsia
- Chronic mesenteric ischemia

Chronic Persistent Pain

- Chronic pancreatitis
- Malignancy

As in the evaluation of acute abdominal pain a good clinical history is essential. A careful history of chronology, location, character, aggravating and relieving factors often narrows the differential diagnosis.

Pain that occurs within 30 minutes of eating and persisting for hours in an elderly signifies mesenteric ischemia. Epigastric pain aggravated by eating and radiating to back indicates chronic pancreatitis as the probable cause. Pelvic pain at monthly interval suggests endometriosis. Weight loss suggests malignancy or malabsorption. Fever, weight loss and diarrhea may be a clue to abdominal tuberculosis.

Physical Examination

The evaluation includes a careful abdominal examination and a systemic examination for extra-abdominal manifestation of underlying disease. Jaundice may be associated with hepatic or biliary cancer. A lump in the right iliac fossa may indicate tuberculosis or Crohn's disease. Perianal lesions are suggestive of inflammatory bowel disease.

Lab Investigations

Lab studies should include CBC, CRP (C-reactive protein), LFT, RFT, blood sugar, stool fat and stool occult blood.

Anemia, raised ESR and CRP may suggest tuberculosis, Crohn's disease or malignancy.

Stool fat may be positive in chronic pancreatitis and malabsorptive diseases. Stool occult blood may indicate malignancy or IBD.

Imaging

Plain X-ray: May reveal calcifications in chronic pancreatitis.

Ultrasound: First line of investigation in pancreatitis, gallstones, liver masses: Lymphadenopathy, abdominal masses and ascites can be made out.

CT Abdomen

This investigation is extremely useful in delineating thickened bowel loops, abdominal lumps, lymphadenopathy as in abdominal tuberculosis and Crohn's disease. CT also gives valuable information in chronic pancreatitis and its complications like pseudocysts and pancreatic masses. In mesenteric ischemia CT may reveal vascular thrombus and thickening of bowel loops.

Mesenteric Angiography

This is a useful modality in suspected in cases of mesenteric ischemia .

Endoscopic Evaluation

Upper GI Scopy and Colonoscopy

Upper GI endoscopy is invaluable in diagnosing peptic ulcers. Endoscopic evaluation is essential in the evaluation of inflammatory bowel disease, abdominal tuberculosis and GI malignancy.

Management

Proton pump inhibitors (PPIs) in peptic ulcer, *H.pylori eradication*. Treatment of underlying cause; e.g., aminosalicylates, steroids and immunosuppressives in inflammatory bowel disease, antituberculous treatment in tuberculosis. Analgesics and pancreatic enzyme replacement therapy in chronic pancreatitis.

In cases where no effective treatment is available as in advanced malignancy palliation should be the aim.

Pharmacologic – analgesics, antidepressants. The dose should be titrated to get pain relief.

Chemical or surgical nerve ablation: Celiac ganglion blockade.

Endoscopic or percutaneous biliary decompression is used in advanced malignancy and biliary obstruction.

Address Physical and Psychologic Symptoms

A multidisciplinary approach involving psychiatrist, physiotherapist and medical social workers is needed in most cases.

SUGGESTED READING

1. Gastroenterology problems – the academy collection by Martin S. Lipsky.
2. JSP Lumley. Hamilton Bailey's Physical signs – Demonstration of physical signs in clinical surgery; 18th edition.
3. S. Das. A manual on clinical surgery. 5th edition, 2000.
4. Michael Swash; Hutchinson's clinical methods; 21st edition, 2002.
5. Hyams JS. Irritable bowel syndrome, functional dyspepsia, and functional abdominal pain syndrome. Adolesc Med Clin 2004; 15: 1-15.
6. Drossman DA. Chronic functional abdominal pain. Am J Gastroenterol 1996; 91:2270-81
7. Drossman DA, Whitehead WE, Camilleri M. Irritable bowel syndrome. A technical review for practical guideline development. Gastroenterology 1997; 122:2120-37.

6

Varghese Thomas

Peptic Ulcer in the Era of *H. pylori*

INTRODUCTION

The discovery of *H. pylori* has revolutionized the management of peptic ulcer disease. There is a very strong correlation between the presence of peptic ulcer disease and *H. pylori* infection. It is now mandatory to check for *H. pylori* infection in all cases of peptic ulcer. At present peptic ulcer disease is classified as *H. pylori* related, NSAID related and those due to miscellaneous causes.

Aims of Management of Peptic Ulcer

- To provide symptomatic relief
- To induce healing of ulcers
- To prevent complications
- To prevent recurrence.

Diagnosis of Peptic Ulcer Disease

The gold standard for diagnosis of peptic ulcer is upper GI endoscopy (Figs 6.1 and 6.2). In the case of gastric ulcer, four-quadrant biopsy is mandatory to rule out neoplasm and in the case of duodenal and gastric ulcer, biopsy from the antrum is mandatory to look for *H. pylori* infection.

HOW TO DIAGNOSE *H. pylori* INFECTION?

Serology Tests

These tests detect IgG antibodies against *H. pylori*. Tests on the whole blood as well as serum are available but these tests are almost as expensive as endoscopy

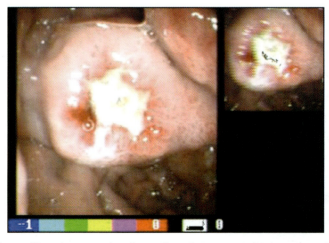

Fig. 6.1: Upper GI endoscopy showing active ulcer on greater curvature of stomach

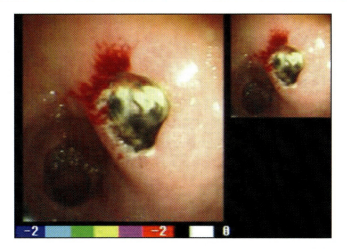

Fig. 6.2: Upper GI endoscopy showing active ulcer in first part of duodenum

test. IgG antibodies test confirms only the presence of past infection and it is of no use to find out whether there is current infection. This test has only limited value in assessment of response to treatment The sensitivity and specificity of these tests range from 80 to 95% depending upon the assay used.

Rapid Urease Test

This test is done on endoscopic biopsies of antral mucosa. Urease test detects the presence of urease enzyme of HP. False negative tests occur soon after antibiotic therapy as well as in patients receiving proton pump inhibitors (PPI). Therefore this test is to be done at least after two weeks of stopping PPI or antibiotics. This is a quick test and therefore this test is widely used by endoscopists.

Histopathology of Gastric Mucosa

Special staining on gastric mucosal biopsies with Warthin Starry or Giemsa stains helps in the detection of *H. pylori* infection. This is a very useful test in the hands of expert pathologists. Histologic identification of organisms is considered the gold standard of diagnostic tests.

Culture for *H. pylori*

Though an ideal test to detect infection, success rate is not very high with this technique. Culture and sensitivity tests became extremely useful in the management of recurrent or relapsed *H. pylori* infection because it helps us to know the pattern of drug sensitivity/resistance of the organisms.

Urea Breath Tests (^{14}C or ^{13}C)

Urea breath test is a noninvasive technique of detecting *H. pylori*. Hence it has very high acceptance among the patients and it is used for the detection of current *H. pylori* infection as well as for assessing response to treatment. Recent use of as well as antibiotics will give a false negative result. The sensitivity and specificity of this test ranges from 94 to 98%.

Detection of ELISA Antigen in Stool

This test detects the antigen of *H. pylori* by using ELISA technique and it requires further validation before it is to be put to routine use.

Indications for Testing *H. pylori* Infection

1. All cases of duodenal ulcers and gastric ulcers confirmed by either endoscopy or barium meal or surgery.
2. All cases of carcinoma stomach and gastric lymphoma.
3. All first degree relatives of patients with carcinoma stomach.
4. Chronic ulcer negative dyspepsia.

Indications for Eradication of *H.pylori*

The only treatment, which will alter the natural history of ulcer, is by eradication of *H. pylori*. It may look superfluous to define criteria for eradication of *H. pylori*. This dilemma is because we are not sure whether the *H. pylori* infection detected in a particular case is due to pathogenic or non-pathogenic strains. The indications for *H. pylori* eradication are:

1. All cases of *H. pylori* positive gastric or duodenal ulcers.
2. All cases of operated carcinoma stomach (*H. pylori* positive).
3. First degree relatives of patients with carcinoma stomach and who are *H. pylori*-positive.
4. Prophylactic eradication in a patient who is to be put on NSAIDS on a long-term basis.
5. Gastric maltoma.

Maastricht 2-2000-Key Management Strategies

1. Test and treat approach—all dyspeptics below 45 years.
2. Diagnosis is based on Urea breath test or stool antigen.
3. Check success by urea breath test or stool antigen test.
4. In uncomplicated duodenal ulcer, no further antisecretory treatment is given after *H. pylori* eradication.
5. Those patients on long term maintenance or on demand therapy are tested for *H. pylori* and treated if found positive.

Standard Regimes—Triple Therapy or Quadruple Therapy

Like in antituberculous treatment, multiple drugs are used to eradicate the bacteria in view of widespread drug resistance Single antibiotic treatment is useless because it induces development of drug resistance faster.

Triple Drug therapy

Conventional regimes (Bismuth based) x two weeks: 30%-80% eradication rate

1. Tetracycline 500 TID, metronidazole 500 mg TID, bismuth 240 mg BID
2. Amoxicillin 750 mg TID, metronidazole 500 mg TID and bismuth 240 mg BID

   Tinidazole 500 mg BID can be used to replace metronidazole in all regimes

Newer Triple Therapy (PPI based) Regimes x two weeks-85-90% eradication rate

1. AOC—Amoxicillin 1gm BID, omeprazole 20 mg BID, clarithromycin 500 mg BID.

2. MOC—Metronidazole 500 mg BID, omeprazole 20 mg BID, clarithromycin 500 mg BID.
3. MOA—Metronidazole 500 mg BID, omeprazole 20 mg BID, amoxicillin 1 gm BID – 80%.
4. Regimes containing metronidazole 500 mg TID and clarithromycin 250 mg BID or amoxicillin 750 mg BID with omeprazole 20 mg BID are also quite effective (85%). Omeprazole can be replaced by lansoprazole 30 mg BID. Metronidazole can be replaced by tinidazole 500 mg BID.

   PPI based regimes with 10-day schedule also has been found to give eradication rate of about 90 %. Although PPI based triple therapy regime for one week is widely promoted by pharmaceutical firms, its efficacy has been found to be about 70% only and hence it cannot be recommended in Indian conditions.

Quadruple Drug Therapy for Two Weeks

Addition of bismuth compounds to the newer triple drug regimes increases the therapeutic efficacy to above 95%. However it is not favoured routinely as compliance comes down with more number of drugs and with high costs of treatment.

Indian Scenario

Due to the wide spread use or misuse of antibiotics in India, resistance to metronidazole and clarithromycin is quite common. Resistances to amoxicillin and bismuth compounds are less common. However, large studies in India using metronidazole/tinidazole containing regime with omeprazole for two weeks have found eradication rates to be around 90%. It has been recommended to give triple or quadruple drug regime for a minimum period of 2 weeks in India (2nd National workshop on *H. pylori* 1999, Thrissur, India). Patient compliance is the single most important deciding eradication of *H. pylori*. Based on current evidence, *H. pylori* eradication is of no use in the routine management of non-ulcer dyspepsia.

The Indian recommendation is to treat for a minimum period of 14 days.

Side Effects of *H. pylori* Eradication Therapy

* Gastrointestinal side effects, insomnia, antibiotic associated colitis.
* Renal involvement due to bismuth therapy, neuropathy.

Economics of *H. pylori* Eradication

A patient with ulcer disease usually gets repeated exacerbation of symptoms for a period upto 10 to 12 years requiring multiple visits to doctors, and multiple investigations repeatedly. Surgical complications will add to the morbidity, mortality and expenses. It has been observed that with conventional therapy, the ulcer recurrence rate is almost 80% at the end of first year after treatment. By eradicating *H. pylori*, this trend can be reversed and the risk of recurrence can be reduced to 20% at the end of first year as well in subsequent years. Therefore eradication of *H. pylori* saves a lot of money for the patient as well as the exchequer and also saves lot of working hours.

Management of Duodenal Ulcer

The history of NSAID intake is to be meticulously noted and *H. pylori* status assessed. In *H. pylori* positive duodenal ulcer disease, initially Hp eradication therapy is to be given for a period of two weeks and this is to be followed by two weeks of standard dose PPI. In most uncomplicated cases this treatment will induce ulcer healing. In patients with complicated ulcer disease, PPI therapy is to be continued for 6-8 weeks and it is worthwhile to check for eradication of *H. pylori* after initial treatment. If *H. pylori* is found to be persisting, drug sensitivity profile of *H. pylori* is to be found out by culture.

Management of Gastric Ulcer

All gastric ulcers in addition to routine testing for *H. pylori* infection should undergo four quadrant biopsy and histopathological examination to rule out malignancy. In benign gastric ulcers, which are *H. pylori* positive, initial *H. pylori* eradication treatment is to be given for a period of two weeks and this is to be followed by PPI therapy for 8-12 weeks. A repeat endoscopy is to be done at the end of the treatment period to confirm ulcer healing. In complicated cases, *H. pylori* eradication is also to be confirmed after treatment.

Management of NSAID Induced Ulcers

If the ulcer disease is likely to be NSAID related, we have to advise the patient to stop the offending drug and start treatment with PPI in standard dose for a period for 6 to 8 weeks. If the NSAID is to be continued, try to switch over to gastric friendly drugs. Low dose aspirin may be replaced with clopidogrel. However if the patient has diseases like rheumatoid arthritis, which require prolonged use of NSAIDs, it will be safe to administer PPI in full dose as long as the NSAID is administered. If there is history of NSAID intake and if *H. pylori* is positive, we have to start treatment with *H. pylori* eradication therapy and follow it up with standard dose of PPI. Prophylactic administration of H_2 blockers have not been found to be effective in preventing occurrence of NSAID related ulcer disease.

Management of Refractory Ulcer

If the ulcer fails to heal even after three standard courses of treatment, we have to consider it refractory and search for other causes. Undetected NSAID intake, failure to eradiate *H. pylori* (false negative tests), smoking and presence of Zollinger-Ellison syndrome are some common causes. Very rarely the ulcer could be due to tuberculosis or Crohn's disease. In the absence of specific causes, double dose therapy with PPI may be administered for 8 to 12 weeks.

Management of Anastomotic Ulcers

Surgery for peptic ulcer is seldom done now-a-days except in cases of complications. If anastomotic ulcer develops, it suggests incomplete vagotomy. Ideally vagotomy is to be completed in such cases. However many patients prefer life long maintenance therapy with PPI in standard doses. *H. pylori*, if found to be positive, needs eradication.

Maintenance Treatment

This form of treatment was in vogue in the pre *H. pylori* era. The earlier indications for maintenance treatment are indications for eradication of Hp at present. In a patient with complicated ulcer disease, if *H. pylori* cannot be eradicated despite repeated attempts either due to drug intolerance or due to resistant bacteria, maintenance treatment can be planned. However, on stopping the treatment, the patient continues to have the same risk of ulcer recurrence. Other indications for drug maintenance are:

1. Complicated ulcer (bleeding, intractability) requiring surgery, but the risks of surgery are extremely high due to co-morbid conditions – *H. pylori* negative.
2. Frequent recurrences—*H. pylori* negative—not fit for surgery due to co-morbid conditions.

Conventional maintenance regimes use half the therapeutic dose of ranitidine or famotidine for indefinite period. If the patient continues to smoke, full dose H_2 blockers will be required. Prophylaxis with PPI (standard or even double dose) is advised if there is refractory ulcer. The rate of break through ulcer is 25% per year. Each acute exacerbation, while on maintenance, is to be treated like active ulcer disease. If the indication for maintenance treatment is in a patient who had a potentially life threatening complication, PPI in the standard/ double dose may be prescribed. At present data on prolonged use of PPI is limited.

Gastric Carcinoma and MALToma

H. pylori infection has been known to progress to gastric carcinoma or gastric MALT (mucosal associated lymphoid tissue) lymphoma (MALToma). This is one important reason for advocating the eradication of *H. pylori* infection.

SUGGESTED READING

1. Chan FK. Helicobacter pylori and nonsteroidal anti-inflammatory drugs. Gastroenterol Clin North Am 2001; 30:937-52.
2. Saad R, Diagnosis and management of peptic ulcer disease. Clin Fam Pract—2004; 6; 569-87.
3. Shiotani A. Pathogenesis and therapy of gastric and duodenal ulcer disease. Med Clin North Am 2002; 86: 1447-66.
4. Marshall B. The relation of Helicobacter pylori to gastric adenocarcinoma and lymphoma: pathophysiology, epidemiology, screening, clinical presentation, treatment, and prevention. Med Clin North Am—2005; 89; 313-44
5. Suerbaum S., Michetti P. Helicobacter pylori infection. N Engl J Med 2002; 347: 1175-86.
6. Walsh J. H., Peterson W. L. The Treatment of Helicobacter pylori infection in the management of peptic ulcer disease. N Engl J Med 1995; 333:984-91.

7

Prem Nair
Rajiv Mehta

The Management of Upper Gastrointestinal Bleed

INTRODUCTION

Upper gastrointestinal (GI) hemorrhage is one of the most common medical emergencies, which carries hospital mortality in excess of 10%. Upper GI bleeding is arbitrarily defined as gastrointestinal hemorrhage from a source proximal to the ligament of Treitz. A multidisciplinary approach involving medical, surgical and interventional radiology teams improves the efficiency of care for patients with acute upper gastrointestinal hemorrhage. There are many causes of upper gastrointestinal bleeding, peptic ulcer and varices being the most important. In this article, the approach to upper GI bleeding is discussed with special emphasis on hemorrhage related to varices and peptic ulcer.

DEFINITIONS

Patients with upper gastrointestinal bleeding can present in four ways:
- *Hematemesis* is vomiting of red blood or "coffee-ground" material.
- *Melena* is black, tarry, foul-smelling stool.
- *Hematochezia* is passage of bright red or maroon blood from the rectum.
- *Occult GI bleeding* is identification of GI bleeding in the absence of overt bleeding by special examination of the stool (e.g. Guaiac testing).

CAUSES

The two most important causes of major life threatening acute gastrointestinal bleeding are peptic ulcer and esophagogastric varices (Table 7.1). In case of peptic ulcer, significant hemorrhage is due to erosion of an underlying artery. *H. pylori* infection and ingestion of non-steroidal anti-inflammatory drugs (NSAID) are two most common causes of peptic ulcer.

Esophagogastric varices secondary to portal hypertension is the most common cause of upper gastrointestinal bleeding in India. Cirrhosis is the most common cause of portal hypertension and is caused by both increased outflow resistance and increased portal venous inflow. The most common site for such collaterals is the gastroesophageal junction, where they form submucosal varicose veins called varices. Prognosis in variceal bleeding is related to the severity of liver disease as well as the magnitude of bleeding. Even without intervention, bleeding ceases in up to 50% of the patients.

Mallory-Weiss tears, which are usually on the gastric side of the gastroesophageal junction, are usually associated with alcohol abuse. Bleeding from these tears stops spontaneously in 80% to 90% of patients and recurs in only up to 5%.

A range of vascular anomalies such as large or multiple arteriovenous malformations (AVMs), gastric antral vascular ectasia (GAVE) and Dieulafoy's lesions may be responsible for upper GI bleeding.

Esophagitis is a common finding in elderly patients who present with "coffee ground" hematemesis. Bleeding usually stops with conservative supportive therapy with proton pump inhibitors.

Hemorrhagic gastritis and duodenitis are often associated with NSAID use and *Helicobacter pylori* infection. Hemodynamic support, stopping NSAIDs, and *H. pylori* eradication are required.

Portal hypertensive gastropathy (PHG) is due to venous congestion of the gastric mucosa secondary to portal hypertension. Majority of times, it causes mild bleeding.

Aortoduodenal fistula should be considered in patients who present with major upper gastrointestinal bleeding after aortic graft insertion. Bleeding occurs from the second part of the duodenum.

Esophagogastric tumors are a relatively uncommon cause of acute upper gastrointestinal hemorrhage. Carcinomas and lymphomas of the stomach tend to present with other upper gastrointestinal symptoms and with iron deficiency anemia rather than acute bleeding.

Causes of Acute Upper Gastrointestinal Bleeding

1. Peptic ulcer disease.
2. Variceal bleeding related to portal hypertension.
3. Mallory-weiss tear.
4. Arteriovenous malformation.
5. Esophagitis.
6. Duodenitis/gastritis/erosions.
7. Portal hypertensive gastropathy.
8. Aortoduodenal fistula.
9. Esophagogastric tumors.

Resuscitation

In any patient with a significant gastrointestinal hemorrhage, history taking, physical examination, and resuscitation need to proceed simultaneously. The principles of "ABC (airway, breathing, and circulation)" apply in the resuscitation of patients with upper GI bleeding. An immediate assessment of hemodynamic status and picked red cell transfusion requirements must be made before detailed history and physical examination. It is very much vital to look for postural tachycardia and postural hypotension to assess blood loss. Hypotensive patients require to be placed in a head-down position to maintain cerebral perfusion. It is crucial to recognize cardiopulmonary co-morbidity in patients with peptic ulcer bleeding, since most deaths are due to decompensation of general medical diseases precipitated by the bleed. Central venous pressure monitoring is useful in the elderly and in patients with cardiac disease to optimize decisions concerning fluid replacement. Crystalloids (principally normal saline) are used to normalize blood pressure and urine output; colloids (such as Hemaccel) are often used in the presence of major hypotension. If the hemoglobin concentration is less than 10 g/dl in a patient with postural hypotension, it is advisable to transfuse, as the hemoglobin will continue to drift downwards after crystalloid infusion.

Differentiation of Upper from Lower GI Bleeding

Hematemesis indicates an upper GI source of bleeding (above the ligament of Treitz). Melena indicates that blood has been present in the GI tract for at least 12 hours. Hematochezia usually indicates a lower GI source of bleeding, although brisk upper GI bleeding may cause hematochezia. Since the sensitivity of nasogastric tube aspiration is low and less tolerated, it is not usually recommended to insert it patients with upper GI bleeding.

Role of Endoscopy

Upper endoscopy can distinguish between variceal bleeding and non-variceal bleeding, as the management strategies are different. Early upper endoscopy in patients hospitalized with upper gastrointestinal hemorrhage results in a shorter hospital stay, reduced risk of recurrent hemorrhage, and reduced requirement for surgical intervention. Optimum resuscitation must be done before endoscopy since endoscopy is dangerous in the hemodynamically compromised or hypoxic patient. Endoscopy must be undertaken within 24 hours after admission since "low risk" patients can be then safely discharged from hospital on the same day.

Endoscopy has three purposes:
1. Accurate diagnosis.
2. Risk stratification.
3. Control of bleeding .

Risk Stratification

The risk of death after admission to hospital for upper GI bleeding depends on host factors like age, co-morbid illness, and presence of shock, endoscopic features and the underlying diagnosis. Early endoscopy permits accurate risk stratification. Morbidity and mortality are higher in those with re-bleeding and 95% of re-bleeding occurs within the first 72 hours of hospitalization. Risk of mortality in variceal bleeding is related to Child –Pugh score of decompensated cirrhosis liver and presence of shock at the time of admission. Risk of mortality in non-variceal bleeding is related to major stigmata of bleeding during upper endoscopy (Table 7.1), associated co-morbidity and presence of shock at admission.

Table 7.1: Modified Forrest criteria of stigmata of recent hemorrhage in peptic ulcer bleeding

Endoscopic findings	% Re-bleeding
1. Actively bleeding ulcer	
1a. Spurting	80
1b. Oozing	50
2. Non-actively bleeding ulcer	
2a. Non-bleeding visible vessels	33
2b. Ulcer with adherent clot	30
2c. Ulcer with flat spot	7
3. Ulcer with clean base	3

MANAGEMENT

Endoscopic hemostasis is the cornerstone in the management of patients with upper GI bleeding. Endoscopic management depends on whether bleeding is variceal or non-variceal. With the advances in therapeutic endoscopy, around 80% to 90% bleeding can be controlled by endoscopy. Treatment algorithm for the management of acute upper gastrointestinal bleeding is given in Fig. 7.1.

Management of Non-variceal Bleeding

The commonest cause of upper gastrointestinal hemorrhage is peptic ulcer disease. Around 50% of patients will have a clean-based ulcer and an uncomplicated presentation requiring no further treatment after endoscopy (See fig. 6.1).

Pharmacological Treatment

Mucosal fibrinolytic activity is enhanced in patients with bleeding gastroduodenal ulcers. Acid suppressive therapy decreases this increased

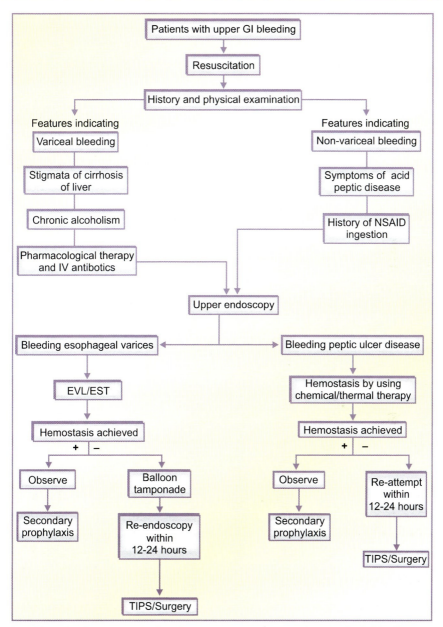

Fig. 7.1: Management algorithm for acute upper gastrointestinal bleeding

fibrinolytic activity. Thus, high dose intravenous omeprazole, after endoscopic treatment of bleeding peptic ulcers, has shown a reduction in re-bleeding rate and surgery.

Endoscopic Therapy

Endoscopic hemostasis for non-variceal therapy is principally based upon clinical trials for peptic ulcer hemorrhage. Main aim of endoscopic hemostasis is to seal the arterial defect created by the ulcer. This can be done by either injection, thermal or mechanical therapy. Recent literature has showed that combination therapy, including injection and thermal, is better than either alone. Mechanical devices like endoclip, which is more costly, has equal results as combination of injection and thermal therapies. Complications of endoscopic therapy are remarkably infrequent. The major concern is aspiration pneumonia during procedure. Perforation and fibrous stricturing at the endoscopically treated point is infrequent. Various modalities of endoscopic hemostasis shown below can be used either singly or in combinations (Table 7.2)

Re-bleeding occurs in 15%–20% of cases after initial successful endoscopic

Table 7.2: Various modalities of endoscopic hemostasis in non-variceal bleeding

Injection	Thermal	Mechanical
Adrenaline (1:10000)	Heater probe	Hemoclip
Absolute alcohol	Bicap probe	Banding
Polidocanol	APC*	Staple device
Ethanolamine oleate	Laser therapy **	Endoloop
Sodium morrhuate		
Fibrin glue		

NB: * Argon plasma coagulation ** Argon/ Nd: YAG laser

Endosopic therapy for re-bleeding

Re-bleeding occurs 15-20% of cases after initial successful and 50% a hemostasis, usually within first 72 hours. Re-bleeding depends on endoscopic findings of ulcer base (Table 7.1). Management of re-bleeding is often difficult and is, to a large extent, based upon clinical judgment and local expertise. If adequate hemostasis is achieved by endoscopic re-treatment, an expectant policy is reasonable, but further bleeding is an absolute indication for operative intervention or radiological emobolization of bleeding vessels.

Secondary Prophylaxis

Avoidance of NSAID or using COX-2 inhibitors and eradication of *H. pylori* infection are the main strategy for secondary prophylaxis.

Management of Variceal Bleeding

Even though bleeding ceases in up to 50% of the patients with variceal bleeding, endotherapy is required in all patients to prevent re-bleeding. Management includes control of bleeding, prevention of re-bleeding and treating complications associated with variceal bleeding in cirrhosis liver like aspiration, pneumonia, sepsis, and hepatic encephalopathy (Figs 7.2 and 7.3)

Control of Bleeding

There are various modalities to control bleeding:
1. Pharmacologic therapy includes vasopression, somatostatin and its analogue,octreotide.
2. Endotherapy includes endoscopic sclerotherapy (EST), endovariceal ligation (EVL), and endoloop therapy.
3. Balloon tamponade.
4. TIPS (Transjugular intrahepatic portosystemic shunt)
5. Surgery includes devascularization.

Pharmacological Therapy

Vasopressin causes splanchnic and systemic vasoconstriction directly and decreases portal venous flow. Vasopressin achieves hemostasis in about 55% of patients but ischemic side effects like myocardial ischemia, cerebral ischemia and acrocyanosis occur in around 20 to 30% of patients. These complications markedly decreased the state of use of vasopressin for variceal hemorrhage.

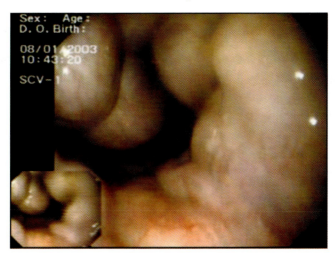

Fig. 7.2: Upper GI endoscopy showing large dilated tortuous venous channel in lower esophagus suggestion of esophageal varices

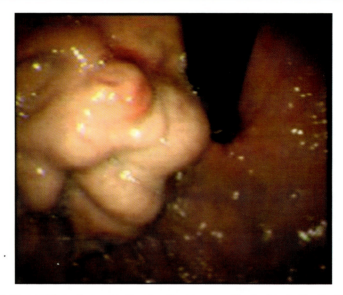

Fig. 7.3: Upper GI endoscopy showing large grape like lesion in the fundus of stomach indicating gastric varices.

Somatostatin and its analogue octreotide inhibit the secretion of various vasodilator hormones, such as glucagon and vasoactive intestine peptide (VIP). They are as effective as vasopressin in the control of variceal bleeding and are associated with virtually no side effects.

Endoscopic Therapy

Combination of endotherapy and pharmacological therapy has been found to be superior to either alone. EST is an effective method for the control of active bleeding from esophageal varices (70% to 90% hemostasis rate). Both intravariceal and paravariceal injections are equally effective. EST carries a 10% to 30% complication rate like stricture formation, ulceration, perforation, pleural effusion and odynophagia.

Endoscopic variceal ligation achieves hemostasis in 90% of cases and is considered preferable to EST because of lower re-bleeding rates and fewer complications. The EVL procedure involves deploying 5 to 10 bands on varices in a circumferential fashion in the esophagus.

Balloon Tamponade

Balloon tamponade achieves short-term hemostasis in 60% to 90% of all variceal hemorrhages. Three types of balloons have been used: (1) the standard

Sengstaken-Blakemore tube, (2) the Minnesota tube, and (3) the Linton-Nachlas tube. Once in place the balloons should be deflated after a maximum of 24 hours to re-evaluate bleeding status. Prolonged use (>24 hours) can produce pressure necrosis and other complications like aspiration, pneumonia, nasopharyngeal bleeding and esophageal rupture.

Transjugular Intrahepatic Portosystemic Shunt (TIPS)

Endoscopic or pharmacologic treatment is ineffective in 10% to 20% of patients with acute variceal bleeding, who require either surgical shunts or non-surgical shunts (TIPS). TIPS is placed by angiographic methods, which usually take 1 to 2 hours, and is technically successful to achieve hemostasis in greater then 90% of subjects. TIPS thrombosis occurs in 3% to 10% of all cases, which may present with recurrent variceal hemorrhage. Regular monitoring of stent patency and function is mandated after TIPS placement.

Surgical Treatment

Surgical treatment includes portosytemic shunts or devascularization. Shunt operations may be classified as nonselective (total or partial), or selective shunts. Nonselective shunts decompress the portal systems by diverting all portal flow away from the liver. Portosystemic encephalopathy occurs in around 40% to 50% of patients following nonselective shunts. Selective shunt,e.g. distal splenorenal shunt, decompresses the gastroesophageal junction and preserves hepatopetal flow. Thus, incidence of portosystemic encephalopathy is low but it cannot be used in patients with ascites since it does not reduce sinusoidal hypertension.

Prevention of Re-bleeding

The risk of re-bleeding is greatest in first 5 days and then declines, reaching a plateau by 6 weeks. Untreated, 70% of patients experience recurrent variceal hemorrhage within one year and 70% die within the first year. Non-selective β-blockers (propranolol, nadalol) reduce the risk of re-bleeding by approximately 40% and mortality by 20%. Since EVL has fewer complications than EST, band ligation is the endoscopic treatment of choice for long-term management of variceal hemorrhage. The combination of non-selective β-blockers and EVL has not been well studied.

SUGGESTED READING

1. American College of Gastroenterology Practice Parameters Committee. Am J Gastroenterol 1997; 92:1081-91.
2. Management of gastrointestinal bleeding. Clin Fam Pract 2004; 6(3); 631.
3. Non-variceal upper gastrointestinal bleeding. Gastroenterol Clin North Am 2003; 32(4): 1053-78
4. Oh D. Management of upper gastrointestinal bleeding. Clin Fam Pract 2004; 6; 631-45.
5. Ghosh S, Watts D, Kinnear M. Management of gastrointestinal haemorrhage. Postgrad. Med. J. 2002; 78: 4-14.
6. Arasaradnam R P and Donnelly M T. Acute endoscopic intervention in non-variceal upper gastrointestinal bleeding. Postgrad. Med. J. 2005; 81: 92—98.
7. Palmer K. Management of haematemesis and melaena. Postgrad. Med. J. 2004; 80: 399-404.

8

Rajiv Mehta

Chronic Diarrhea

INTRODUCTION

Chronic diarrhea is a common problem in day-to-day practice. With a broad ranging differential diagnosis and dozens of diagnostic tests to choose, every physician feels some trepidation in evaluating these patients. Systematic approach to chronic diarrhea is usually rewarded by a correct diagnosis and effective treatment. Diarrhea in HIV positive patients has been discussed separately in another chapter.

DEFINITION

Diarrhea is defined as an increase in the frequency and fluidity of stools. Since stool weight depends on dietary intake, stool weight by itself is an imperfect criterion to define diarrhea. Acute diarrhea refers to an illness of less than two weeks duration. Chronic diarrhea refers to an illness of greater than two weeks duration.

PATHOPHYSIOLOGY

Normally, 9 to10 liters of fluid composed of ingested fluid and secretions from salivary glands, stomach, pancreas, bile ducts and duodenum pass the ligament of Treitz. The jejunum absorbs approximately 6 L and the ileum 2.5 L, leaving about 1 to 1.5 L to pass into the colon each day. The colon removes 90% of this load, and so stool water represents only about 1% of the fluid entering the gut each day. Reduction of water absorption by as little as 1% can result in diarrhea. Reduction of net water absorption may be due to a reduced rate of water absorption by the mucosa, stimulation of secretions, or increased intestinal motility, thereby reducing the time for absorption to take place.

Osmotic diarrhea: Unlike renal tubules, the intestine cannot maintain an osmotic gradient between luminal contents and the plasma because of its high permeability of water. Thus, retention of solute molecules within the bowel lumen generates osmotic forces that retard the normal absorption of water. Ingestion of magnesium salts, lactose ingestion by lactase deficient individuals, excessive lactulose intake, and ingestion of artificial sweeteners like sorbitol, cause osmotic diarrhea.

Secretory diarrhea: Secretory diarrhea occurs by either of two mechanisms: by inhibiting absorption or stimulating secretions. It is usually difficult to ascertain which of the two events is predominant. The most common cause of secretory diarrhea is infection. Bacterial enterotoxins cause diarrhea either affecting c-AMP or c-GMP. Secretory diarrhea is also caused by hormones (gastrin, calcitonin), peptides (VIP), luminal factors (bile acids and fatty acids), and neurotransmitter (serotonin).

Exudative diarrhea: Structural disruption of intestinal wall by inflammation, diffuse ulceration, infiltration and tumors will lead to exudation of cellular debris, mucus, protein and blood into the intestinal lumen.

Intestinal transit and diarrhea: There are some patients in whom intestinal hurry produces chronic diarrhea. Normal oro-cecal transit time is 6 hours. Rapid transit prevents adequate time for absorption; diarrhea results despite intact mucosal absorptive capacity. Intestinal hurry has been linked to post-vagotomy diarrhea, diarrhea predominant-irritable bowel syndrome and diabetic diarrhea.

Clinical Classification of Chronic Diarrhea

Clinical classification of chronic diarrhea can help to organize the physician's thinking about possible causes of chronic diarrhea and direct the evaluation in meaningful ways, thereby avoiding unnecessary investigations.

1. *Osmotic versus secretory diarrhea:* This classification helps to separate the small number of causes of osmotic diarrhea from the much larger number of causes of secretory diarrhea. Osmotic diarrhea usually ceases with fasting. The most useful way to differentiate secretory and osmotic diarrhea is to measure fecal electrolytes and calculate the fecal osmotic gap.
2. *Watery versus fatty versus inflammatory diarrhea:* This is the most useful classification of chronic diarrhea, based on gross appearance of stool and simple laboratory testing.
   - Watery diarrhea is characterized by its fluidity and the absence of blood or pus. It is due to defect in water absorption (secretory diarrhea) or ingesting of poorly absorbed substances (osmotic diarrhea).
   - Fatty diarrhea (steatorrhea) is characterized by greasy, bulky and often light colored stools, due to defective digestion or absorption of fat in the small intestine.
   - Inflammatory diarrhea is characterized by presence of blood and pus, due to inflammatory or neoplastic process in the gut.
3. *Small bowel versus large bowel diarrhea:* Distinction between small bowel and large bowel diarrhea may provide a clue for further diagnostic studies (Table 8.1). However, this classification is unlikely to be useful in condition where extensive involvement of small intestine and colon occur.

Table 8.1: Differences between small bowel and large bowel diarrhea

Features	Small bowel diarrhea	Large bowel diarrhea
Volume of stool	Large	Small
Blood in stool	Absent	May be present
Rectal symptoms	Absent	Present
Steatorrhea	May be present	Absent
Excessive flatulence	May be present	Absent
Pain	Periumbilical	Hypogastric
Protein malabsorption	Present	Usually absent
Smell of stool	Offensive	Non offensive

Table 8.2: Differential diagnosis of chronic diarrhea

Chronic watery diarrhea
*   *Osmotic diarrhea*
    Osmotic laxative (e.g. Mg^{2+}, PO_4^{3-})
    Carbohydrate malabsorption
    Lactose intolerance

Secretory diarrhea
Bacterial toxins
Bile acid malabsorption
Inflammatory bowel disease
Stimulant laxatives
Vasculitis
Disordered motility
*   Diabetic diarrhea
*   Post vagotomy
*   Irritable bowel syndrome
Endocrine diarrhea
*   Gastrinoma
*   Hyperthyroidism
*   VIPoma
*   Carcinoid syndrome
Tumors
*   Colon carcinoma
*   Villous adenoma
Idiopathic secretory diarrhea

Chronic inflammatory diarrhea
Inflammatory bowel disease
Infectious colitis
*   Pseudomembranous colitis
*   CMV infection
*   Tuberculosis
Ischemic colitis
Radiation colitis

Chronic fatty diarrhea
Maldigestion
Pancreatic exocrine deficiency
Inadequate luminal bile acid
Malabsorption
Diffuse mucosal diseases
Short bowel syndrome
Bacterial overgrowth syndrome

Differential Diagnosis of Chronic Diarrhea

Many gastrointestinal and systemic disorders lead to chronic diarrhea. To facilitate the differential diagnosis, chronic diarrhea is divided into watery, inflammatory and fatty diarrhea (Table 8.2).

Approach to a Patient with Chronic Diarrhea

A systematic approach can provide clues to the cause of chronic diarrhea (Fig. 8.1)

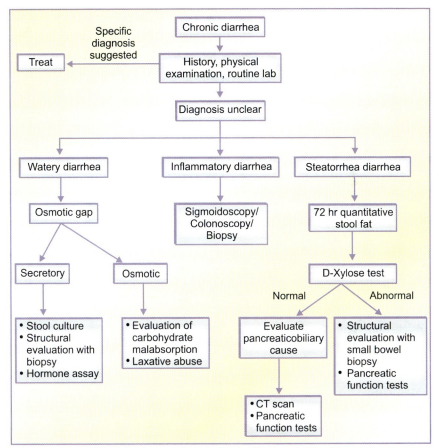

Fig. 8.1: Approach to patient with chronic diarrhea

History

A careful medical history is the key to the evaluation of patients with chronic diarrhea. Following points should be assessed as a part of comprehensive medical history of chronic diarrhea:

1. Onset of diarrhea – congenital, abrupt or gradual.
2. Duration of diarrhea.
3. Whether diarrhea is continuous or intermittent.
4. Diarrhea—watery, bloody or fatty.

5. Pattern of diarrhea—small bowel or large bowel diarrhea (Table 8.1).
6. Presence of abdominal pain suggestive of inflammatory bowel disease, ischemia or irritable bowel syndrome.
7. Fever and weight loss suggest inflammatory bowel disease, lymphoma or infections like tuberculosis.
8. Epidemiological factors like travel history or illness in other family members.
9. Aggravating factors like stress and diet.
10. Previous surgery gastrointestinal tract.
11. History of systemic disease like diabetes, thyroid disease and autoimmune diseases.
12. All current medications, illicit drugs, alcohol, and caffeine used by the patients should be noted.
13. A detailed dietary history with special attention to " artificial sweetener", fiber intake, fruit juices.
14. Because functional disorders are very common and may be associated with diarrhea, factors suggestive of IBS should be sought (Rome II criteria, see chapter on irritable bowel syndrome).
15. Factitious diarrhea caused by surreptitious laxative ingestion should be considered in every patient with diarrhea.

Physical Examination

Physical examination suggests cause of diarrhea only in a few causes. But it gives important information about severity of diarrhea and nutritional status of the patients. Other features of diagnostic significance include presence of flushing or rashes on the skin, mouth ulcers, thyroid swelling, arthritis, edema, ascites, and hepatomegaly. Anorectal examination is very important in inflammatory diarrhea.

ROUTINE LABORATORY TESTS

A complete blood count should be obtained to assess anemia, leucocytosis and eosinophilia. Liver function tests, renal function including electrolytes, should be done in all patients. Blood sugar and thyroid function tests should be done in all patients with chronic diarrhea.

Stool Analysis

Stool analysis is one of the most important investigations in patients with chronic diarrhea. It is either spot stool sample analysis or quantitative stool collection tests.

Spot Stool Analysis

1. Stool leucocytes—Presence of white blood cells by Wright's staining indicates an inflammatory cause of diarrhea.
2. Occult blood—The sensitivity and specificity of the gauiac card test for the detection of inflammatory or neoplastic conditions causing diarrhea has not been properly evaluated.
3. Qualitative fat estimation—The presence of fat can be assessed in a semi-quantitative fashion by means of Sudan III stain. The presence of a positive Sudan stain categorizes the diarrhea as being fatty, and would lead to evaluation for malabsorption problems. Recently developed stool steatocrit test has not been evaluated in patients with chronic diarrhea.
4. Fecal culture—Since bacterial infection rarely causes chronic diarrhea in immunocompetent patients, routine fecal culture is not indicated.
5. Tests for protozoa—Fecal ELISA test for giardia-specific antigen and detection of strongyloides larvae and cysts and ova of E.histolytica.
6. Fecal pH—Fecal pH less than 5.3 indicates carbohydrate malabsorption.
7. Fecal osmotic gap—Fecal electrolyte concentrations are measured in stool water. The osmotic gap of fecal fluid can be used to estimate the contribution of electrolytes and non-electrolytes to retention of water in the intestinal lumen. The osmotic gap is calculated by following formula:

$$\text{Osmotic gap} = 290 - 2\,(Na^+ + K^+).$$

Osmotic gap < 50 mOsm is suggestive of secretory diarrhea and > 125 mOsm is suggestive of osmotic diarrhea.

Quantitative Stool Collection

1. Quantitative fecal fat estimation
   - A 72-hour quantitative stool collection and estimation of fecal fat is the gold standard for evaluating steatorrhea (Van de Kamer test).
   - Steatorrhea is defined as excretion of fat more than 7 g/ 24 hour. In the presence of diarrhea value more than 14 g/ 24 hours is considered significant.
2. Analysis for laxative—Analysis should be done in all patients of diarrhea of unknown origin.

Radiological Investigations

Radiographic studies may play a role in the evaluation of a patient with chronic diarrhea. A plain roentgenogram of the abdomen occasionally is helpful.

Thickened loops of bowel may be an indicator of either small bowel or colonic abnormalities, but this finding is non-specific. Pancreatic calcification, when present, indicates chronic pancreatitis.

Ultrasound examination and abdominal CT scan have a limited role in the evaluation of chronic diarrhea. Ultrasound and CT scan may be useful as a screen to exclude biliary tract obstruction or pancreatic disease, which can cause chronic fat malabsorption. The CT scan also is useful to detect intra-abdominal complications of inflammatory bowel disease, or neuroendocrine tumors.

Upper GI series may help elucidate the cause for chronic diarrhea by showing evidence of prior gastric surgery, (e.g. a small gastric pouch); a fistula, (e.g. between the stomach and the colon); and abnormal small bowel mucosal folds (as may be seen in some small bowel diseases such as Whipple's disease and lymphoma).

A small bowel follow-through examination can be useful to diagnose ileal disease, which cannot be easily detected by endoscopic means. Ileal abnormalities are most commonly seen in Crohn's disease and other causes of ileocolitis; impaired absorption of bile salts leads to fat malabsorption and choleraic diarrhea.

Single or double contrast evaluation of the colon often is used in confirming a diagnosis of cancer or mucosal disease like inflammatory bowel disease, ischemic colitis or radiation colitis.

Role of Endoscopy

Endoscopy usually is more specific than roentgenographic studies because it allows direct inspection of the mucosa, detection of superficial lesions, and the ability to biopsy the mucosa. Upper endoscopy facilitates small bowel mucosal biopsy, which is essential in establishing the diagnosis of proximal small bowel diseases, like Crohn's disease, Whipple's disease, celiac sprue, abetalipro-teinemia and mycobacterium avium complex.

Flexible sigmoidoscopy and colonoscopy permit inspection of the colon and its mucosal biopsy and are especially useful in the evaluation of small volume diarrhea or diarrhea with gross or occult blood. Thus, it can be used to diagnose inflammatory bowel disease, microscopic colitis, ischemic colitis and colorectal cancer.

Special Testing

When the diagnosis of chronic diarrhea remains uncertain, additional special tests can be helpful. Peptide hormone secreting tumors are extremely rare causes of diarrhea. Thus, peptide hormone levels should not be measured in blood without good evidence for a classical syndrome associated with one of these tumors or identification of a tumor by computerized tomography. Carcinoid tumors that cause diarrhea can be discovered with the help of a 24-hour urine collection for 5-hydroxy indoleacetic acid (5-HIAA). Other blood tests that can be of use include thyroid-stimulating hormone, anti-nuclear antibody, anti-gliadin, anti-endomysial antibodies and antibody against tissue transglutaminase for celiac disease, perinuclear antineutrophil cytoplasmic antibodies (p-ANCA) for ulcerative colitis and anti-saccharomyces cerevisiae antibody (ASCA) for Crohn's disease.

Physiologic tests of mucosal absorption and pancreatic exocrine function help in the diagnosis of unusual causes of chronic diarrhea. Proximal mucosal absorption can be assessed by the D-xylose test. Breath hydrogen testing can be of help in evaluating lactase deficiency and bacterial overgrowth in the small intestine. Secretin test remains the most reliable tests for pancreatic exocrine function, but measurement of fecal chymotrypsin or elastase concentration may be a useful screening study.

Treatment

Patients with chronic diarrhea can have such severe diarrhea as to cause fluid- and electrolyte-depletion. In such situations oral rehydration solutions, and intravenous fluids can be lifesaving. So it is very important to correct dehydration before starting evaluation for chronic diarrhea.

When a specific diagnosis is made, specific treatment often can afford a cure of chronic diarrhea. Induction and maintenance of remission is the main goal of therapy in patients with inflammatory bowel disease. This goal can be achieved by using 5-ASA (aminosalicylates) and immunosuppressant drugs. Gluten free diet is the main therapeutic measure in patients with celiac disease. Role of long-term antibiotics in management of tropical sprue is yet not proved, but limited studies showed that 6 months treatment using doxycyclin and folic acid improved diarrhea frequency and malabsorption. The somatostatin analogue, octreotide, is of proven effectiveness in carcinoid tumors and other peptide-secreting tumors, dumping syndrome, and chemotherapy-induced diarrhea. Patients with gastrinoma, and VIPoma can be treated by surgical removal. Cholestyramine is of little use in most patients with chronic diarrhea, unless bile acid malabsorption is causing the diarrhea.

Empiric therapy can be provided: a) as a temporizing measure during evaluation, b) when there is a failure to reach a diagnosis in a patient with chronic diarrhea, or c) when a diagnosis is made, but is not specifically treatable. Antimotility agents and opiates are the most effective empiric therapy for diarrhea. They not only relieve symptoms of frequency and urgency, but also reduce stool weight. Many patients respond to diphenoxylate or loperamide. Anti-secretory drugs like Rececadotril, a new anti-enkephalinase inhibitor, can also be used to reduce the frequency and output of the stool. Role of bismuth in chronic diarrhea is unproven. Fiber supplements may improve stool consistency, but tend to increase stool weight.

SUGGESTED READING

1. Fine KD, Schiller LR. AGA technical review on the evaluation and management of chronic diarrhea. Gastroenterology 1999; 1166:1464-86.
2. Wilcox CM, Rabeneck L, Friedman S. AGA technical review: malnutrition and cachexia, chronic diarrhea, and hepatobiliary disease in patients with human immunodeficiency virus infection. Gastroenterology 1996; 111:1724-52.
3. Lee SD, Surawicz CM. Infectious causes of chronic diarrhea. Gastroenterol Clin North Am. 2001; 30:679-92.
4. Donowitz M., Kokke F. T., Saidi R. Evaluation of Patients with Chronic Diarrhea. N Engl J Med 1995; 332:725-729
5. Thomas PD, Forbes A, Green J, Howdle P, Long R, Playford R, Sheridan M, Stevens R, Valori R, Walters J, Addison GM, Hill P, and Brydon G Guidelines for the investigation of chronic diarrhoea, 2nd edition Gut, Jul 2003; 52: 1-15.,
6. Susan Hicks and Alan D Phillips chronic diarrhoea in AIDS. Gut, pp 1997; 41: 417.
7. Chronic diarrhea Lawrence R. Schiller Gastroenterology 2004 p287 to p293 American Gastroenterological Association medical position statement: Guidelines for the evaluation and management of chronic diarrhea. Gastroenterology 1999
   • Number 6 146;1463
8. Management of infectious diarrhoea. Casburn-Jones A C and Farthing M J G. Gut, 2004; 53: 296—305.

9

Vinayakumar KR

Pathogenesis and Management of Acute Diarrhea

INTRODUCTION

Acute diarrhea is the number one killer disease in infants and young children in the developing countries. It is estimated that about 5 to 8 million individuals succumb to acute diarrhea every year. It accounts for about 7.1 lakh deaths in India of which 4 to 5 lakh are under five years of age. Often it occurs in epidemic proportions causing severe dehydration and death.

DEFINITION

Acute diarrhea is defined as a diarrhea of acute onset and lasting for 5 to 6 days and not more than 14 days.

Persistent diarrhea is diarrhea of acute onset and lasting for more than 14 days. It causes severe malnutrition and morbidity.

ETIOPATHOGENESIS

Acute diarrheal disease is usually infective and is bacterial in adults and older children whereas viruses predominate in young children under two years. The transmission is usually feco-oral; but person to person transmission can also occur. It is mainly due to poor sanitation, over-crowding and lack of safe drinking water. Other causes include food intolerance, drug toxicity and poisons.

INFECTIVE DIARRHEAS

It may be viral, bacterial (mostly), protozoal or metazoal (helminths). Rota virus is responsible for up to 50% of diarrhea in under two years age group. Other viruses which can cause diarrhea are norwalk, calici, astra and small round viruses. Common bacterial agents in diarrhea are *E.coli, V. cholera, Salmonella, Yersinia, Campylobacter, S. aureus, Clostridium, Welchic and Bacillus Cereus*. Systemic infections such as atypical pneumonia, legionnaires disease, typhoid fever, urinary infection and brucellosis can also cause diarrhea.

E.coli

There are five different diarrheal subtypes. Enterotoxigenic *E. coli* has an exotoxin, which stimulates cyclic GMP. Enteroinvasive type presents as acute dysentery and is responsible for outbreaks in newborn nurseries. Enteropathogenic variety produces small outbreaks in schools and nurseries affecting small children and enteroadhesive type leads to persistent diarrhea. Enterohemorrhagic

E. coli (O157:H7) may be associated with hemolytic uremic syndrome. It is a zoonosis and is contracted primarily through contaminated beef.

Cholera

Vibrio cholerae is the major cause for large epidemics with high fatalities especially in the third-world countries. It can occur in pandemic proportion also. The cholera agent may be classical or El tor (depending on microbiologic properties). Now the seventh pandemic of cholera is in progress, which is of El tor strain and this epidemic started in Indonesia. Cholera has a somatic antigen; but the recent isolates from around the Bay of Bengal has have no O antigen and is termed O139 strain. It is detected in epidemics from South India also.

Kerala is an endemic area for cholera and there was a major epidemic in 1996.

V. cholera elaborates an exotoxin, which has two components—A and B. B component has five sub units and it binds the vibrio to the enterocyte. The component A has two sub units and in the host enterocyte stimulates c AMP, which opens the Cl-channels leading to watery diarrhea. Diarrhea can be very severe at the rate of 10 to 15 ml/kg and rapidly lead to fatal dehydration in 4 to 6 hours. Relapse is a phenomenon which the author has noted during the 1996 epidemic. The relapse tends to be more serious than the initial presentation and is associated with higher mortality.

Salmonella

There are more than 2000 species, which could be pathogenic to humans. Human specific salmonella is *S. typhi* and *S. paratyphi* causing typhoid and paratyphoid fever respectively. Other species rarely invade the intestinal mucosa and the usual clinical picture is that of acute diarrhea (*e.g. S. suis, S. typhimurium, S. enteritides,* etc.)

Shigella

The clinical presentation is with acute dysentery. There are mainly four species: *S. dysenteriae, S. sonnei, S. flexneri* and S. boydii. The infection can be severe with septicemia. Hemolytic uremic syndrome (HUS) is a complication.

Campylobacter

C. jejuni, fetus and fecalis are capable of both mucosal invasion and stimulation. The clinical picture is that of acute diarrhea, which is sometimes bloody and associated with abdominal pain. Water-borne infections are common.

Yersinia

It usually involves the iliocecum and presents like acute appendicitis. Mesenteric lymphadenitis and diarrhea may also be seen. It is rarely seen in India.

Potozoal Diseases

Giardia lamblia is a common cause of acute and chronic diarrhea in endemic areas. It frequently infects the immunocompromised hosts. Isospora, cryptosporidia and microsporidia are also protozoa infecting the immuno compromised such as in AIDS and invade the enterocytes. They can also be isolated in community-acquired diarrhea.

Non-infective Causes

Drugs are the commonest in this group. Antibiotics (pseudomembranous colitis), non-steroidal anti-inflammatory drugs, colchine, salazopyrine, antidepressants, antihypertensives, anti-arrhythmics and neostigmine are classic examples.

Acute exacerbation of inflammatory bowel disease, food intolerance, food allergies, alcohol and poisoning (mushroom, organophosphrus, copper sulphate, arsenic etc.) can also produce acute diarrhea.

CLINICAL SUBTYPES

Acute Watery Diarrhea

The basic mechanism in this type is secretory diarrhea due to the toxins stimulating cAMP and cGMP. Cholera is the prototype of this group. Enterotoxigenic *E. coli* is the commonest cause of watery diarrhea world over. *Giardia, Salmonella, Cryptosporidium, Yersinia*, HIV, etc. can also induce enterocyte secretion. The main danger is dehydration.

Acute Bloody Diarrhea

The mechanism here is mucosal invasion by the organism. There is mucosal destruction and inflammatory cell infiltration. There is mainly cytokines-mediated B cell type of response. There is ultimately an exudative diarrhea characterized by fecal leucocytes and RBCs. The classical example is shigella. Invasive *Salmonella, Yersinia, Campylobacter, E.histolytica* and cytomegalovirus can also cause acute dysentery by this mechanism. The main dangers apart from dehydration are intestinal damage and sepsis.

Persistent Diarrhea

An acute diarrhea lasting for more than 14 days is usually due to enteroadhesive type of *E. coli* and leads to severe malnutrition. It can also predispose to non-enteric infections.

Diarrhea with Severe Malnutrition

Malnutrition predisposes the child to diarrhea, which in turn precipitates further malnutrition and thus it forms a vicious cycle. The main dangers are severe systemic infections, dehydration, heart failure and vitamin and mineral deficiency.

Food Poisoning

Usually presents with severe vomiting, diarrhea and abdominal pain. Several members who have consumed the suspected food item may be affected. There are two types of food poisoning—toxin type and infection type. In toxin type preformed toxin in the food is responsible for the manifestations and hence is seen within a few hours of the exposure (e.g. *Staph aureus, Clostridium welchi,* etc). In infection type, the organisms multiplying in the food infects the gut before the symptoms start and hence is delayed by 2 to 3 days (e.g. salmonella food poisoning)

Acute Diarrheal Disease—A Clinical Approach

An infective etiology may be considered always in endemic areas. Watery diarrhea with dehydration should raise the suspicion of cholera. Rota virus is likely in under two age group. Bloody diarrhea may be due to shigella, especially in children and young adults. Tourists returning from endemic areas require expert advice based on the epidemiologic data (e.g. cyclospora cayatenensis diarrhea in tourists from Nepal). AIDS patients require evaluation for giardia, isospora, microsporidia, coccidia and CMV infection. Epidemics should be investigated promptly and appropriate treatment guidelines may be issued. A careful food history and the number of persons involved are important in food poisoning.

Drug history (antibiotics, NSAIDS, etc.) extraintestinal manifestations (IBD), diabetes and hypertension (ischemic bowel disease) may all be important.

Patient may be carefully evaluated for dehydration in watery diarrhea, for evidence of toxicity in invasive diarrhea as in shigellosis, and for underlying conditions such as malnutrition, diabetes and HIV infection. Metabolic and renal status should be assessed in all severe cases.

INVESTIGATIONS

Stool examination with methylene blue can detect fecal leucocytes, which indicates mucosal invasion. Fresh stool specimen can be examined for giardia and vegetative forms of amoeba. Hanging drop preparation can detect *V. cholera* quickly and ZN stain can detect oocyst of isospora. Stool can be cultured for *Salmonella, Shigella, and Cholera*. Special media are required for campylobacter and yersinia. Clostridium difficile toxin in antibiotic associated diarrhea can be detected in the stool by bioassay or ELISA.

The blood counts may indicate bacterial invasion and septicemia. The renal parameters and electrolytes may be closely monitored especially in more serious cases. Serological tests are available for typhoid and yersinia.

Sigmoidoscopy and colonoscopy are important investigations in IBD, antibiotic colitis and ischemic colitis. Higher investigations such as spiral CT of the abdomen may be required when IBD or bowel ischemia are suspected.

MANAGEMENT

The most important lethal factor in acute diarrhea is dehydration and hence fluid management is the key factor especially in watery diarrhea. It is given separately.

Antibiotics

Most of the diarrheas are self-limiting and antibiotics are not required. However antibiotics are indicated in bloody diarrhea, extremes of age, when patient has other debilitating problems such as severe diabetes or when cholera is suspected. In salmonellosis inadvertent antibiotic use can promote bacterial invasion of the gut. The antibiotic selection is very important. Quinolones (ciprofloxacin, ofloxacin, etc.) are preferred in shigellosis since the organisms are sensitive and resistance is rare. Tetracycline, doxycycline, trimethoprim and quinolones are recommended in cholera. Diarrhea in AIDS may be referred to specialized centers for management.

Antibiotic-associated diarrhea may be managed symptomatically after promptly withdrawing the offending agent. Oral vancomycin is the drug of choice in severe cases. Metronidazole and bacitracin are also effective. Recurrence is a major problem and can be reduced if the above drugs are withdrawn under the cover of cholestyramine. Cholestyramine binds the C difficile toxin.

Symptomatic Treatment

Antiemetics and antidiarrheals are not generally recommended. They can have an adverse effect also. Antidiarrheals such as loperamide or diphenoxylate can precipitate toxic megacolon. Vomiting is often due to electrolyte disturbances and subsides when it is corrected. Antispasmodics like hyoscine are also seldom required.

Specific Situations

Management of acute exacerbation of IBD, ischemic bowel disease or guidelines for poisoning are beyond the scope of this book and the reader is advised to consult the references given at the end.

Community Level Management

Acute infective diarrhea is a public health problem, which should be addressed at the community level. It is feco-orally transmitted and is due to lack of safe drinking water and inadequacies in sewage disposal. Hence it is a major problem in the developing countries where it often occurs in epidemics. Large outbreaks occur in seasonal pilgrimage centres and during monsoons. Health education, improvement in the living standards and effective health policies are required for community level control.

Prevention

Individual level protection can be obtained from the use of safe drinking water and effective hand washing. Vaccines are available for many agents such as rota virus, cholera and shigella. It may be helpful for the tourists to the endemic areas, during epidemics and for high risk individuals.

Fluid Management in Secretory Diarrhea

As already emphasized correction of dehydration saves life in severe watery diarrhea and physicians are advised to meticulously follow the WHO guide lines, which are frequently updated.

Since severe diarrhea can be rapidly fatal (often within 4 to 6 hours), the treatment should begin early in the household itself. Parents with an awareness can be encouraged to initiate fluid therapy (Plan-A).

If the diarrhea continues, oral rehydration solution (ORS) treatment can be initiated with the help of a trained health worker (Plan-B).

If there is any problem such as vomiting, dehydration, severe diarrhea, the patient may be referred to a centre with facility for intravenous fluid therapy (Plan-C).

Assessment of Dehydration

Fluid management policies are based on the hydration status and hence dehydration should be carefully assessed. The WHO guidelines are given in the chart below. If there is no clinical dehydration, the fluid loss is less than 7% if there is some dehydration the fluid loss may be 7 to 10% and in severe dehydration the fluid loss is more than 10%. More than 12 to 15% fluid loss could be fatal.

Table 9.1: Assessment of diarrhea patients for dehydration

1. Look at			
Condition	Well, alert	Restless*, irritable*	Lethargic*, floppy
Eyes	Normal	Sunken	Very sunken and dry
Tears	Present	Absent	Absent
Mouth, tongue	Moist	Dry	Very dry
Thirst	Drinks normally, not thirsty	Thirsty*, drinks eagerly*	Drinks poorly* or not able to drink*
2. Feel Skin pinch	Goes back quickly	Goes back slowly*	Goes back very slowly*
3. Decide	No signs of dehydration	If there are 2 or more signs including a * sign there is some dehydration	If there are 2 or more sign including a * sign, there is severe dehydration
4. Treat	Plan A	Plan B	Plan C—Urgent

Other Factors to be Considered

- Presence of blood in the stool
- Fever, cough or other systemic symptoms
- Immunization status
- Nutritional status.

Management Objectives

- Prevent dehydration if there are no signs of dehydration
- Treat dehydration when it is present
- Prevent nutritional damage by feeding during and after diarrhea.

Treatment Plan A – Home Therapy

Mothers should be taught how to prevent dehydration at home by giving the child more fluid than usual during diarrhea. They should also know the signs when they should take the child to the health worker.

What Fluids to give in Plan A?

Most fluids, which the child normally take can be given (salted drinks such as salted rice water, or salted yoghurt or soup); or, salt can be added to unsalted drinks (plain water, green coconut water, weak tea, fresh fruit juice). ORS can be made available at home especially during an epidemic.

Fluids to be avoided include soft drinks, sweetened fruit juices, sweetened tea and coffee.

How much Fluid to give?

As a general rule give as much fluid as the patient wants. Children may be given half to one cup of fluid after each episode of diarrhea.

Feeding

Continue to feed during diarrhea. This helps to prevent malnutrition. Infants should continue breast-feeding. Cereals, vegetables and other usual foods can be permitted. Well-cooked and mashed food will be easy to digest. Fish, egg and meat can also be given if appetite is good. Potassium rich foods such as banana or tender coconut may be encouraged.

Plan B

The child is taken to a health worker for ORS treatment.

Oral Rehydration Solution

ORS is the universal solution in the treatment of diarrhea since it can be used to prevent and treat dehydration

Table 9.2: Composition of ORS			
Sodium chloride	3.5 gm/L	Na	90 mmol/L
Bicarbonate	2.5 gm/L	HCO_3	30 mmol/L
Potassium chloride	1.5 gm/L	K	20 mmol/L
Glucose	20 gm/L		111 mmol/L

How much ORS is Needed?

Depends on the degree of dehydration, age and body weight.(see table 9.3). If the child wants, more ORS can be given provided there is no evidence of over hydration.

Table 9.3: ORS amount in the first 4 hours in severe dehydration						
Age	Less 4/12	4-11 mon	12-23 mon	2-4 yrs	5-14 yrs	>15 yrs
Weight	<5 kg	5-7.9 kg	8-10.9 kg	11-15.9 kg	16-29.9 kg	>30 kg
ORS in ml	200-400	400-600	600-800	800-1200	1200-2200	2200-4000

How to give ORS?

ORS may be given in a cup and the patient may be encouraged to sip it slowly. A teaspoon can be used in small children. ORS can be stopped temporarily if the patient vomits and can be restarted after 5 to 10 minutes.

Reassess the patient after 4 hours and plan further treatment.

Plan C – Intravenous Fluid Therapy

Use Ringer lactate solution.
Indications:
- When there is severe dehydration
- When there is continuous vomiting and ORT is impossible
- Severe diarrhea
- Abdominal distention

Table 9.4: Guidelines for intravenous fluid therapy		
Age	Give first 30ml/kg in	Subsequent 70ml/kg in
Under 12 months	1 hour	5 hours
Older patients	30 minutes	2½ hrs (150 mts)

Reassess the patient after 6 hours (infants) or 3 hours (older) and plan further treatment.

Other Types of ORS

- Rice based ORS which contains 50 gm/one of rice powder instead of glucose. It reduces the stool output faster.
- Citrate ORS, where citrate is used instead of bicarbonate. It increases the shelf life.

SUGGESTED READING

1. Harrison's Principles of Internal Medicine, 15th Ed, 2001.
2. WHO – The treatment of diarrhea (A manual for the physicians) 2001
3. Cheney CP, Wong RK. Acute infectious diarrhea. Med Clin North Am 1993; 77: 1169-96
4. Ilnycky j A. Clinical evaluation and management of acute infectious diarrhea in adults. Gastroenterol Clin North Am 2001; 30:599-609.
5. Park SI, Giannella RA. Approach to the adult patient with acute diarrhea. Gastroenterol Clin North Am 1993; 22:483-97.
6. Powell DW, Szauter KE. Nonantibiotic therapy and pharmacotherapy of acute infectious diarrhea. Gastroenterol Clin North Am. 1993;22:683-707pp.
7. Salazar-Lindo E, Santisteban-Ponce J, Chea-Woo E, Gutierrez M. Racecadotril in the treatment of acute watery diarrhea in children. N Engl J Med 2000; 343: 463-67
8. Pierce N F, Fontaine O, Sack R B, Ramakrishna BS, Binder H J Amylase-Resistant Starch plus oral rehydration solution for cholera. N Engl J Med 2000; 342: 1995-96

10

Sobhana Devi R

Inflammatory Bowel Disease—What is New?

INTRODUCTION

Inflammatory bowel disease (IBD) comprises those conditions characterised by a tendency for chronic or relapsing immune activation and inflammation within the gastrointestinal tract. Crohn's disease and ulcerative colitis are the two major forms.

Crohn's disease is a condition of chronic inflammation, potentially involving any location of the alimentary tract, from mouth to anus; discontinuous along the longitudinal axis of the gut, but involving all layers from mucosa to serosa.

Ulcerative colitis is an inflammatory disorder that affects the rectum and extends proximally to affect a variable extent of the colon.

EPIDEMIOLOGY

Crohn's disease and ulcerative colitis are more common in industrialized western countries. Increasing prevalence is now being reported from the developing countries also. Prevalence of ulcerative colitis is 1.8 to 15 per 100,000 person years and that of Crohn's disease is 0.8 to 11 per 100,000 person years. Increasing prevalence of Crohn's disease, in comparison with ulcerative colitis, is seen.

Peak incidence is in the second or third decade, though in ulcerative colitis, a bimodal presentation is seen. Females are more affected than males in Crohn's disease, but such gender preference is not seen in ulcerative colitis.

Caucasian race, especially Jews are at high risk. High prevalence is seen in South Asian migrants to western countries. Low prevalence is seen in Asia Pacific region.

IBD is usually reported to be seen in persons of high socio-economic status.

ETIOLOGY AND PATHOGENESIS

Smoking habit is high in persons with Crohn's disease, whereas, ulcerative colitis is seen in ex-smokers. Probably smoking confers protection against ulcerative colitis. Childhood infection, oral contraception, NSAID use, highly refined diet, breast feeding, hygiene, pollution, and stress have all been cited as etiologically significant.

Genetics: Ethnic and familial predilection is seen in IBD. Family members of index cases, especially, first-degree relatives have forty per cent chance of developing the disease. Concordance is seen in monozygotic twins. Genetic anticipation, that is, earlier onset of the disease, is seen in the immediate next generation. NOD-2 gene in chromosome-16 is the susceptibility gene in Crohn's disease.

Microbiology

E. coli, Mycobacterium paratuberculosis and *Listeria* are implicated. Antibiotics and fecal stream diversion benefit IBD.

Auto-immunity

Immune response in IBD is appropriate but ineffective. Antigen triggers are microbial antigens. Mucosal T cells, especially T helper cells, become activated, leading to imbalance in production of cytokines such as *interleukins, tumor necrosis factor (TNF) and transforming growth factor (TGF),* with resultant inflammation. Soluble mediators such as, prostaglandins, nitric oxide, growth factor, short chain fatty acids, free oxygen radicals and adhesin molecules play important role in inflammation.

Evaluation of critical proinflammatory mediators such as TNF, interleukins and adhesins involved in final inflammatory cascade has led to development of effective methods to control inflammation.

Clinical Presentation

Symptoms and signs are nonspecific. Extra intestinal manifestations are unique to IBD. Usually affects the young, between second and third decade.

Features	Crohn's disease	Ulcerative colitis
Abdominal pain	Common	Rare
Diarrhea	Common	Uncommon
Blood in stools	Occasional	Always
Abdominal mass	Yes	Rare
Perianal disease	Common	Rare
Fistulas, Abscesses	Common	Rare
Recurrence after surgery	Common	Nil
Toxic megacolon	No	Can occur
Smoker	Yes	Ex smoker
Old appendicectomy	Yes	Rare
p-ANCA	No	60% to 80%
ASCA	60% to 80%	No
Distribution of disease	Anywhere in GIT, discontinuous	Colon with terminal ileum. Continuous

Ulcerative colitis can be proctitis, proctosigmoiditis, left sided colitis or pancolitis. The disease may be mild, moderate or severe depending on the number of stools (mild < 4, moderate, severe > 6 or fulminant > 10) and presence of blood (mild +, severe +++). Systemic signs such as fever, tachycardia and anemia are seen in severe and fulminant types only. Dilated colon, (>6 cm) is seen in toxic megacolon.

Crohn's disease can affect the entire gastrointestinal tract from mouth to anus. Abdominal pain and systemic signs are more commonly seen in Crohn's disease. Crohn's disease can be classified based on (a) age at diagnosis (A1–< 40 yrs, A2–> 40 yrs), (b) location (L1 – terminal ileum, L2 – colon, L3 – ileocolon, L4 – upper GI), or its behaviour (B1 – non stricturing, non penetrating, B2 – stricturing, B3 – penetrating).

Diagnosis is by symptoms, endoscopy, imaging and histopathology (Figs 10.1 and 10.2)

Endoscopic Differentiation

Endoscopic finding	Crohn's disease	Ulcerative colitis
Distribution	Rectal sparing, skip lesions	Diffuse: from rectum
Inflammation	Focal, asymmetric, cobble stoning	Diffuse with mucosal granularity and friability
Ulcer	aphthoid ulcers, linear ulcers	Small ulcers
Colonic lumen	Strictures common	Strictures rare

Histology

Histology	Crohn's disease	Ulcerative colitis
Mucosa	Focal inflammation, sub mucosal or transmural involvement, granuloma, fissuring.	Goblet cell depletion, crypt distortion, crypt abscess

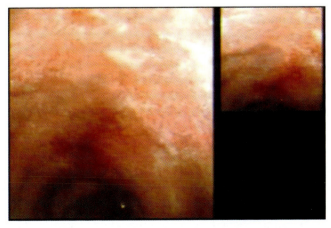

Fig. 10.1: Colonoscopy showing granular, friable colonic mucosa with loss of vascularity suggestive of active ulcerative colitis

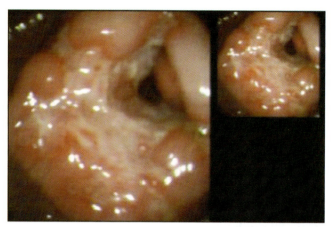

Fig. 10.2: Colonoscopy showing ulceration with narrowing of colonic lumen suggestive of Crohn's disease

Extraintestinal Manifestations

Arthritis, ankylosing spondylitis, osteoporosis, erythema nodosum, pyoderma gangrenosum, aphthous stomatitis, iritis, uveitis, episcleritis, primary sclerosing cholangitis, fatty liver, gall stones, renal calculi.

Differential Diagnosis

Infections – *E. coli, Salmonella, Shigella, Entamoeba histolytica*, tuberculosis.

Diverticulosis, drug induced, radiation enterocolitis, ischemia and vasculitis.

Imaging Techniques

Plain film of abdomen to assess for intestinal obstruction in Crohn's disease and toxic megacolon in ulcerative colitis.

Enteroclysis (small bowel enema) is employed to diagnose small bowel Crohn's. Enteroscopy or capsule endoscopy are other newer modalities to detect small bowel lesions. Barium meal follow through or colonoscopy may show aphthoid ulcers, rose thorn ulcers, deep fissures with cobble-stoning, bowel wall thickening, strictures and skip areas.

Barium enema in ulcerative colitis shows granularity, deep collar-stud ulcers, shortening of colon (lead pipe colon) (Fig. 10.3)

Computed tomography helps to demonstrate abscess, fistulae and assess disease activity

Scintigraphy using labelled white cells may help to assess disease activity.

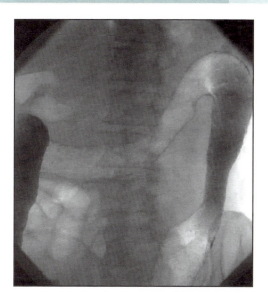

Fig. 10.3: Double contrast braium enema showing granular colonic mucosa with superficial ulceration and featureless colon suggests chronic active ulcerative colitis.

Disease markers—ESR, C-reactive protein and serum albumin. pANCA test is positive in 60 to 80% of ulcerative colitis and ASCA in 60 to 80% of Crohn's disease cases. Genetic markers *Nod 2 Gene* on *chromosome 16 is* seen in 20 to 30% of Crohn's disease patients. Markers are used to monitor disease activity and the effect of treatment; to differentiate between ulcerative colitis and Crohn's disease, especially in children, and to assess the natural history.

Medical Treatment

Aminosalicylates

Sulphasalazine (salicylazosulphapyridine) – 4 g to 6 g/day in active disease and 2 g to 4 g/day to maintain remission. Side effects are anemia, sperm abnormalities, rash, agranulocytosis.

Many of the newer preparations do not contain the sulpha moiety, thus avoiding the side effects of sulpha compounds.

Mesalamine (5ASA)(this is aminosalicylate without the sulphua moiety) – 2 g to 4 g/day. Side effects are nausea, diarrhea and pancreatitis.

Olsalazine (5ASA dimer) – 1.5 g to 3 g/day

Balsalazide (5ASA + carrier) 2 g to 6 g/day
Topical mesalamine enemas and suppositories.
Corticosteroids are the mainstay of treatment to induce remission.

Oral: Prednisolone, budesonide.

Parenteral: Hydrocortisone, methyl-prednisolone,budesonide.

Topical: Hydrocortisone, prednisolone, budesonide.

Antimicrobials: Metronidazole, quinolones.

Immunomodulators: Azathioprin, 6-mercaptopurine, methotrexate, cyclosporine.

Immunomodulators are mainly used for their steroid sparing effect in IBD.

Intravenous cyclosporine is used in fulminant colitis to salvage the colon from immediate surgery.

Biological Therapy

Anti tumor necrosis factor alpha (anti TNF a – Infliximab). This is a chimeric monoclonal antibody against human TNF alpha. Mainly useful in fistulizing Crohn's disease, severe Crohn's disease and fulminant ulcerative colitis at a dose of 5 µg to 10 µg per kg at 0 week, 2 weeks, 6 weeks with maintenance dose at 8 weekly intervals.

Etanercept – Anti TNF alpha (95% Human, 5% Murine) has less chance of antibody formation.

Thalidomide also has anti -TNF alfa activity, but not safe in pregnant women and in children.

Other anti inflammatory cytokines: Recombinant human interleukins, antisense oligoneucleotide against intercellular adhesion molecule, monoclonal antibody against lymphocyte adhesion molecule and human growth hormone, have been tried effectively.

Other drugs: Nonfractionated heparin, rosiglitazone, glutamine, fish oils, short chain fatty acids—all have been used with variable results in IBD.

Ulcerative Colitis—Medical Treatment

Proctitis: Topical therapy is more effective. Mesalamine suppositories or enemas daily till remission, followed by twice or thrice weekly as maintenance. Topical steroids may be needed if response is poor. Oral aminosalicylates and oral steroids also are useful in severe cases.

Left sided or distal colitis: Mesalamine enemas are preferred. If response is poor, add steroid enemas. Oral salicylates and steroids are used in severe cases.

Pancolitis: Oral amino salicylates at higher dose and to maintain remission at lower dose. Prednisolone orally at 30 to 60 mg till remission and then taper and stop over a few weeks.

Severe and fulminant cases: Intravenous corticosteroids—hydrocortisone 100mg every six hours for seven days. If no improvement is seen add intravenous cyclosporine. If nonresponsive or toxic megacolon develops, surgery is indicated.

Crohn's Disease—Medical Management

Mild to moderate cases respond to salicylates. If no improvement is seen, add metronidazole or ciprofloxacin. Corticosteroids are used if poor response is seen to the above.

Maintenance of remission is by oral mesalamine. In steroid-dependent Crohn's, maintain remission with azathioprin or 6 mercaptopurine. Non healing fistulae and sinuses heal with Infliximab.

Surgery in Inflammatory Bowel Disease
Indications

Ulcerative colitis: Failure of medical treatment, cancer risk, fulminant colitis, toxic megacolon, perforation, hemorrhage. Surgery done is total proctocolectomy with continent ileostomy or ileoanal pouch anastamosis.

Crohn's disease: Failure of medical treatment, intestinal obstruction, intra abdominal abscess, hemorrhage, perforation, perianal abscess. Surgeries done are resection and anastamosis, resection with stoma, stricture plasty, intestinal bypass, fistulectomy, closure of fistula, drainage of abscess. General principle in Crohn's – minimal resection.

IBD in Children

Twenty percent of patients develop symptoms in childhood. There is potential for growth failure and delayed sexual maturation. It is important to exclude enteric infections. Treatment regimes are similar to adults with more emphasis on steroid sparing regiments and nutritional interventions to minimize growth failure.

IBD and Pregnancy

IBD in remission during conception tends to remain in remission throughout pregnancy. Active disease during conception may worsen during pregnancy.

Key principle in management is that greatest risk to pregnancy is not active therapy but active disease. Mesalamine, corticosteroids, and topical preparations are safe during pregnancy and breast-feeding. Immunosuppressives are not safe in pregnancy. Infliximab is safe during pregnancy.

Nutritional Management in IBD

Enteral nutritional supplements such as elemental diet hasten remission in active Crohn's disease. Total parenteral nutrition is used as adjunctive treatment in exacerbation of Crohn's disease. Correction of anemia, vitamin and mineral deficiency, especially calcium, is mandatory.

Cancer Risk in IBD

Ulcerative colitis and Crohn's disease predispose to increased risk of gastrointestinal malignancy.

Ulcerative colitis: risk of carcinoma colon is 6%. Risk is low up to eight years after which it increases to 58 times by the fourth decade.

Surveillance for malignancy: Proctitis only screen as in general population.

In pancolitis, without sclerosing cholangitis, colonoscopy every three years for twenty years, then two yearly for ten years followed by annual colonoscopy.

With sclerosing cholangitis, annual colonoscopy. Risk of cholangiocarcinoma is high.

Crohn's disease: Risk of cancer is 1.1% to 26 %. Surveillance is more difficult due to presence of strictures and fistulae preventing ready access to endoscope.

SUGGESTED READING

1. Russel D Cohen. Inflammatory bowel disease-diagnosis and therapeutics. Humana Press. New Jersey 2003.
2. Miguel D Regueiro MD. Gastroenterology clinics of North America. Inflammatory bowel disease Saunders. March 2002;31(1), 5a.
3. Podolsky D. K. Medical Progress: Inflammatory bowel disease. N Engl J Med 2002; 347:417-429
4. Sutherland L, Roth D, Beck P. Alternative to sulfasalazine: A meta-analysis of 5-ASA in the treatment of ulcerative colitis. Inflamm Bowel Dis 1997; 3: 665-78
5. Present DH, Rutgeerts P, Targan S, et al. Infliximab for the treatment of fistulas in patients with Crohn's disease. N Engl J Med 1999; 340: 1398-405
6. Comerford LW et al. Treatment of luminal and fistulizing Crohn's disease with infliximab. Gastroenterol Clin North Am 2004; 33(2): 387-406
7. Janet Harrison, Stephen BH. Medical treatment of Crohn's disease. Gastroenterol Clin N Am 2002; 31: 167-184
8. Judge TA. Treatment of fistulizing Crohn's disease. Gastroenterol Clin North Am 2004; 33: 421-54

11

Sobhana Devi R

Intestinal Tuberculosis

INTRODUCTION

Tuberculosis can be rightly termed India's national disease. Abdomen is the most common site of extra pulmonary involvement. A steady decline in the late twentieth century has suffered a set back due to resurgence secondary to AIDS, changes in epidemiological and clinical profile.

EPIDEMIOLOGY

One third of all tuberculosis cases in the world are in India of which abdominal tuberculosis accounts for 0.2 to 5%. Prevalence is 500 per 1 lakh population in developing countries and 36 per 1 lakh population in Asians migrated to developed countries. Seventy five percent of intestinal tuberculosis is primary. Presence or absence of pulmonary disease is a poor predictor of intestinal disease.

PATHOGENESIS AND PATHOLOGY

Infection occurs by swallowing of infected sputum, ingestion of contagious milk, hematogenous spread from active pulmonary tuberculosis or direct extension from adjacent organs. Tuberculosis can affect any region from mouth to anus. Predilection for ileocecum is due to abundance of lymphoid tissue, physiologic stasis, minimal digestive activity with greater contact between organism and mucosal surface.

Tuberculous lesions can be ulcerative, hypertrophic, ulcerohypertrophic, or fibrous strictures.

CLINICAL FEATURES

Females are more affected than males in the ratio of 5.8:4.2. Usually occurs in the third and fourth decades. Symptoms last more than six months. Common symptoms are abdominal pain, fever, diarrhea, abdominal mass, ascites and features of intestinal obstruction. Symptoms are usually non-specific.

DIAGNOSIS

- Isolation or demonstration of *Mycobacterium tuberculosis*
- Mycobacterial DNA or RNA detection
- Biopsy showing caseating or non-caseating granuloma with giant cells
- Granulomas with radiologic findings and serologic positivity.

RADIOLOGY

- Chest X-ray shows changes in 25% cases
- Barium contrast studies show pulled-up cecum, strictures, dilatations, ulcerations
- CT abdomen to identify peripancreatic, porta hepatis, mesenteric, omental, or retroperitoneal lymph nodes and thickening of the mesentery or bowel wall
- Ultrasound abdomen shows presence of fluid, omental thickening, inter-loop ascites.

IMMUNODIAGNOSIS

- Manteux test considered positive if induration is more than 15 to 20 mm.
- Elisa test has 90% specificity and 80% sensitivity.

BACTERIOLOGICAL DIAGNOSIS

- Usual culture will take 4 to 6 weeks.
- Rapid culture techniques are available and the results will be available in two weeks.
- Biopsy specimen can be evaluated for identifying mycobacterial DNA by PCR, DNA or RNA amplification.

COLONOSCOPY

Fifty to 65% of intestinal tuberculosis have terminal ileal and colonic involvement. These can be viewed and biopsied.

Enteroscopy can be used to visualize small intestinal lesions.

DIFFERENTIAL DIAGNOSIS

- Crohn's disease
- Diverticular disease
- Ischemic enterocolitis
- Malignancy

TREATMENT OF INTESTINAL TUBERCULOSIS

Standard antituberculous drugs are combination of INH, rifampicin and ethambutol and pyrazinamide for two months, followed by the former three drugs alone for another 9 to12 months. According to new recommendation, a total period of treatment of 6 months is adequate

Response to medical treatment with standard antituberculous treatment is good. Bacillary burden is lower in intestinal tuberculosis and penetration of drugs is adequate.

Clinical trials have shown effectiveness of standard 12 month, short course or intermittent regimes. End point of treatment is difficult to define in intestinal tuberculosis.

Six month short course therapy is most preferred. There should be careful monitoring for compliance and complications.

Treatment in Special Situations

- HIV co-infection—short course is preferred. Rifampicin is an enzyme inducer. Hence rifabutin is preferred
- Hepatic disease—avoid hepatotoxic drugs such as INH, rifampicin, pyrazinamide or their combinations
- Multi drug resistant strains

Use five first line drugs for three months followed by INH, rifampicin, ethambutol for five months. If resistance to INH and rifampicin is seen, use pyrazinamide, ethambutol and streptomycin for 12 to 18 months. If resistance to all first line drugs is seen, use one injectable and any three of PAS, quinolones, ethionamide, cycloserine, for two years.

Steroids

Corticosteroid administration for first few weeks may be beneficial in miliary tuberculosis with toxemia. Steroids may reduce fibrosis but this has to be substantiated in studies.

Surgery

Indicated only in presence of complications such as obstruction, perforation, fistulae or massive bleed. Surgery is mainly conservative, preserving as much of bowel as possible.

SUGGESTED READING

1. VK Kapoor, Abdominal tuberculosis. The Indian contribution. Indian J Gastro 1998; 17:141-47.
2. A K Jain. Diagnosis of Abdominal Tuberculosis. Gastroenterology Today 1998; II, 21-26.
3. John B Marshall. Tuberculosis of the Gastrointestinal Tract and Peritoneum. American J gastroenterol 1993; 88:989-98.
4. Intestinal Tuberculosis. Return of an Old Disease: Karen D Horvath and Richard I Whelan. American J gastroenterol 1998, 93, 692-96.
5. V K Kapoor. Abdominal Tuberculosis. Postgrad Med J 1998; 74:459-67.

12

Subhalal N

Acute Appendicitis—
Do's and Don'ts

INTRODUCTION

Appendicitis is the most common acute surgical condition of the abdomen. Approximately 7% of the population will have appendicitis in their lifetime, with the peak incidence occurring between the ages of 10 and 30 years. It has protean manifestations, generous overlap with other clinical syndromes, and significant morbidity, which increases with diagnostic delay. No single sign, symptom, or diagnostic test accurately makes the diagnosis of appendiceal inflammation in all cases. Despite technologic advances, the diagnosis of appendicitis is still based primarily on the patient's history and the physical examination. Prompt diagnosis and surgical referral may reduce the risk of perforation and prevent complications. The mortality rate in nonperforated appendicitis is less than 1%, but it may be as high as 5% or more in young and elderly patients, in whom diagnosis may often be delayed, thus making perforation more likely.

PATHOGENESIS

The appendix is a long diverticulum that extends from the inferior tip of the cecum. Its lining is interspersed with lymphoid follicles. Most of the time, the appendix has an intraperitoneal location (either anterior or retrocecal) and, thus, may come in contact with the anterior parietal peritoneum when it is inflamed. Up to 30% of the time, the appendix may be "hidden" from the anterior peritoneum by being in a pelvic, retroileal or retrocolic (retroperitoneal retrocecal) position. The "hidden" position of the appendix notably changes the clinical manifestations of appendicitis.

Obstruction of the narrow appendiceal lumen initiates the clinical illness of acute appendicitis. Obstruction has multiple causes, including lymphoid hyperplasia (related to viral illnesses, including upper respiratory infection, mononucleosis, and gastroenteritis), fecoliths, parasites, foreign bodies, Crohn's disease, primary or metastatic cancer and carcinoid syndrome. Lymphoid hyperplasia is more common in children and young adults, accounting for the increased incidence of appendicitis in these age groups.

HISTORY AND PHYSICAL EXAMINATION

Abdominal pain is the most common symptom of appendicitis. In multiple studies, specific characteristics of the abdominal pain and other associated symptoms have proved to be reliable indicators of acute appendicitis. A thorough review of the history of the abdominal pain and of the patient's recent genitourinary, gynecologic and pulmonary history should be obtained.

Anorexia, nausea and vomiting are symptoms that are commonly associated with acute appendicitis. When vomiting occurs, it nearly always follows the onset of pain. Vomiting that precedes pain is suggestive of intestinal obstruction, and the diagnosis of appendicitis should be reconsidered. The classic history of pain beginning in the periumbilical region and migrating to the right lower quadrant occurs in only 50% of patients. Duration of symptoms exceeding 24 to 36 hours is uncommon in nonperforated appendicitis. Approximately 2% of patients report duration of pain in excess of two weeks. Diarrhea or constipation is noted in as many as 18% of patients and should not be used to discard the possibility of appendicitis.

Common symptoms of appendicitis

Common symptoms	Frequency (%)
Abdominal pain	~100
Anorexia	~100
Nausea	90
Vomiting	75
Pain migration	50
Classic symptom sequence (vague periumbilical pain to anorexia/nausea/unsustained vomiting to migration of pain to right lower quadrant to low-grade fever)	50

A careful, systematic examination of the abdomen is essential. While right lower quadrant tenderness to palpation is the most important physical examination finding, other signs may help confirm the diagnosis. The abdominal examination should begin with inspection followed by auscultation, gentle palpation (beginning at a site distant from the pain) and, finally, abdominal percussion. The rebound tenderness that is associated with peritoneal irritation has been shown to be more accurately identified by percussion of the abdomen than by palpation with quick release.

When the appendix is hidden from the anterior peritoneum, the usual symptoms and signs of acute appendicitis may not be present. Pain and tenderness can occur in a location other than the right lower quadrant. A retrocecal appendix in a retroperitoneal location may cause flank pain. In this case, stretching the iliopsoas muscle can elicit pain. The psoas sign is elicited in this manner: the patient lies on the left side while the examiner extends the patient's right thigh .In contrast, a patient with a pelvic appendix may show no abdominal signs, but the rectal examination may elicit tenderness in the cul-de-sac. In addition, an obturator sign (pain on passive internal rotation of the flexed right thigh) may be present in a patient with a pelvic appendix.

Common Signs of Appendicitis

- Right lower quadrant tenderness on palpation (the single most important sign)
- Low-grade fever (38°C [or 100.4°F])—absence of fever or high fever can occur
- Peritoneal signs
- Localized tenderness to percussion
- Guarding
- *Other confirmatory peritoneal signs* (absence of these signs does not exclude appendicitis)
- Psoas sign—pain on extension of right thigh (retroperitoneal retrocecal appendix)
- Obturator sign—pain on internal rotation of right thigh (pelvic appendix)
- Rovsing's sign—pain in right lower quadrant with palpation of left lower quadrant
- Dunphy's sign—increased pain with coughing
- Flank tenderness in right lower quadrant (retroperitoneal retrocecal appendix)
- Patient maintains hip flexion with knees drawn up for comfort.

Differential Diagnosis

The differential diagnosis of appendicitis is broad, but the patient's history and the remainder of the physical examination may clarify the diagnosis. Because many gynecologic conditions can mimic appendicitis; a pelvic examination should be performed on all women with abdominal pain. Given the breadth of the differential diagnosis, the pulmonary, genitourinary and rectal examinations are equally important. Studies have shown, however, that the rectal examination provides useful information only when the diagnosis is unclear and, thus, can be reserved for use in such cases (Table 12.1)

Laboratory and Radiologic Evaluation

If the patient's history and the physical examination do not clarify the diagnosis, laboratory and radiologic evaluations may be helpful. A clear diagnosis of appendicitis obviates the need for further testing and should prompt immediate surgical referral.

Laboratory Tests

The white blood cell (WBC) count is elevated (greater than 10,000 per mm³]) in 80% of all cases of acute appendicitis. Unfortunately, the WBC is elevated in up

Table 12.1: Differential diagnosis of acute appendicitis		
Gastrointestinal	**Gynecologic**	**Pulmonary**
Abdominal pain, cause	Ectopic pregnancy	Pleuritis
unknown	Endometriosis	Pneumonia (basilar)
Cholecystitis	Ovarian torsion	Pulmonary infarction
Crohn's disease	**Pelvic inflammatory**	**Genitourinary**
Diverticulitis	**disease**	Kidney stone
Duodenal ulcer	Ruptured ovarian cyst	Prostatitis
Gastroenteritis	(follicular, corpus	Pyelonephritis
Intestinal obstruction	luteum)	Testicular torsion
Intussusception	Tubo-ovarian abscess	Urinary tract infection
Meckel's diverticulitis	**Systemic**	Wilms' tumor
Mesenteric	Diabetic ketoacidosis	**Other**
lymphadenitis	Porphyria	Parasitic infection
Necrotizing	Sickle cell disease	Psoas abscess
enterocolitis	Henoch-Schönlein	Rectus sheath
Neoplasm (carcinoid,	purpura	hematoma
carcinoma, lymphoma)		
Omental torsion		
Pancreatitis		
Perforated viscus		
Volvulus		

to 70% of patients with other causes of right lower quadrant pain. Thus, an elevated WBC has a low predictive value. Serial WBC measurements (over 4 to 8 hours) in suspected cases may increase the specificity, as the WBC count often increases in acute appendicitis (except in cases of perforation, in which it may initially fall).

In addition, 95% of patients have neutrophilia and, in the elderly, an elevated band count greater than 6% has been shown to have a high predictive value for appendicitis. In general, however, the WBC count and differential are only moderately helpful in confirming the diagnosis of appendicitis because of their low specificities.

A more recently suggested laboratory evaluation is determination of the C-reactive protein level. An elevated C-reactive protein level (greater than 0.8 mg per dL) is common in appendicitis, but studies disagree on its sensitivity and specificity. An elevated C-reactive protein level in combination with an elevated WBC count and neutrophilia are highly sensitive (97 to 100%). Therefore, if all three of these findings are absent, the chance of appendicitis is low.

In patients with appendicitis, a urinalysis may demonstrate changes such as mild pyuria, proteinuria and hematuria, but the test serves more to exclude urinary tract causes of abdominal pain than to diagnose appendicitis.

In all women of reproductive age who present with acute abdominal pain, the serum β-human chorionic gonadotropin level should be measured to rule out uterine or ectopic pregnancy.

Radiologic Evaluation

The options for radiologic evaluation of patients with suspected appendicitis have expanded in recent years, enhancing and sometimes replacing previously used radiologic studies. Plain radiographs, while often revealing abnormalities in acute appendicitis, lack specificity and are more helpful in diagnosing other causes of abdominal pain. Likewise, barium enema is now used infrequently because of the advances in abdominal imaging.

Ultrasonography and computed tomographic (CT) scans are helpful in evaluating patients with suspected appendicitis. Ultrasonography is appropriate in patients in whom the diagnosis is equivocal by history and physical examination. It is especially well suited in evaluating right lower quadrant or pelvic pain in pediatric and female patients. A normal appendix (6 mm or less in diameter) must be identified to rule out appendicitis. An inflammed appendix usually measures greater than 6 mm in diameter, is non-compressible and tender with focal compression. Other conditions such as inflammatory bowel disease, cecal diverticulitis, Meckel's diverticulum, endometriosis and pelvic inflammatory disease can cause false-positive ultrasonography results.

CT, specifically the technique of appendiceal CT, is more accurate than ultrasonography. Appendiceal CT consists of a focused, helical, appendiceal CT after a gastrografin-saline enema (with or without oral contrast) and can be performed and interpreted within one hour. Intravenous contrast is unnecessary. The accuracy of CT is due in part to its ability to identify a normal appendix better than ultrasonography. An inflamed appendix is greater than 6 mm in diameter, but the CT also demonstrates periappendiceal inflammatory changes. If appendiceal CT is not available, standard abdominal/pelvic CT with contrast remains highly useful and may be more accurate than ultrasonography.

Treatment

The standard for management of nonperforated appendicitis remains appendectomy (See Fig 12.1). Because prompt treatment of appendicitis is important in preventing further morbidity and mortality, a margin of error in over-diagnosis is acceptable. When the history and findings on physical examination are consistent with the diagnosis of appendicitis, appendectomy should be performed without further evaluation. Currently, the rate of negative appendectomies is approximately 20%. Some studies have investigated non-operative management with parenteral antibiotic treatment, but 40% of these patients eventually required appendectomy.

Appendectomy may be performed by laparotomy (usually through a limited right lower quadrant incision) or laparoscopy. Diagnostic laparoscopy may be helpful in equivocal cases or in women of childbearing age, while therapeutic laparoscopy may be preferred in certain subsets of patients (e.g., women, obese patients, athletes).

While laparoscopic intervention has the advantages of decreased postoperative pain, earlier return to normal activity and better cosmetic results, its disadvantages include greater cost and longer operating time. Open appendectomy may remain the primary approach to treatment until further cost and benefit analyses are conducted. Laparoscopic appendectomy may be considered if patient prefers and surgeon is experienced.

If the clinical presentation does not suggest the need for immediate surgery the patient may be observed for 6 to 10 hours in order to clarify the diagnosis. This practice may reduce the rate of unnecessary laparotomy without increasing the rate of appendiceal perforation. In this subset of patients the radiological imaging and other investigation may help to confirm or exclude the diagnosis. Diagnostic laparoscopy has been advocated to clarify the diagnosis in equivocal cases and has been shown to reduce the rate of unnecessary appendectomy. It is most effective for female patients, since a gynecologic cause of pain is identified in approximately 10 to 20% of such patients.

Special Considerations

While appendicitis is uncommon in young children, it poses special difficulties in this age group. Young children are unable to relate a history, often have abdominal pain from other causes and may have more nonspecific signs and symptoms. These factors contribute to a perforation rate as high as 50% in this group.

In pregnancy, the location of the appendix begins to shift significantly by the fourth to fifth months of gestation. Common symptoms of pregnancy may mimic appendicitis, and the leukocytosis of pregnancy renders the WBC count less useful. While the maternal mortality rate is low, the overall fetal mortality rate is 2 to 8.5%, rising to as high as 35% in perforation with generalized peritonitis. As in nonpregnant patients, appendectomy is the standard for treatment.

Elderly patients have the highest mortality rates. The usual signs and symptoms of appendicitis may be diminished, atypical or absent in the elderly, which leads to a higher rate of perforation. More frequent perforation combined with a higher incidence of other medical problems and less reserve to fight infection contributes to a mortality rate of up to 5% or more.

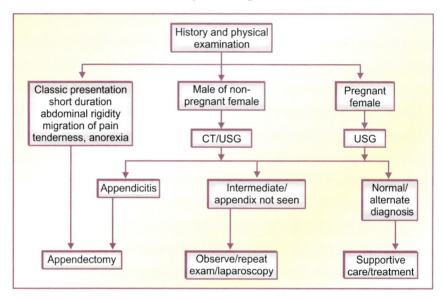

Fig. 12.1: The algorithm for suspected cases of acute appendicitis

SUGGESTED READING

1. Paulson EK, KaladyMF, PappasTN. Suspected appendicitis. N Engl J Med2003; 348; (3):236-42.
2. Wagner JM,McKinnyWP,CarpenterJL. Does this patient have appendicitis? JAMA1996; 276: 1589-94.
3. TelfordGL, WallaceJR. Appendix. Shackelford's surgery of the alimentary tract 5th edition, volume IV, 180-90.
4. Suspected acute appendicitis: trends in management over 30 years. Jones PF. Br J Surg (England), Dec 2001; 88(12):p1570-7.
5. Shelton T, McKinlay R, Schwartz RW. Acute appendicitis. Current diagnosis and treatment. Curr Surg (United States), Sep-Oct 2003; 60(5):p502-5.
6. Terasawa T, Blackmore CC, Bent S, et al. Systematic review: computed tomography and ultrasonography to detect acute appendicitis in adults and adolescents. Ann Intern Med (United States), Oct 5 2004; 141(7):p537-46.
7. Paulson EK, Kalady MF, Pappas TN. N Clinical practice. Suspected appendicitis. Engl J Med (United States), Jan 16 2003;348(3):p236-42.

13

Narayanan VA

Irritable Bowel Syndrome—The Brain Speaks to the Gut

INTRODUCTION

Irritable bowel syndrome (IBS) is a functional disorder of the intestines, clinically characterized by abdominal pain/discomfort, flatulence with either diarrhea or constipation, without any structural bowel disease. Although IBS is a common disorder, it is one of the most poorly understood conditions. The general practitioners are usually hesitant to diagnose the condition and attribute the symptoms of colonic origin such as diarrhea and passage of mucus to intestinal amoebiasis. Also, there is a tendency to dump the symptoms of flatulence and excess gas as psychiatric. This review is an attempt to correct this erroneous concept and to present our current understanding of this condition.

PREVALENCE

IBS is recognized as the most common gastrointestinal malady in Western countries and accounts for 50-70% of cases seen in gastroenterology centers. The situation is not different in India. Out of 230 cases of chronic diarrheas, 60 were diagnosed as irritable bowel syndrome in the All India Institute of Medical Sciences, New Delhi. Studies in Vellore showed 32% of referral cases to gastroenterology clinics were due to IBS. Population surveys carried out in the West have shown the prevalence of the disease in general population to be 8-24%. Recent studies in the USA have estimated the cost of IBS to society as 1.6 billion dollars (primarily due to inpatient hospitalization and clinic visits) and an additional 20 billion dollars due to indirect costs (lost workdays and illness in general).

This disorder affects all ages and both sexes. However, it is unusual for symptoms to start after the age of 50. In adults, there is a female preponderance reported from the West, but studies based in Indian hospitals show a male preponderance. This probably may be a reflection on the pattern of hospital referrals in our country rather than the true prevalence.

SYMPTOMS AND SIGNS

Most patients complain of vague abdominal pain or discomfort and "too much gas". Pain is often in left lower quadrant and is never severe enough to awaken the patient from sleep. Bloating after meal is a common symptom. Pain is temporarily relieved after defecation. In some patients, pain is provoked by eating.

Bowel habits may vary. In Western patients, constipation is predominant. However, the Indian experience is that diarrhea is more common than constipation. Usually, the diarrhea is before 10:00 hours in the morning and after that the patient does not pass stools. Some patients have exaggerated gastrocolic reflex and get the urge to pass stool after meals. Some have pellety or ribbon like stools. Passage of mucus and feeling of incomplete evacuation is a frequent complaint.

The major symptoms of IBS, namely diarrhea, abdominal pain, bloating and constipation can occur in organic structural disorders of the colon also. In view of the above, Manning et al initially analyzed the symptoms and evolved a criteria based on symptoms to diagnose irritable bowel syndrome. Later, two international conventions held in Rome modified the Manning criteria and evolved Rome I and later Rome II criteria for diagnosis.

In the original Manning study, (1) flatulence, (2) pain relieved by defecation, (3) more frequent stools at the onset of pain and (4) lesser stools at the onset of pain along with any two of the above, if passage of mucus and history of feeling of incomplete evacuation are present, makes the diagnosis certain.

However, Rome II criteria is the currently accepted symptom-based criteria. This is based on epidemiological, clinical and factor analytic studies, and is established by multinational consensus.

Rome II Diagnostic Criteria for Irritable Bowel Syndrome

At least 12 weeks (need not be consecutive) of abdominal discomfort/pain in the preceding 12 months with two of the following three features.
1. Relieved with defecation and/or
2. Onset associated with a change in frequency of stool and/or
3. Onset associated with a change in form (appearance) of stool.

A slightly modified ROME III citica has now born proposed.

The physical examination is normal. There may be tenderness in the left flanks and the descending colon may be palpable.

Diagnosis

Although diagnosis requires the exclusion of organic disease, it should be a positive one, based on the typical history and absence of physical findings with normal sigmoidoscopic appearance. Recent interest has focused on "alarm signs" or "red flags" such as weight loss, blood in stools, nocturnal symptoms, abnormal physical examination, anemia or a family history of cancer or inflammatory bowel disease. Thus, the presence of Rome II criteria and the

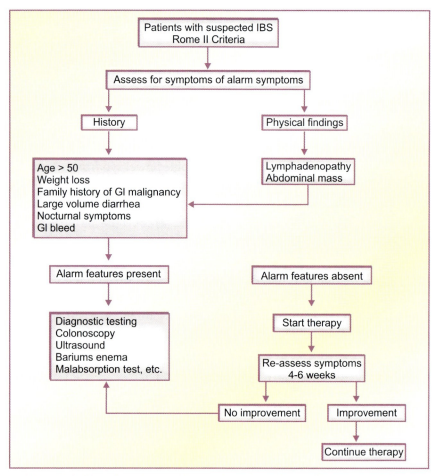

Fig. 13.1: Algorithm showing the workup of a patient with suspected IBS.

absence of red flags reduce the need for detailed investigations and the diagnostic accuracy is 98-100% when patients are screened in this manner (Fig. 13.1). Stool examination, sigmoidoscopy/colonoscopy, ultrasound examination, barium enema in selected cases, and malabsorption work up are carried out to rule out organic structural disease. Barium enema may show increased haustral contractions and at times a spastic segment. Patients should be followed up to ensure that no structural disease has been missed.

Pathogenesis

Sir James Paget, prophesied one hundred years ago, "stammering in whatever organ, appears due to want of concord between certain muscles that must contract for the expulsion of something and others that must at the same time relax to permit the thing to be expelled". This probably is true of IBS and the uncoordinated activity of smooth muscle has been documented in IBS.

The present evidence support that IBS symptom complex results from altered regulation of gastrointestinal motility and epithelial function as well as an altered perception of visceral events.

Motility Disturbances

There are several studies demonstrating motility disturbances in IBS in recent years. The questions posed by these studies are:

a. Is the motility pattern in IBS qualitatively different from that of normal colon or is there any quantitative difference?
b. Is there any specific underlying motility pattern that determines the susceptibility to symptoms?
c. Will improved understanding of the myoelectrical activity and motility patterns lead to improved treatment?

Although these questions are not still answered, a lot of data are emerging.

Visceral Hypersensitivity

Patients with IBS have increased sensitivity to distension of bowel whether this is artificially induced by inflation of balloons or by gas infused into the bowel. They develop pain in response to the gas generated in the colon by normal mechanism or from swallowed air. Precisely how distension causes pain is still not known. It may be a response to tension in muscle wall.

Abnormalities in Brain-gut Regulation

A greater appreciation for the role of the "brain-gut" axis is achieved now and now it is realised that brain-gut interactions play a key role in the modulation of GI functioning in health and disease. Functional neuro-imaging studies using colonic stimulation have demonstrated alterations in regional brain activation in IBS patients compared to healthy control subjects.

Role of Immune or Inflammatory Mediators

A subset of patients with IBS can trace their symptom to an episode of infectious diarrhea and this has been termed as post infectious IBS (PIIBS). Investigators have found increased number of intra epithelial lymphocytes, and EC cells and increased intestinal permeability. When the secreting granules of the EC cells were evaluated, patients with PIIBS had granules containing serotonin.

Enteric nervous system plays a key role in regulation of gut motility and secretion. And serotonin receptors have been found to be important modulators of motor activity.

To summarize, the present pathophysiological concept is a more integrated understanding consistent with a biopsychosocial framework consisting of the physiological components of dismotility, visceral hypersensitivity and abnormalities in brain-gut regulation.

Treatment

Treatment is directed towards
a. Ameliorating symptoms
b. Modifying factors that aggravate the disorder and
c. Helping patient to adapt to the condition (Fig. 13.2).

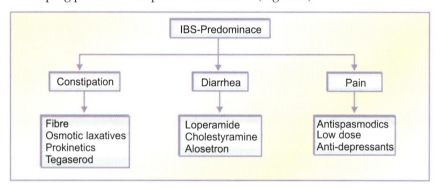

Fig. 13.2: Treatment of IBS

General Approach

The mainstay of management is reassurance. If patients are just factually told that their X-ray and other tests are normal and they have no disease, they are not happy. Once it is explained to them that although their X-rays and tests are normal, disturbances in motility can lead to symptoms, they are satisfied. Also, it has to be pointed out that emotional disturbances and stress also may be involved in producing motility disturbances; once brain-gut regulation is explained to them they accept the same. The most important thing is to listen to the patient and accept his symptoms are real and disturbing to him.

The treatment of predominant pain or discomfort varies with the severity of symptoms. If the pain is mild and meal-related (occurring after a full meal), an anticholinergic or antispasmodic agent like mebaverine can be considered and advised half an hour before meal. If associated with diarrhea, $5HT_3$ antagonist (alosetron) may be useful particularly in females. However, ischemic colitis is an adverse effect. If constipation is predominant, then $5HT_4$ agonist tegaserod may be effective. If pain is more severe, an antidepressant (tricyclic antidepressant) can be prescribed. High fibre diet is effective in constipation-predominant IBS. Isphagulla improves overall well being and bowel dissatisfaction in many patients.

PROGNOSIS

Generally, IBS is a life-long illness, but one can improve the quality of life and reduce the morbidity in majority of patients. Patients should be monitored so that serious illness is not missed. With good rapport with the patient, overall prognosis is good in majority of patients.

CONCLUSION

Although IBS is the most common gastrointestinal disorder, it is one of the most poorly understood, and till recently, one of the most neglected in terms of research. But now, with improved technology, the situation has improved and newer treatment modalities based on pathogenetic mechanisms have evolved.

SUGGESTED READING

1. Talley NJ, Spiller R. Irritable bowel syndrome, a little understood organic bowel disease. Lancet 2002; 360 555-64.
2. Langstreth GF, Drossman DA. New developments in the diagnosis and treatment of irritable bowel syndrome. Current Gastroenterology Rep 2002; 4: 427-34.
3. Drossman DA, Camilleri M, Mayer EA, Whitehead WE. AGA technical review on the irritable bowel syndrome. Gastroenterology 2002; 723: 2108-31
4. Spiller RC. Post infectious irritable bowel syndrome; Gastroenterology 2003; 124: 1662-71.
5. Narayanan V.A. Study of colonic myoelectric rhythm in irritable bowel syndrome. Ind J Gastroenterology 1988; 7 (suppl) II 7.
6. Mathur AK, Tandon BN, Omprakash. Irritable colon syndrome – a clinical and lab study. Journal of Ind Med Association 1966; 46: 651-53.
7. Horwitz B. J., Fisher R. S. Current concept: The irritable bowel syndrome. N Engl J Med 2001; 344:1846-1850.
8. Mertz H. R. Drug therapy: Irritable bowel syndrome. N Engl J Med 2003; 349: 2136-46
9. Camilleri, M. Treating irritable bowel syndrome: overview, perspective and future therapies. Br. J. Pharmacol. 2004; 141: 1237-1248.
10. Viera AJ. Management of irritable bowel syndrome. Am Fam Physician 2002; 66(10): 1867-74.
11. Budavari AI. Psychosocial aspects of functional gastrointestinal disorders. Gastroenterol Clin North Am 2003; 32: 477-506.

14

Sunil Mathai

The Gastrointestinal Tract and HIV

INTRODUCTION

Gastrointestinal and hepatobiliary complications were recognized as universal complications of HIV infection, but after 1996 the protease inhibitors became available and in combination with other antiretroviral medications – termed the highly active anti retroviral treatment (HAART) – viral replication and circulating virus was decreased, the consequence being a change in the frequency of GI disorders. The impact of HAART could be summarized as follows:

1. Increase in CD4 counts to more than 200 / l, the threshold for development of opportunistic infections (OI)
2. Prophylactic medication to OI may be discontinued in persons who respond to HAART
3. HAART may form the primary therapy for OIs that are resistant to standard therapy
4. HIV infected patients showed a substantial reduction in OIs as demonstrated by endoscopic evaluation after institution of HAART
5. HAART is associated with GI and hepatic side effects in more than 10 % and is now the major concern of gastroenterologists.

Symptoms of Gastrointestinal Involvement

The most common symptom is diarrhea occurring in more than 90 % of patients. Odynophagia and dysphagia occur in one third of the patients. Abdominal pain, GI bleeding and anorectal disorders occur with lesser frequency. Hepatomegaly with or without jaundice is seen frequently. While evaluating the symptoms, certain general points have to be emphasized.

1. There is no specificity for signs and symptoms
2. CD4 counts may be used to predict pattern of infection, as this is a reflection of immune status – more than 200/l is usually associated with common bacterial and nonopportunistic infections, and if less than 100/1 CMV, fungi, mycobacterium avium complex and unusual protozoa predominate
3. GI infections exist as a part of systemic infections and identification of a systemic pathogen would obviate the need for a GI evaluation
4. Multiple infections are common.

Evaluation of Diarrhea

Alteration in the mucosal immune system in AIDS predispose to intestinal infection. It may lead to untreatable infection by organisms that typically produce self-limited infection in an otherwise healthy host, or it may predispose to a virulent course of a common enteric infection. In AIDS a differential diagnosis could be formulated based on the clinical presentation and the degree of immunodeficiency. Table 14.1 summarizes the differential diagnosis of diarrhea in AIDS.

Table 14.1: Differential diagnosis of diarrhea in AIDS		
Protozoa	*Bacteria*	*Fungi*
Cryptosporidium	Salmonella	Histoplasmosis
Microsporidium	Shigella	Cryptococcosis
Isospora belli	Campylobacter	Coccidioidomycosis
Cyclospora	MAC (*Mycobacterium avium* complex)	Candida albicans
Giardia lamblia		
Entamoeba histolytica		
Viruses	*Gut Neoplasms*	*Drug Induced*
CMV (Cytomegalovirus)	Lymphoma	HAART
HSV (Herpes simplex virus)	Kaposi's sarcoma	
HIV		
Others		
AIDS enteropathy		
Pancreatic insufficiency		

Protozoal Diarrhea

Cryptosporidium is the most frequent cause of protozoal diarrhea in HIV infected patients. The manifestations depend on the degree of immunocompromise, from a transient illness to a florid chronic diarrhea with short survival. The small bowel is affected, with the patient complaining of severe borborygmi and periumbilical pain. A right hypochondrial pain suggests an uncommon biliary involvement. The organism resides on the surface of the enterocyte, inciting only a modest inflammatory response, unless a high parasite burden occurs. Diagnosis is made by AFB staining of stool where the organism appears as bright red spherules. Multiple stool examinations are required. Small bowel and rectal biopsies may also reveal the organism. Apart from symptomatic treatment for diarrhea, i.e., fluid support and antidiarrheal agents, the agent that has shown efficacy against the organism is paromomycin, an oral aminoglycoside. A more effective therapy would be HAART.

Microsporidium has emerged as one of the common infections in AIDS. There are two species – Enterocytozoon bienusi and Encephalitozoon intestinalis. The frequency of infection ranges from 15–30%. Infection is associated with severe immunodeficiency with median CD4 counts of less than 100/l. The organism is very small and is visualized with the electron microscope as a merozoite vacuole near the enterocyte nucleus. Tissue inflammation is minimal. Transmission is through water. Light microscopy could identify the tissue with special stains like Brown Brenn or Gram stain but electron microscopy is more definite and PCR analysis is considered highly accurate. HAART is most effective, though symptomatic improvement is seen with metronidazole and atovaquone. Albendazole is effective in E. intestinalis.

Giaridia lamblia and *Entamoeba histolytica:* Unless it is endemic, is not a common infection in AIDS. The reason for this is not known. Helminthiasis has been described with abdominal pain and eosinophilia.

Viral Diarrhea

CMV is the most frequent cause of chronic diarrhea in AIDS. It occurs in the severely immunocompromised with CD4 counts of less than 100/l. The commonest site of infection is the colon, followed by esophagus, stomach or small bowel. Mucosal ischemia, due to vascular involvement and activation of local proinflammatory cytokines are proposed as pathogenetic mechanisms. Clinical manifestations vary from asymptomatic state to peritonitis, perforation and bleeding. Chronic diarrhea and abdominal pain are most common. Endoscopy would show subepithelial hemorrhages and mucosal ulceration. Demonstration of inclusion bodies and cultures are used for diagnosis. Specific drugs used for treatment of CMV include IV ganciclovir, valganciclovir orally, foscarnet, and cidofovir. Combination therapy of ganciclovir and foscarnet has been used. Cidofovir has a long half-life and is given once a week. Treatment has to be given for several weeks and relapse is common after withdrawal. HAART is to be instituted alongwith anti-CMV drugs. Opthalmologic examination is recommended for all persons to exclude retinitis, and a close follow up is required in order to prevent blindness.

The role of other viruses is minimal. HIV itself is implicated in the pathogenesis of diarrhea. *Idiopathic enteropathy* of AIDS is proposed as a cause when no diarrheal pathogen is detected. Mucosal atrophy impairing small bowel absorption and permeability, and HIV effects on the autonomic nerves altering the motility seem to be the pathogenesis inducing diarrhea. Management of these diarrheas would be symptomatic therapy and HAART.

Bacterial Diarrhea

Increased frequency and virulence are the features of bacterial diarrhea, which includes organisms like *Salmonella, Shigella* and campylobacter. In an HIV positive patient, recurrent salmonella infection establishes the diagnosis of AIDS. The presentation is similar to otherwise healthy patients and diagnosis would rest on stool and tissue cultures.

The choice of antibiotic is determined by sensitivity tests. Quinolones, either ciprofloxacin or ofloxacin is recommended for empirical therapy. Clostridium difficile may produce diarrhea due to the greater antibiotic use than being an OI. Treatment with metronidazole and vancomycin is effective. Small bowel bacterial overgrowth is uncommon, but occurs due to gastric achlorhydria and motility impairment.

Mycobacterium tuberculosis or MAC may involve the intestines leading to diarrhea. Duodenal involvement is seen commonly with MAC. Diagnosis is made by endoscopic mucosal biopsies. AFB stain shows the tissue teeming with the organisms. There is a poorly formed inflammatory response and granulomas are rarely present. Multidrug regimens are given for treatment, including rifampicin, ethambutol, amikacin, ciprofloxacin, and clarithromycin. Eradication is rarely achieved and institution of HAART may hasten resolution and prevent relapse. In contrast to MAC, Mycobacterium tuberculosis generally responds to standard ATT.

Fungal Infections

GI histoplasmosis has most commonly been described in association with pulmonary and hepatic disease. Diffuse colitis, diarrhea and ulceration are the presentations. Diagnosis is achieved with a fungal smear and culture of infected tissue or blood. Intravenous amphotericin B is given initially followed by long-term suppressive therapy with Itraconazole. Coccidioidomycosis and cryptococcosis have been described producing GI and liver involvement.

Drug Induced Diarrhea

The components of HAART, especially the protease inhibitor nelfinavir may cause diarrhea in up to 20% of patients. Though the mechanism is unknown symptomatic therapy is effective.

In the setting of negative results of the investigations and severe diarrhea, the role of an empirical antibiotic trial arises. The antibiotics recommended are ciprofloxacin and metronidazole. Spontaneous resolution occurs in 20–35%. HAART holidays may also be effective.

Table 14.2: Evaluation of diarrhea in AIDS

History
- Lactose intolerance
- Food intolerance

Laboratory evaluation
- Stool tests
- Leucocytes
- Ova and parasites
- AFB
- Clostridium difficile toxin

Endoscopic evaluation
- Sigmoidoscopy/colonoscopy
- Biopsy, culture, PCR of tissue
- Upper G.I. endoscopy
- Small bowel mucosal biopsy
- Electron microscopy

Evaluation of Odynophagia and Dysphagia

One third of patients with AIDS report esophageal complaints. HAART has changed the spectrum of the illness and now non AIDS related diseases such as GERD is on the increase.

Table 14.3: Differential diagnosis of dysphagia and odynophagia in AIDS

Candida albicans
CMV
Idiopathic ulcerations
Herpes simplex
MAC
Neoplasms
GERD
Pill induced

Candida esophagitis occurs in about 64% of patients, frequently in association with oral thrush. Diagnosis is fairly easy with endoscopy showing typical plaques and biopsy revealing yeast forms. Fluconazole 200 mg as a loading dose followed by 100 mg/day is recommended. Itraconazole and ketaconazole are effective. Relapse was common before the HAART era.

CMV esophagitis is less frequent. Endoscopy reveals extensive ulcerations, and mucosal biopsy shows viral cytopathic effects and inclusion bodies. Immuno-histochemical stains confirm the diagnosis. Intravenous ganciclovir, foscarnet and cidofovir are used.

The idiopathic ulcer syndrome is diagnosed considering the following criteria:

1. Endoscopic and histopathologic ulcer
2. Viral cytopathic effect is absent
3. No clinical or endoscopic evidence of GERD

These ulcers respond to oral corticosteroids 40 mg tapered off in 4 weeks. Thalidomide is also effective.

Herpes simplex esophagitis is uncommon with AIDS. Endoscopy reveals discrete ulcers and they respond to acyclovir.

HAART has altered the long-term survival of these patients. CMV esophagitis carried a survival rate of 7.6 months, which has been improved after institution of HAART.

Evaluation of Abdominal Pain

Abdominal pain in AIDS may be secondary to HIV and its consequences like OI s or neoplasms, or it may arise due to common causes seen in the general population (Table 14.4).

Perforation of the bowel occurs most often with CMV infection, frequently in the distal small bowel or colon, and is the commonest cause of acute abdomen in AIDS. *Obstruction* may arise from neoplasms or intussusception from lymphomatous infiltration. Infectious enteritis or colitis may lead to dull aching pain. Infectious or nonspecific *peritonitis* can occur, with tuberculosis or fungal infections.

Pancreatitis may arise as result of drugs or infections. Macroamylasemia can occur in AIDS. Dideoxyinosine or pentamidine can cause a 5% incidence of pancreatitis. Antiretroviral drugs may cause hyperlipidemia and lead to pancreatitis. Neoplastic infiltration of pancreas, lymphoma and Kaposi's sarcoma (KS) have been described.

Management of patients falls on similar lines of a non-HIV patient. Radiological studies like USG, CT, MRI and barium studies are used in appropriate manner. Endoscopic evaluation is done wherever required. Surgery carries a higher mortality due to poor health, malnutrition and underlying infections, especially CMV. Lymphoma and Kaposi's sarcoma may respond to chemotherapy or radiation. Pancreatitis is managed on similar lines as in a non-HIV patient.

TABLE 14.4: Differential diagnosis of abdominal pain in AIDS

Area	Cause
Stomach Gastritis, ulcer, outlet obstruction	CMV, lymphoma, KS (Kaposi's sarcoma)
Small bowel Enteritis, obstruction, perforation	CMV, lymphoma, MAC, KS
Colon Colitis, obstruction, perforation, appendicitis	CMV, lymphoma, KS, cryptosporidium
Biliary tract Cholecystitis, papillary stenosis	CMV, cryptosporidium, microsporidium, KS
Pancreas Inflammation and tumor	CMV, drugs, lymphoma, tuberculosis
Mesentery, peritoneum MAC, tuberculosis, histoplasmosis, cryptococcosis, toxoplasmosis	

Table 14.5: Anorectal lesions in HIV

Infections

Bacterial	*Viral*
Chlamydia trachomatis Neisseria gonorrhea Lymphogranuloma venereum	HSV, CMV
Protozoal Entamoeba histolytica Leishmania donovanii	*Fungus* Candida Albicans Histoplasma
Neoplasms Lymphoma, squamous cell carcinoma Condyloma acuminatum Kaposi's sarcoma	

Anorectal Diseases

The frequency of these illnesses are quite high, infections, fistula, abscesses and neoplasms being the presentation. Anorectal carcinoma is seen in homosexual men and is secondary to infection with human pappilloma virus 16 and 18. Table 14.5 lists the differential diagnosis of anorectal lesions in HIV positive patients.

All patients with anorectal disease should undergo anoscopy, sigmoidoscopy and biopsy. Culture studies and imaging studies should be done appropriately. Healing of these lesions depend on stage of HIV infection. Patients with AIDS are likely to have a poor outcome.

Gastrointestinal Bleeding

As a symptom this occurs in less than 1% of patients and is associated with a reduced survival. Mucosal ulceration, ischemia, and infarction are the causes identified. Endoscopic hemostasis, angiographic embolization and surgery are all employed with supportive blood component therapy.

Liver Involvement in HIV

Liver may be involved either as parenchymal disease or biliary disease. Apart from the OIs, drugs used in HAART, and the hepatotropic viruses B, C and D produce liver disease.On clinical examination hepatomegaly is a frequent finding, and mild LFT alterations without significant jaundice is detected in many patients.

Drug induced liver injury has emerged as the most prevalent cause of LFT abnormality. Sulfonamides and the protease inhibitors especially zidovudine is implicated as the major drugs responsible. Indigenous medications in the form of herbal remedies are also reported to cause LFT derangements. The immune upgradation by HAART may cause flare up of underlying viral hepatitis. Liver biopsy in drug induced injury shows a hepatocellular pattern. In sulphonamide injury granuloma with eosinophilic infiltration is seen. Zidovudine, ddI and stavudine are now recognised to produce a syndrome of hepatomegaly, steatosis, lactic acidosis and liver failure. This may revert with stopping the drug, but is often fatal and liver transplantation is recommended in such cases.

MAC infection in AIDS is manifested by granulomas and plenty of AFB may be seen even without granulomas. In contrast to MAC, *Mycobacterium tuberculosis* occurs prior to development of profound immunocompromised state. Tubercular abscess and bile duct granulomas are rarely seen. Liver biopsy, tissue culture and PCR are employed for diagnosis.

CMV involvement of the liver is seen in around 20–25% of liver biopsies. Typical viral inclusion bodies are seen, with mononuclear cell infiltration and occasional granuloma.

The hepatitis viruses have altered clinical and histological manifestation in the presence of HIV co-infection.

HBV and HIV: The seroprevalence of HBV markers in AIDS is approximately 90%. In spite of immune anti-HBs levels, reappearance of HBsAg has been described. Accelerated loss of anti HBs, re-infection and reactivation in the face of immunodeficiency are all cited as causes for recurrence of HBsAg. There is an increased prevalence of HBe Ag expression and HBV DNA titres. A large proportion of patients develop a highly infectious chronic state as compared to non-HIV infected patients. An interesting observation is that in spite of chronicity, the severity of biochemical and histological parameters are attenuated. This is explained by the diminution of lymphocyte mediated hepatocellular injury. HBV has no independent effect on survival of patients with HIV. Vaccination is ineffective regardless of stage of immunocompromise. When HAART is instituted immune reconstitution occurs. Antibody production directed against infected hepatocytes lead to an acute flare manifested as acute hepatitis or even fulminant hepatic failure. Seroconversion is also reported. Hence it is now suggested that lamivudine should be added to HAART therapy if there is co-infection with HBV. Screening for all patients for active or past infection is recommended prior to instituting HAART. Delta hepatitis behaves in a similar way to HBV in HIV co-infected patients from the observations of a limited number of patients.

HCV and HIV: Intravenous drug users and hemophiliacs have the highest co-infection rate ranging from 52 to 89%. In non-drug users the prevalence is 1-11 %.HCV RNA has to be detected to assess the true prevalence, as HCV antibody may be lost in immunodeficiency. In contrast to HBV, disease process worsens rapidly in HCV infection with biochemical and histological parameters showing rapid progression to cirrhosis and liver failure. Rapid elevations of HCV RNA levels occur with progressive HIV illness. The mechanism of this rapid course is unknown. However, like HBV, HCV does not cause progression of HIV disease. Treatment of HCV with interferon alone is less effective. Combination therapy with ribavirin is more effective and clearance rate of up to 50% has been documented. Institution of HAART has produced variable effects in HCV. Some reports suggest attenuation of biochemistry and histopathology while some reports have shown a flare up of illness.

Fungal infections of liver: Histoplasmosis is seen in association with pulmonary infection, biopsy revealing caseating granuloma along with the fungus. Cryptococcosis and coccidioidomycosis may occur as a part of systemic infection, but candida infection is rare in spite of high prevalence of mucosal disease.

Neoplasms in liver: Kaposi's sarcoma arises from the lymphocyte endothelial cell and is triggered by infection by human herpes virus 8 (HHV 8). Otherwise known as kaposi's sacoma associated herpes virus (KSHV). Ten to 15% of liver biopsies carry the tumor. Histologically, it appears as violaceous or hemorrhagic masses in the hepatic parenchyma. Hodgkin's lymphoma of liver may be the presenting manifestation and may appear as a primary site manifestation. It is usually aggressive, spreads rapidly and prognosis is related to the degree of immunocompromise.

Bartonella infection may be associated with *peliosis hepatis*. LFT reveals a raised alkaline phosphatase and liver biopsy demonstrates the organisms under special stains. Prolonged or lifelong treatment with erythromycin or tetracycline is reported to be effective.

AIDS cholangiopathy: This is characterized by a syndrome comprising of sclerosing cholangitis and papillary stenosis. Raised alkaline phosphatase and minimal elevation in transaminases are noted. ERCP detects extrahepatic strictures and intra hepatic ductular changes. The etiology is infectious as cryptosporidium, microsporidium and CMV have been demonstrated in the bile and biliary epithelium. Endoscopic sphincterotomy relieves symptoms in papillary stenosis.

Acalculous cholecystitis has been demonstrated in AIDS patients, frequently caused by CMV.

Neoplastic lesions like primary biliary lymphoma and Kaposi's sarcoma have been reported. At present biliary tract disease from non-HIV related diseases is as frequent as those associated with AIDS.

SUGGESTED READING

1. Sleisenger and Fordtran, Gastrointestinal Manifestation of the Acquired Immunodeficiency Syndrome; Gastrointestinal and Liver Disease, 6th Edition, 2002;387-409.
2. Prevalence of enteric pathogens in homosexual men with and without acquired immunodeficiency syndrome. Gastroenterology 1988;94:984
3. Intestinal infections in patients with AIDS .Dig. Dis. Sci. 1989;34:773.
4. Gastrointestinal CMV disease. Ann . Intern. Med> 1993;119:924.
5. Efficient management of diarrhea in AIDS. Ann. Intern. Med 1990;112:942.
6. Hepatic disease in patients with AIDS. Hepatology 1987;7:925.
7. HBV infection in AIDS. Ann. Intern. Med 1986;101:795.
8. Talal AH, Weiss LM, Vanderhorst C. Molecular diagnosis of gastrointestinal infections associated with HIV infection. Gastroenterol Clin North Am 1997; 26:417-44.
9. Lew EA, Poles MA, Dieterich DT. Diarrheal diseases associated with HIV infection. Gastroenterol Clin North Am. 1997;26:259-90.
10. Poles MA, Lew EA, Dieterich DT. Diagnosis and treatment of hepatic disease in patients with HIV. Gastroenterol Clin North Am 1997;26:291-321.

15

Sudheer OV

Anorectal Disorders

INTRODUCTION

It is essential to have a good understanding of anorectal anatomy and physiology in the diagnosis and management of the anorectal disorders and their management.

The rectum begins where sigmoid colon ends; the tenia coli end at this point. For uniformity in definition, the rectum is considered to extend up to 12 cm from the anal verge.

The surgical anal canal is approximately 4 cm long and extends from anal verge to anorectal ring, which is defined as the proximal level of the levator external anal sphincter complex.

Anal sphincters: The internal anal sphincter is a condensation of the lower end of circular smooth muscle of the rectum. The external sphincter is a complex plate of striated muscles surrounding the anal canal. The function of both sphincters is related to defecation and continence. The longitudinal smooth muscles of rectum continues into anal canal within the intersphincteric space, traverses the internal sphincter and is attached to the epithelium and skin. It probably acts as a suspensory ligament for the epithelium of the anal canal.

SYMPTOMS OF ANORECTAL DISORDERS

Bleeding

Loss of blood from anal lesions occurs characteristically at the time of defecation and appears as a bright red streak or smear on the surface of the stool. It can be in drops or a jet of bleeding before or after defecation in case of hemorrhoids. Bleeding from a rectal lesion as a malignant disease of rectum would be mixed with stools or as passage of blood and mucus per rectum. This may also be the case in inflammatory bowel disease. Large quantities of blood in conjunction with or independent of stool passage usually mean that the bleeding is higher in the gastrointestinal tract.

Pruritus

Many anorectal conditions that cause persistent discharge, such as fistula and hemorrhoids can cause pruritus.

Pain

As the mucosa above the dentate line is insensitive, mucosal lesion at this level may not cause pain. At the same time the skin below the dentate line is very sensitive and the disease involving this part of the anal canal can have excruciating pain. Perianal abscess and the fissure in ano can also lead to severe pain.

Swelling or Lump

Patient might report to the clinician with complaints of a swelling prolapsing from the anal canal during defecation. The swelling which might appear on straining or defecation might be prolapsing rectum or anal canal, hemorrhoids or polyp. A persistent lump may be indicative of a growth.

Discharge

There are three types of discharge.

Fecal soiling: Usually the result of either distortion of the anal anatomy, say by tumor, or of incontinence.

Mucoid: Changes in the mucosa of the rectum and or proximal anal canal which are commonly inflammatory, but may imply a mucus secreting tumor.

Purulent: Almost always associated with sepsis.

HEMORRHOIDS

The exact prevalence of hemorrhoids is difficult to estimate. Patients attribute any anorectal condition to hemorrhoids, which should be carefully investigated and diagnosed by an experienced clinician.

The submucosa of the anal canal is not a continuous ring but a discontinuous series of vascular cushions. The three main anal cushions are found in left lateral, right anterior and right posterior positions. These cushions are rich in blood vessels and muscular fibres. The muscular fibres are responsible for adherence of mucosal and submucosal tissues to the internal sphincters and blood vessels of submucosa.

The deterioration of the supportive tissues to the vascular cushions in anal canal produces venous distension, erosion, bleeding and thrombosis. There is congestion and hypertrophy of anal cushions, prolapse and downward displacement and abnormal dilatation of the venous plexuses in the anal cushions. Other factors such as heredity, age, anal sphincter tone, diet, occupation, constipation and pregnancy also have been implicated in the causation of hemorrhoids.

CLASSIFICATION

Hemorrhoids are classified according to its location and degree of prolapse.

The internal hemorrhoid is above the dentate line. External hemorrhoids are below the dentate line and the mixed internoexternal hemorrhoids are both above and below.

Hemorrhoids are classified according to the degree of prolapse.

First degree: Cushions located above the pectinate line that doesn't descend on straining. They are usually associated with bleeding at the time of defecation.

Second degree: Cushions that protrude below the pectinate line during straining but return spontaneously to within the anal canal once the straining stops

Third degree: Cushions that prolapse to the exterior of anal canal during straining or defecation and requiring manual reduction back into the anal canal.

Fourth degree: Cushions that are irreducible and remain constantly prolapsed independent of straining or defecation.

DIAGNOSIS

A detailed history is essential. The bleeding usually occurs at the time of defecation, is bright red in color, in spurts or drops after defecation, or at other times of exertion. Mucous discharge or fecal soiling could be due to incomplete closure of anal canal due to hemorrhoids. Uncomplicated hemorrhoids do not cause pain. It occurs when hemorrhoids get thrombosed ulcerated or infected.

Digital examination and proctoscopy are essential in patients with perianal symptoms. Colonoscopy or limited sigmoidoscopy has to be done in cases of rectal bleeding in order to rule out more proximal lesions and importantly colorectal malignancy.

At proctoscopy the appearance of hemorrhoids vary from a slight increase in size of normal anal cushions to large internoexternal hemorrhoids apparent on inspection of the anal verge. The external component of the second and third degree hemorrhoids comprise the perianal skin and hair depending on prolapse. There is always a groove between the hemorrhoidal masses corresponding to anal valves.

Conditions that are related to hemorrhoids and which may cause diagnostic confusions are anal skin tags, fibrous polyps, prolapse rectum and thrombosis in perianal skin (perianal hematoma).

MANAGEMENT

Conservative management of hemorrhoids can be accomplished in the majority of patients. Because of the tendency to constipation advice about ensuring a more regular bowel habit such as increased intake of fluids, vegetables, fruits and addition of bulk laxatives is encouraged. Neglecting the first urge to defecate, spending prolonged time in toilet and straining are common defecation errors. A high fibre diet is associated with an improvement in bowel habits and reduction in constipation. Furthermore, the addition of bulk forming agents to normal diet can minimize the amount of trauma to anal canal epithelium caused by hardened stools therefore the likelihood of ulceration and bleeding. The use of sitz bath and warm soaks is commonly advised to lessen the perianal discomfort.

Topical Preparations

These include a variety of ingredients, which include topical steroids, local anesthetics and antibiotics. The efficacy of such preparations is yet to be proved. Some symptomatic relief of hemorrhoidal disease can be achieved with their use.

TREATMENT DIRECTED AT HEMORRHOIDS

Injection Sclerotherapy

Injection of sclerosing agents like phenol in vegetable oil, sodium morrhuate, and sodium tertradecyl sulfate causes fibrosis of vascular cushions and therefore obliterates hemorrhoids. However sclerotherapy is contraindicated in management of external hemorrhoids, thrombosed or ulcerated internal hemorrhoids as well as in the presence of inflammatory or gangrenous piles. This procedure is useful in actively bleeding piles.

Cryotherapy

The principle of cryotherapy is based on rapid freezing followed by thawing. This procedure is associated with profound foul smelling discharge and irritation. In addition to pain and low healing rate, the inappropriate use of cryotherapy can cause necrosis of internal anal sphincters resulting in anal stenosis and incontinence. Due to this, cryotherapy is now losing its popularity.

Infrared Coagulation

Infrared light penetrates the tissues and cause tissue destruction. The primary benefit is in individuals with smaller hemorrhoids and when the bleeding is not amenable to rubber band ligation. It is an office procedure and no anesthesia is needed.

Rubber Band Ligation

Now this method has replaced surgical hemorrhoidectomy for approximately 80% of patients. It is a simple inexpensive office based procedure that can be applied to most patients with bleeding and or prolapsed hemorrhoids. It is ideal for the treatment of second and third degree hemorrhoids. Multiple ligations at three or four weeks' intervals may be required. Sixty to 70% are cured in a single session; if symptoms persist after 3 or 4 session's treatment, surgical hemorrhoidectomy should be considered. Rubber band ligations may be considered as a procedure of choice for the management of first through third degree hemorrhoids.

Operative Treatment

Surgical hemorrhoidectomy should be considered in the presence of an external component, ulceration, gangrene, extensive thrombosis, hypertrophied papillae, associated fissure or failure of rubber band ligation.

Hemorrhoidectomy is of two types.

Closed method: After ligation and excision the mucocutaneous defect is closed by suture with the objective of primary healing

Open method: After excision the wound heals by granulation and reepithelialization.

Both of these procedures aim to excise as much redundant epithelium and vasculature as possible.

Stapled Hemorrhoidectomy /Stapled Hemorrhoidopexy

Rationally the stapled hemorrhoidopexy is based on the concept that interruption of superior and middle hemorrhoidal vessels and upward lifting of the prolapsed anorectal mucosa and repositioning of vascular cushions back into anal canal cause the hemorrhoidal tissue atrophy. Stapled hemorrhoidopexy has been mainly advocated for third and fourth degree internal hemorrhoids.

Residual external hemorrhoids may partially or completely be drawn into the anal canal with PPH and would atrophy and become asymptomatic. Stapled hemorrhoidectomy is a relatively painless procedure, but is done under anesthesia in operating room. The procedure is gaining wide acceptance as it is painless and there is no residual wound.

FISSURE IN ANO

Fissures are ulcers consequent to tears of the mucosa at the anal margin which extend into pecton.

Etiology

The cause is not obvious. Constipation and passage of hard stools might initiate the problem. Self-digital evacuation of stools, trauma at childbirth may also be responsible in some cases. Most patients have sustained hyper tonicity of the internal anal sphincter and sphincture spasm. A vicious cycle is set up consequently pain-> sphincter spasm-> constipation-> greater difficulty on defecation which makes the local condition worse.

The common site is posteriorly in the midline but it may be anterior or lateral. Depth may range from a simple superficial break in the epithelium to a chronic lesion with exposure of the fibers of the internal sphincture. Chronic lesions may have an associated skin tag, the so-called sentinel pile, an anal polyp of varying size and undermining edges.

Pain

Pain occurs during defecation and may be severe. It may continue for some time but usually is eased before the passage of next stool; when the cycle may be repeated.

Pain may be common and severe with acute fissure and some chronic indolent fissures may be relatively pain free.

Constipation may be the consequence of the patient's unwillingness to defecate because of pain. Bleeding can occur but it is not usually severe and may stain on the sides of stools. Sometimes discharge of pus might occur. It is often possible to see the lower end of the fissure by separating the buttock and asking the patients to strain. In an acute fissure there is tenderness posteriorly at the site of fissure and digital examination is extremely painful which is better avoided.

In chronic fissure a sentinel tag is usually seen. A digital examination can normally be done and reveals thickening at the anorectal ring and varying amount of tenderness although this is not usually very severe. Proctoscopy shows a lesion of varying depth in which fibres of external sphincters may be visible; there is granulation tissue and small amount of bleeding.

Management

Medical treatment is most likely to be effective in patients with acute fissure. The main stay of medical treatment is avoidance of hard stools. Bulk laxatives might help. Warm sitz bath are recommended to alleviate pain.

Nitric oxide temporarily reduces the internal sphincter tone. Topical application of 0.2% glyceryl trinitrate two or three times daily helps in reduction of sphincter tone and thereby epithelialization and healing of fissure. Glyceryl trinitrate has been shown to be effective in both acute and chronic fissure and is now considered as first line treatment. The side effect of glyceryl trinitrate is headache about which the patients should be warned of. Another agent, which has shown reduction in sphincter tone and aids in healing of fissure, is the calcium channel blocker diltiazem. Topical 2% diltiazem has been found to be effective in up to 50% of patients.

Other symptomatic measures of treatments are use of local anesthetics, 1% lignocaine, warm sitz bath, bulk laxatives and use of analgesics.

Surgical Therapy

Surgical therapy is reserved for the patients who have failed medical therapy. The surgical procedure is aimed at disruption of internal sphincter. Maximal anal dilatation, which was done under anesthesia, is losing its popularity due to the complication of incontinence.

Closed or open lateral internal sphincterotomy is the surgical method of choice. The internal sphincter muscle is divided upto the uppermost part of the fissure. The whole of the internal sphincter is not divided as it might increase the chance of partial incontinence.

Anorectal Abscess

Anorectal abscess is an acute inflammatory condition with acute presentation due to severe pain. Usually it results in or is associated with anal fistula. Most of the anorectal abscesses are due to nonspecific causes but certain conditions such as foreign body, instrumentation, trauma, malignancy, radiation, tuberculosis, actinomycosis, and Crohn's disease also can result in anorectal abscess.

The cause of nonspecific abscess is thought to be due to the obstruction of anal glands.

Abscesses occur more commonly in males, in 3rd and 4th decades.

Types of Abscesses

Four presentations of anorectal abscesses have been described.
1. Perianal
2. Ischiorectal
3. Intersphincteric
4. Supralevator.

Perianal Abscess

Perianal abscess presents as a superficial tender mass outside the anal verge. It is the most common type of anorectal abscess. The patient presents with short history of pain and swelling in the perianal region, which is exacerbated by defecation, and sitting. Proctosigmoidoscopic examination is difficult to perform due to pain. Occasionally anoscopy can show pus exuding from the base of the crypt.

Treatment
A perianal abscess should be drained in a timely manner. If the abscess is superficial it may be drained in the office setting under local anesthetic. If it is too tender for physical examination drainage in operation room may be needed. Antibiotics have no major role in treatment. It may be used in special situations such as immunosuppressed, extensive cellulitis, or diabetes.

Ischiorectal Abscess

Ischiorectal abscess may present as a large erythematous, tender mass of the buttock or may be virtually inapparent, the patient complaining only of severe pain. Waiting for the abscess to mature unnecessarily prolongs the patient's sufferings. Proctoscopy and sigmoidoscopy may be done later as it might be too painful.

Treatment
The drainage needs some planning, as this type of abscess is the result of transsphincteric fistula or might result in a transsphincteric fistula in ano. The

drainage should be done close to the anal verge. After drainage a wick is placed in the wound loosely to prevent early closure of the wound.

Intersphincteric Abscess

This condition arises from an infected crypt in the anal canal and burrows in the intersphincteric space. This is rare and represents 2-4% of anorectal abscesses. Rectal examination may show a tender submucosal mass and can be confused with thrombosed internal piles. An anal fissure is associated with the abscess in 25% cases.

Treatment

This abscess should be drained under general or regional anesthesia. The abscess is drained through the internal sphincter removing the associated crypt bearing area. Patient is advised sitz baths.

Supralevator Abscess

Supralevatorabscess is comparatively rare representing less than 2.5% of cases. Perianal and buttock pain are the common presenting complaints. Most patients are febrile and have leukocytosis.

Many patients with supralevator abscess have a pelvic inflammatory condition such as Crohn's disease, diverticulitis, salpingitis, or have had recent abdominal surgery. Supralevator abscess may also occur as a cephalic extension of transsphincteric or intersphincteric abscess.

Treatment

The etiology of the abscess determines the therapy transrectal or transvaginal drainage for abscess caused by pelvic sepsis or external drainage for abscess secondary to transsphincteric fistula. These patients need detailed evaluation under anesthesia.

ANAL FISTULA

Formation of a Fistula

The fistula follows an acute nonspecific inflammation. The pus from an abscess burrows in two directions into and through the wall of the anorectal canal and emerge distal to the mucocutaneous junction. Two openings are formed—internal and external, and the track that connects them is lined with granulation tissue. One or both of these openings may be closed at any time, and if both seal, further abscess develops. Repeated episodes of this kind may cause further and more complex tracks.

Fistula in the vast majority of cases arises from the preexisting abscesses. Other etiologies of anal fistulae include superficial fistulae associate with anal fissure, anorectal Crohn's disease and tuberculosis of anal canal are other causes of fistula in ano.

Patients with fistula may present with either pain or sepsis. The commonest type of presentation of fistula is with drainage of pus or blood in the perianal region unrelated to defecation.

Classification of Fistula

Classification is in relation to the anal musculature. There are two main types of fistulae-inter-sphincteric and trans-sphincteric

1. **Intersphincteric fistula:** All the inflammatory tracts remain medial to the striated muscles
2. **Transsphincteric:** There is a primary track across the external sphincter, which may be at any level from just below puborectalis to the lowest fibers of the external sphincter.

Identification of Fistula Tract

A number of methods are applied to identify the fistulous tract. The basic principle is to include the Goodsall's rule, careful physical examination, probing of the tract by a variety of injection technique and usage of imaging modalities as magnetic resonance imaging.

Goodsall's rule: when the external opening lies anterior to the transverse plane, the internal plane tends to be located radially. Conversely when the external opening lies posteriorly the internal opening is usually located in the posterior midline. Careful physical examination may show the fistulous track as an induration if it is a low fistula. Failure to identify this implies that it is a deep transsphincteric fistula and more detailed examinations are needed to characterize the tract as by passing a probe and fistulogram using a radioopaque contrast medium.

Magnetic Resonance Fistulogram

Magnetic resonance fistulogram is a recently employed method of investigation. The fistulous tract, its side branches, multiple tracks, and the relationship to the anal sphincters is more clearly delineated with this method.

Surgical Treatment

The fistulous tract should be incised completely into the anal canal through the internal opening. Care should be taken not to create a false passage. All the side branches should be identified and should be laid open.

Fistulectomy has no additional benefit over fistulotomy except it provides a good biopsy specimen. Fistulectomy might delay the healing of fistula. In fistulotomy as well, a biopsy specimen should be obtained from the fistulous tract.

In high fistulas the concern is the injury to the external sphincter leading to incontinence. This should be avoided at any cost. In high fistulas the preferred treatment is passage of a setori through the fistulous tract and keeping it tightened. The ligature passed will gradually cut through the sphincter without retraction of the cut ends, avoiding the possibility of incontinence.

Rectal Prolapse

Rectal prolapse usually occurs in extremes of life. The two types of presentations are complete and incomplete or partial prolapse. The latter may be incomplete and may be circumferential or may involve only a portion of rectal mucosa.

Etiology

The etiological factors believed to produce rectal prolapse may be congenital or acquired. Poor bowel habits, especially constipation, neurological disorders, patulous anus, chronic debility and lack of fixation of rectum to the sacrum are described as causes for rectal prolapse. In infants prolapse may be caused by lack of skeletal support and by excessive intraabdominal pressure from above. Patients from psychiatric hospitals are not uncommonly afflicted with this disorder. Most of these patients have an abnormal behavior.

Clinical Features and Evaluation

The patient's chief complaint is the prolapse itself. Problems with bowel regulation and incontinence are also common presenting features. Almost one half of the patients have history of constipation. Significant bleeding is rarely seen.

Fecal incontinence associated with prolapse is a frequent complaint. When the patient's symptoms are suggestive of rectal prolapse, some times the only way to visualize the prolapse is to make them sit on a toilet and ask them to strain, even though it is not a pleasant experience.

Treatment

Infants and children: In infants, the straight downward course of rectum predisposes for the prolapse. As the child grows and the sacral curve develops the prolapse usually corrects by itself. Till then the mother is taught to reduce the prolapse by gently pushing it in by a lubricated finger.

Treatment in adults: Partial prolapse: Submucosal injections of phenol in almond oil occasionally are successful in cases of early prolapse.

Excision of prolapsed mucosa: The prolapsed mucosa can be excised and the cut ends reapproximated with absorbable sutures. Hemorrhoidal staplers can achieve the same results.

Complete Prolapse

Most often surgery is required in prolapse rectum. The operation can be performed via the perineal or abdominal approach. Whenever possible an abdominal rectopexy is recommended, but when the patient is elderly or very frail or is suffering from injury, a perianal operation is indicated.

SUGGESTED READING

1. Lembo A., Camilleri M. Current concept: Chronic constipation. N Engl J Med 2003; 349:1360.
2. Kaiser AM. Anorectal anatomy. Surg Clin North Am 2002; 82: 1125-38
3. Thorson AG. Anorectal physiology Surg Clin North Am 2002; 82: 1115-23
4. Rao SS. Constipation: evaluation and treatment. Gastroenterol Clin North Am 2003; 32: 659-83.
5. Gopal DV. Diseases of the rectum and anus: a clinical approach to common disorders. Clin Cornerstone 2002; 4: 34-48.
6. Judge TA. Treatment of fistulizing Crohn's disease. Gastroenterol Clin North Am 2004; 33: 421-54.

16

Mathew Philip

The Management of Lower Gastrointestinal Bleeding

INTRODUCTION

Lower GI bleeding is defined as an abnormal intraluminal blood loss from a source distal to the ligament of Treitz. Incidence of lower GI bleed is higher in men and increases with age.

Etiology varies according to the age of the patient. Mortality rates are reportedly 10-20%. Despite improvement in diagnostic imaging and procedures, 10-20% of patients with lower GI bleeding have no demonstrable bleeding source. The bleeding may be massive or trivial, occult (hidden) or overt (obvious).

TERMINOLOGY

Hematochezia: Bright red or maroon blood per rectum suggests a lower GI source; however, 11-20% of patients with an upper GI bleed will have hematochezia as a result of rapid blood loss.

Melena: Black tarry and mostly foul smelling stools. Melena is due to degradation of blood to hematin or other hemochromes by bacteria. Mostly the source is upper gastrointestinal tract but also can be from the proximal portions of lower GI tract. Sticky, black, foul-smelling stools suggest a source proximal to the ligament of Treitz, but it can also result from bleeding in the small intestine or proximal colon. Fifty to 100 ml of blood is necessary to make a melenic stool.

Occult bleeding: Refers to bleeding that is not obvious to the patient and indicates small amounts of bleeding. This is detected by fecal occult blood test. Most tests for fecal occult blood become positive when more than 2 ml of blood are lost per day.

Obscure GI bleeding: In up to 5% of patients with overt GI bleeding, the source of bleeding remains unidentified after readily identifiable causes have been ruled out by endoscopic procedures like upper GI endoscopy and colonoscopy. Obscure bleeding can be either occult or obvious.

The Causes of Lower GI Bleeding in Adults

1. Colonic diverticulosis
2. Vascular ectasia
3. Colonic neoplasia
4. Benign anorectal diseases (hemorrhoids, fissure in ano)
5. Inflammatory bowel disease
6. Infectious colitis
7. Ischemic colitis/mesenteric vascular insufficiency

8. Radiation colitis
9. Portal colonopathy/colonic/rectal varices
10. Dieulafoy's lesions
11. Colonic ulcers/solitary rectal ulcer syndrome
12. Diversion colitis
13. Vasculitides
14. Small intestinal lesions like ulcers, tumors, diverticula, aortoenteric fistula
15. Endometriosis
16. GI bleeding in runners

Common Causes of Acute Lower GI Bleeding in Children and Adolescents

- Intussusception
- Polyps and polyposis syndromes
- Inflammatory bowel disease
- Meckel's diverticulum

Clinical Evaluation

The principles of evaluation and management are
1. Determine the source of bleed
2. Stop active bleeding
3. Treat underlying pathology
4. Prevent recurrent bleed

The severity of blood loss and hemodynamic status should be assessed immediately. Initial management consists of resuscitation with colloidal or crystalloid solutions and other blood products if necessary. The source of bleeding should be sought while the patient is being resuscitated. The duration and quantity of bleeding are assessed; however, the duration of bleeding is often underestimated and the quantity is often overestimated.

Risk factors that may have contributed to the bleeding should be assessed, such as the use of nonsteroidal anti-inflammatory drugs, anticoagulants, history of preexisting disease like hemorrhoids, polyps or diverticulosis.

Associated Findings

Abdominal pain may result from ischemic bowel, inflammatory bowel disease, or a ruptured aortic aneurysm. Malignancy may be indicated by a change in stool caliber, anorexia and weight loss. Painless, massive bleeding suggests vascular bleeding from diverticula, angiodysplasia or hemorrhoids. Bloody diarrhea suggests inflammatory bowel disease or an infectious origin. Bleeding with rectal pain is seen with anal fissures, hemorrhoids, and rectal ulcers. Chronic constipation suggests hemorrhoidal bleeding. New onset constipation or thin stools suggests a left-sided colonic malignancy. Blood on the toilet paper or dripping into the toilet water after a bowel movement suggests a perianal source. Blood coating the outside of stool suggests a lesion in the anal canal. Blood streaking or mixed with the stool may result from a polyp or malignancy in the descending colon. Maroon colored stools often indicate small bowel and proximal colon bleeding.

Physical Examination

The physical examination must include careful inspection and examination of the oropharynx, nasopharynx, abdomen, and anal canal. Place a Foley catheter to monitor urine output. Careful digital rectal examination, anoscopy, and rigid proctosigmoidoscopy should exclude an anorectal source of bleeding. However a benign anorectal lesion need not rule out a serious disease proximally. Orthostatic hypotension (i.e., a blood pressure fall of >10 mm Hg) is usually indicative of blood loss of more than 1000 ml.

Nasogastric aspirates usually correlate well with upper gastric hemorrhage proximal to the Treitz ligament; therefore, insert a nasogastric tube to confirm the presence or absence of blood in the stomach. If necessary, perform gastric lavage with saline to look for bilious aspirate.

INVESTIGATIONS

Lab Studies

Appropriate blood tests include CBC count, blood group and sample for cross match, coagulation profile including activated partial thromboplastin time (aPTT), prothrombin time (PT), platelet count, and bleeding time.

Imaging Studies

Colonoscopy has an important role in diagnosis and treatment of lower GI bleeding. Rapid colonic lavage clears the intraluminal blood, clot, and stool, providing an adequate environment for visualization of the lower GI mucosa and lesions. The best candidates for colonoscopic evaluation are patients who are bleeding slowly or who have already stopped bleeding. Perform the urgent colonoscopy in the operating room or endoscopy suite on hemodynamically stable patients. If patients become unstable or colonoscopy reveals an active fulminant inflammation, abort the procedure.

Tagged Red Blood Cell Scintigraphy

The role of nuclear scintigraphic imaging in the diagnosis and treatment of patients who present with lower GI bleeding remains controversial. Many investigators recommend that scintigraphic imaging be used primarily as a screening examination to select patients for mesenteric angiography.

Technetium Tc 99m–labeled red blood cell scanning is the preferred technique because its half-life is longer. Although nuclear scintigraphy is sensitive enough to diagnose ongoing bleeding at a rate as low as 0.1 mL/min, it is not highly accurate in locating the bleeding point because of the high false localization rate (10-60%) of the bleeding site. Recently, cinematic technetium Tc 99m red blood cell scan (real-time scanning) has been described as a noninvasive alternative to mesenteric angiography.

Angiography

The value of mesenteric angiography in the diagnosis and management of lower GI bleeding has been well established. The extravasation of contrast material indicates a positive study. Mesenteric angiography can detect bleeding at a rate of more than 0.5 mL/min. Once the bleeding point is identified, angiography offers potential treatment options such as selective vasopressin drip and embolization.

Other Tests

Double-contrast barium enema examinations can be justified only for elective evaluation of unexplained lower GI bleeding. Do not use barium enema examination in the acute hemorrhage phase because it makes subsequent diagnostic evaluations including angiography and colonoscopy, impossible.

Elective contrast radiography of the small bowel and/or enteroclysis is often valuable in investigation of long-term, unexplained lower GI bleeding.

Esophagogastroduodenoscopy has been used to variable degrees in the evaluation of lower intestinal bleeding. In a large study where all subjects underwent initial upper GI endoscopy, 11% were found to have lesions in the stomach and duodenum that were responsible for hematochezia.

Enteroscopy like push or Sonde type, double balloon enteroscopy, capsule endoscopy or laparoscopy assisted panenteroscopy (LAPE) is beneficial in selected cases of small bowel bleed especially obscure bleed.

Spiral CT scan is seldom used for evaluation of lower GI bleed, but detect bowel related neoplasms, pseudoaneuryms or other vascular lesions in cases with recurrent bleed.

TREATMENT

The spontaneous remission rate for acute gastrointestinal bleeding, even if massive, is 80%. No source of bleeding can be identified in 12%, and bleeding is recurrent in 25%. Bleeding ceases by the time the patient presents with hematochezia.

The fundamental principle of management of gastrointestinal bleed is immediate assessment and stabilization of patient's hemodynamic status (Fig. 16.1).

After stabilizing the hemodynamic status the most important goals of management are to stop active bleeding and prevent further bleed. No specific pharmacological therapy is available for acute lower GI bleed.

The different forms of treatment modalities are:

1. Endoscopic
2. Angiographic
3. Surgery

Endotherapy

Colonoscopy has become the first choice of diagnostic modality following rapid purge with volume cathartics. Therapeutic interventions can be performed through colonoscope. Endoscopic coagulation of angiodysplasias is becoming a treatment of choice using either heater probe or lasers such as Nd: YAG and argon. Argon plasma coagulation is an effective form of therapy for superficial and mucosal bleeding lesions. Injection therapy with 1:20000 adrenaline controls bleeding lesions especially ulcer or diverticular bleed. Hemoclips are used effectively for active bleeding in conditions like ulcer bleed and post polypectomy bleed. Endoscopic therapy for lower GI bleeding is a minimally invasive and viable option in carefully selected patients.

Angiographic Therapy

Once the bleeding source is identified in angiography, hemostasis can be achieved by intra arterial infusion of vasoconstrictive agents like vasopressin or superselective embolisation.

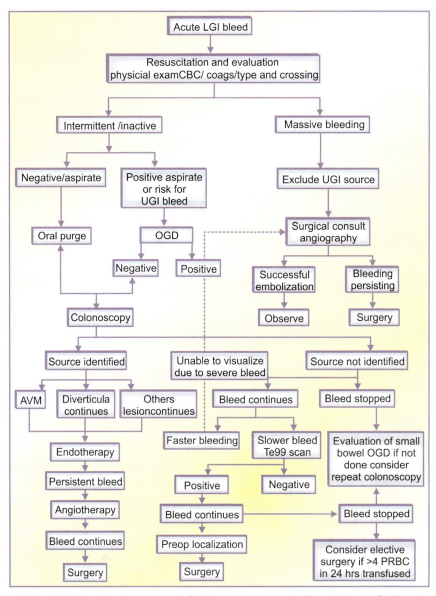

Fig. 16.1: Algorithmic approach for the management of acute lower GI bleeding

During vasopressin infusion, monitor patients for recurrent hemorrhage, myocardial ischemia, arrhythmias, hypertension, and volume overload with hyponatremia. Nitroglycerine paste or drip can be used to overcome cardiac complications.

Autologous clot, gelfoam, polyvinyl alcohol, microcoils, ethanolamine, and oxidized cellulose can be used as embolic agents. Embolization involves superselective catheterization of the bleeding vessel to minimize necrosis, the most feared complication of ischemic colitis. Overall bleeding control is 83% with a re-bleeding rate of 11%. Complications were observed in 20%, and bowel injury and perforation were observed in 12%.

Surgical Therapy

An emergency operation is required in approximately 10% of patients with lower GI bleeding. When the bleeding point is localized, a limited segmental resection of the small or large bowel is performed.

If the patient is hemodynamically unstable because of ongoing hemorrhage, perform an emergency operation before any diagnostic study. In these cases, make every attempt to diagnose the bleeding point intraoperatively. Intraoperative endoscopy, surgeon-guided enteroscopy, and colonoscopy may be helpful in diagnosing previously undiagnosed massive GI bleeding. If the bleeding point cannot be diagnosed following a thorough intraoperative endoscopy or examination, and if evidence points to colonic bleeding, subtotal colectomy is done as a last resort.

SUMMARY

Acute lower gastrointestinal bleeding is less common than upper GI bleed. The most common cause of acute significant bleeding is diverticular bleed and minor intermittent hematochezia is hemorrhoidal bleeding. The best diagnostic test would be colonoscopy while angiography and surgery are important modalities of management. Multispecialty approach comprising of gsatrophysician, surgeon and radiologist is essential for successful care of these patients.

SUGGESTED READING

1. Zuckerman GR, Prakash C. Acute lower intestinal bleeding: part I: clinical presentation and diagnosis. Gastrointest Endosc 1998; 48: 606-16.
2. Zuckerman GR, Prakash C. Acute lower intestinal bleeding: part II: etiology, therapy, and outcomes. Gasgtrointest Endoscop 1999; 49: 228-38.
3. Farrell JJ, Priedman LS. Gastrointestinal bleeding in the elderly. Gastrointestinal Clin N Am 2001; 30: 377-407.
4. Jenson DM, Machicado GA. Colonoscopy for diagnosis and treatment of sever lower gastrointestinal bleeding. Routine outcomes and cost analysis. Gastrointest Endosc Clin N Am 1997; 7: 477-98.
5. Jensen DM. Endoscopic diagnosis and treatment of severe hematochezia. Techniques in Gastroint Endosc 2001; 3: 177-84.

17

Rajeendranath T

Constipation

INTRODUCTION

Constipation is one of the most frequently encountered problems in day-to-day practice. As there are wide variations among individuals in their bowel habits, the exact prevalence of constipation is hard to determine. However, it is definitely higher in children and the elderly. Though a high female preponderance is highlighted among western population, a gender difference is not striking among our patients. Owing to the misconception regarding "normal bowel habits", use of over the counter laxatives still continues and self-administered enema are common especially among the elderly.

Constipation, like diarrhea, is hard to define with precision since normal bowel habits show wide individual variations.

A working group proposed the following criteria for diagnosis of constipation referred to as Rome II Criteria.
1. Straining
2. Lumpy or hard stool
3. Sensation of incomplete evacuation
4. Sensation of anorectal obstruction/blockade
5. Fewer than three bowel actions per week

Constipation is defined by two or more of the above symptoms persisting for at least 12 weeks, not necessarily consecutive, in the preceding 12 months.

Etiology and Pathophysiology

Constipation results from a variety of disorders both local and systemic. When there is an identifiable cause for constipation it is referred to as secondary constipation. Common causes of secondary constipation are:
1. Structural—Colonic/anorectal. e.g., colon cancer, stricture due to diverticulitis, tuberculosis, Crohn's disease, ischemia, radiation injury, prior surgery, hemorrhoids, fissure in ano, etc.
2. Drugs – (see Table 17.1)
3. Endocrine – Diabetes mellitus, hypothyroidism
4. Metabolic – Hypokalemia, hypercalcemia, uremia
5. Infiltrative disorders – Scleroderma, amyloidosis
6. Neurological – Parkinson's disease, spinal cord disease, autonomic neuropathy
7. Psychological

Table 17.1: Drugs causing constipation

Antacids, calcium and aluminium compounds	
Analgesics	Anticholinergics
Anticonvulsants	Antihypertensives
Antiparkinsonian drugs	Antidepressants
Diuretics	Iron supplements
Opiates	NSAIDs
	Laxatives (chronic use)

When investigations fail to reveal any specific cause, constipation may be regarded as functional/idiopathic. Conceptually this may be regarded as disordered movement of fecal contents through the colon or rectum.

The common functional constipation syndromes are:

1. Constipation predominant irritable bowel syndrome (IBS).
2. Slow transit constipation.
3. Abnormal anorectal function – outlet dysfunction constipation.

Constipation Predominant IBS

Also referred to as spastic colon, this is the commonest cause of functional constipation among young and middle-aged persons. It is accompanied by abdominal pain and a feeling of incomplete evacuation. The exact pathophysiology of this condition is uncertain, although decreased number of propagating contractions and delay in colonic transit time have been documented in many patients.

Slow Transit Constipation

It is a clinical syndrome characterized by intractable constipation and delayed colonic transit. Colonic inertia refers to a severe form of slow transit constipation marked by lack of contractile response to feeding or to stimulants.

The pathophysiology of slow transit constipation is poorly understood. The proposed mechanisms include excessive sigmoid colonic phasic motor activity, a reduced colonic contractile response to a meal or fewer colonic high amplitude propagated contractions (HAPC). A subset of patients with slow transit constipation may have disturbed visceral perception and marked reduction of nerve fibres and interstitial cells of Cajal in the colon.

In some patients with slow transit constipation the above abnormalities may be localized only to rectosigmoid segment – hindgut dysfunction.

Outlet Dysfunction Constipation

This is characterized by a number of anatomic and functional abnormalities that result in symptoms of excessive straining at stool. The pathophysiology of outlet dysfunction constipation includes pelvic floor dyssynergia (failure of co-coordinated relaxation of puborectalis muscle and external anal sphincter), weak expulsion forces and redirection of expulsion forces, as may occur with a large rectocele. Many patients with outlet dysfunction constipation have no demonstrable mechanism to account for their symptoms (unexplained rectal dysfunction).

CLINICAL ASSESSMENT

History

A detailed history is mandatory in all patients presenting with a history of constipation. A general assessment of the life style, any psychological stress, diet, physical activity, etc. are of value in diagnosing functional constipation. A very short duration of the symptom, anorexia, presence of weight loss or blood in the stool will give a clue regarding a serious organic disease. A history of various drugs consumed by the patient is important as many commonly used drugs are known to produce constipation. Since metabolic disorders can result in constipation, an enquiry should be made into the history of diabetes or thyroid dysfunction.

A history of cerebrovascular accident, peripheral neuropathy, symptoms of parkinson's disease or any spinal cord injury are important clues to the abnormal bowel habits.

Physical Examination

Must include careful exclusion of systemic and neurological disorders. Emaciation, pallor and signs of nutritional deficiency point to a serious disorder which warrants detailed evaluation. A search should be made in the abdomen for mass, tenderness, hepatomegaly or ascites. Digital examination of the rectum should always be considered as an extension of physical examination and should never be omitted. It provides important information regarding anal sphincter tone, rectal prolapse and any obstruction or painful lesion of anal canal.

Investigations

Acute constipation occurring as a result of sudden decrease in physical activity (e.g., during travel, hospitalization for surgery or other acute illness) does not require any specific investigations. It often responds to fibre supplement and judicious use of laxatives.

Constipation persisting and not responding to simple measures warrant further investigations to exclude an obstructive/structural cause or a systemic disorder.

Initial Screening Investigations

- A complete hemogram, stool examination for ova or cysts of parasites, blood sugar and X-ray chest. Sigmoidoscopy with a rigid instrument is an easy outpatient procedure and should be done in all patients with constipation to exclude lesions up to 25 cm in the rectosigmoid.
- Barium enema, flexible sigmoidoscopy and colonoscopy to exclude an obstructive lesion or other pathological conditions in the large gut
- Biochemical tests for hypothyroidism, hypocalcaemia and hypokalemia

When no obvious cause could be identified after clinical assessment and investigations, the patient may be considered to be suffering from idiopathic/functional constipation.

Additional Tests

1. Whole gut and colonic transit time
2. Anorectal manometry
3. Anal sphincter electromyography
4. Defecating proctography
5. Balloon expulsion techniques.

Whole gut/colonic transit time is measured by ingesting 30 radio opaque markers (Sitz Mark Capsule) and taking abdominal X-ray on day five. If transit function is normal, at least 80% of the ingested markers should not be visible on the X-ray. Scattered markers throughout the colon suggest colonic inertia and markers localized to the recto sigmoid, a hindgut dysfunction.

Pressure changes in the rectum and anal canal and electromyographic recordings from the external anal sphincter can distinguish patients with outlet dysfunction constipation from those with slow transit constipation. As symptoms alone cannot distinguish between constipation resulting from pelvic floor dysfunction and slow transit constipation, pelvic floor function should be assessed in all patients with refractory constipation. Moreover, presence of delayed colonic transit is not sufficient to diagnose slow transit constipation as colonic transit is often delayed in patients with pelvic floor dysfunction.

Defecography is useful in assessing completeness of rectal evacuation and can demonstrate abnormalities like rectocele, mucosal prolapse and paradoxical pelvic floor motions.

MANAGEMENT

General Measures

Reassurance and education regarding normal bowel habits are important. Patient should be advised to set aside a regular time for defecation and the need for always responding to a defecatory urge should be stressed. Activity should be encouraged in those who are inactive. The effect of exercise on colon transit and constipation have been studied and the result generally supports a slightly decreased transit time without any significant increase in stool weight and frequency of bowel movements.

Psychological support is essential for those patients in whom constipation is a manifestation of stress or emotional disturbances.

In those who consume a poor calorie diet, the deficiency should be rectified since adequate caloric intake often restores colonic transit. Patient should be encouraged to take plenty of fluids as dehydration and salt depletion may lead to increased salt and water absorption by the colon.

The results of increasing fibre in the diet for constipation are often disappointing. Though fibre may increase stool weight and accelerate colonic transit, stool weight may still be below normal. However, patients with constipation should be advised to increase the dietary fibre intake by consuming common foods containing high fibre, especially fine fibre, content. (e.g., unpolished rice, wheat, ragi, maize, legumes, dals)

Table 17.2: Classification of Laxatives		
I. Bulk	Methyl cellulose	
	Plant gum	
II. Stimulant	Castor oil	Cascara
	Bisacodyl	Senna
	Phenolphthalein	Danthron
III. Osmotic	Sodium picosulfate	Sorbitol
	Dioctylsulfosuccinate	Polyethyleneglycol
	Lactulose	
IV. Saline	Milk of magnesia	
	Sodium phosphate	
V. Emollient	Docusate sodium	
VI. Lubricant	Mineral oil	

The Use of Laxatives

Four major classes of laxatives are in common use for increasing the stool frequency – bulk laxatives, osmotic laxatives, saline laxatives and stimulant laxatives (See Table 17.2).

Bulk Laxatives

Bulk laxatives contain non-digestible unabsorbed polysaccharides either natural or semi synthetic. In the gut, they swell to form a viscous gelatinous mass. The bulk thus created is believed to stimulate peristalsis. Large number of preparations available in the market incorporate isapghula which is derived from dried ripe seeds of plant plantago ovata. Standard dose is 12-15 gm/day. Flatulence and bloating are the main side effects, which often subside over time.

Osmotic Laxatives

They are non-digestible disaccharides, which are hydrolyzed to organic acids and provide osmotically active particles to sitmulate intestinal fluid secretion and motility.

The main side effects include bloating and abdominal cramps (standard dose of lactulose is 15 to 30 ml once or twice daily).

Stimulant Laxatives

These compounds produce fluid and electrolyte accumulation in the colon and distal ileum after being converted into active metabolites by colonic bacteria. Some agents in this group (phenolphthalein and bisacodyl) can directly stimulate the myenteric plexuses of the colon and can inhibit water and glucose uptake. These agents are to be preferred when the effect is needed within 24 hours.

Saline Laxatives

These contain non-absorbable cation/anion mixtures of sulfates, phosphates or citrates. They draw fluid osmotically into the lumen, stimulate cholecystokinin release, and accelerate colonic transit.

Other Pharmacological Agents used in Constipation

a. Cisapride: Being a panprokinetic, this agent has an effect on colonic transit. Eight to 12 weeks of treatment in patients with chronic constipation progressively increased the quality and frequency of stools.

b. Sodium picosulfate: It is a stimulant laxative, which acts by promoting accumulation of water and electrolytes in the colonic lumen and stimulating intestinal motility. The onset of action is within 10-14 hours. It is well tolerated without any systemic side effects. The standard dose is 10 mg at bedtime.

c. Selective serotinin reuptake inhibitors (SSRI)

d. Fluoxetine, sertraline, citalopram: They tend to cause diarrhea as side effects and hence may be tried in patients of constipation predominant IBS. They are less sedating than tricyclic anti-depressants with fewer side effects.

e. Tegaserod: It is a new drug now available for treating constipation predominant IBS. It is a partial agonist of serotonin 5HT4 receptors. The drug acts by simulating peristalsis and increasing intestinal secretions. The optimal dose in 6 mg given twice daily.

Behavioral Therapy

Habit training in children and bedridden patients is useful in relieving constipation and is found to be successful in about 80% of patients.

Biofeedback therapy is the mainstay in managing patients with outlet dysfunction constipation. The principle involves making the patient watch a visual display of a normal response of electromyograph activity of rectum and anal canal. The patient is then instructed to normalize his own recording by trial and error.

Controlled studies of these techniques are few and the results are not always predictable.

Surgery

When all measures fail, patients with refractory slow transit constipation may be considered for a subtotal colectomy with ileorectal anastamosis after excluding pelvic floor dysfunction.

Surgical repair of a rectocele relieves constipation when this anatomical abnormality has been demonstrated to be the sole cause for constipation.

SUGGESTED READING

1. Wald A. Outlet dysfunction constipation; Curr. Treat opt. Gastroenterol 2001; 4:293-7
2. Barucha AE, Phillips SF. Slow transit constipation; Curr. Treat opt. Gastroenterol (selected papers) 2001;2:51-7.
3. Locke GR, Pemberton JH, Phillips SF. Technical review on constipation. Gastroenterology 2000;119:1766-78.
4. Sleisenger Fordtran's. Gastrointestinal and liver disease. 7th edition.
5. Rao SS. Constipation: evaluation and treatment. Gastroenterol Clin North Am 2003; 32: 659-83.
6. Lembo A., Camilleri M. Current concept: Chronic constipation. N Engl J Med 2003; 349:1360-68.
7. Mertz H, Naliboff B, Mayer E. Physiology of refractory chronic constipation. Am J Gastroenterol 1999;94:609-15.

18

Musthafa CP

Functional Gastrointestinal Disorders—All in the Mind?

DEFINITION

The functional gastrointestinal disorders (FGID) are syndromes causing chronic or recurrent symptoms attributable to the GI tract, unexplained by any structural or biochemical abnormalities. Patients with FGIDs report a wide variety of symptoms affecting different regions of the gastrointestinal tract. These symptoms have in common disturbances in sensory and/or motor gastrointestinal function, which may overlap across anatomic regions. Irritable bowel syndrome is described in a separate chapter.

CLASSIFICATION

The FGIDs are classified by anatomic region; there can be several disorders, each with specific clinical features.

Primary Functional GI Disorders

A. **Esophageal disorders**
   A1. Globus
   A2. Rumination syndrome
   A3. Functional chest pain of presumed esophageal origin
   A4. Functional heartburn
   A5. Functional dysphagia
   A6. Unspecified functional esophageal disorder
B. **Gastroduodenal disorders**
   B1. Functional dyspepsia
      B1a.   Ulcer-like dyspepsia
      B1b.   Dysmotility-like dyspepsia
      B1c.   Unspecified(non-specific) dyspepsia
   B2. Aerophagia
   B3. Functional vomiting
C. **Bowel disorders**
   C1. Irritable bowel syndrome
   C2. Functional abdominal bloating
   C3. Functional constipation
   C4. Functional diarrhea
   C5. Unspecified functional bowel disorder
D. **Functional abdominal pain**
   D1. Functional abdominal pain syndrome
   D2. Unspecified functional abdominal pain

E. **Biliary disorders**
    E1. Gall bladder dysfunction
    E2. Sphincter of Oddi dysfunction
F. **Anorectal disorders**
    F1. Functional fecal incontinence
    F2. Functional anorectal pain
        F2a. Levator ani syndrome
        F2b. Proctalgia fugax
    F3. Pelvic floor dyssynergia
G. **Functional pediatric disorders**

Functional Dyspepsia

Functional dyspepsia is one of the most common disorders seen in general practice and by gastroenterologists. Functional dyspepsia is defined as persistent or recurrent pain or discomfort centered in the upper abdomen, without evidence of organic disease or relation between dyspeptic symptoms and bowel movements. Rome II committee classified functional dyspepsia into ulcer-like (pain is the dominant symptom), dysmotility-like (discomfort symptoms are the dominant symptom), and unspecified (none of the previous). Most of these patients have no identifiable cause by standard diagnostic tests. Patients with predominant heartburn should be excluded.

Pathophysiology

Pathophysiology of functional dyspepsia is still unclear. Some of the proposed mechanisms are delayed gastric emptying, hypersensitivity to gastric distention, impaired accommodation of the proximal stomach to a meal, helicobacter pylori infection, abnormal duodenojejunal motility, duodenal hypersensitivity to acid or nutrients, and central nervous dysfunction.

Delayed gastric emptying in dyspepsia is associated with postprandial fullness, nausea, and vomiting. In patients with functional dyspepsia *impaired accommodation* of food and abnormal distribution of the food within the stomach have been demonstrated, with a relatively higher proportion of a meal residing in the antrum, rather than in the proximal stomach; this can cause early satiety and weight loss. *Hypersensitivity to gastric distention* was observed in 34% of the patients with functional dyspepsia and this can be associated with postprandial epigastric pain, belching, and weight loss.

In patients with functional dyspepsia postprandial symptoms are very common and many claim exacerbation of their symptoms after a fatty or rich meal. A high proportion of patients with functional dyspepsia demonstrate increased gastro duodenal sensitivity to meals of high energy or lipid content.

The role of acid in the pathophysiology of functional dyspepsia is unclear. The gastric acid secretion is normal in most of these patients and the gastric mucosa does not seem to be abnormally sensitive to acid or duodenal contents. Manometry studies in functional dyspepsia have revealed antral hypo-motility to be a common feature.

In functional dyspepsia the role of *H. pylori* infection is less clear. A recent systematic review of the epidemiologic evidence on the relationship between *H. pylori* infection and functional dyspepsia found no evidence for a strong association. According to the authors, however, there was not enough evidence to rule out a modest association.

Clinical presentation and diagnosis: The most prevalent symptom complaints in patients with functional dyspepsia seen at a referral center are postprandial fullness and bloating, followed by epigastric pain, early satiety, nausea, and belching. There is also a huge overlap between functional dyspepsia and IBS. In a referral center 46% of patients with functional dyspepsia were proved to have concomitant IBS. Psychologic symptoms are also common in patients with functional dyspepsia.

DIAGNOSIS

A careful clinical evaluation and history taking are essential features to make a correct diagnosis of dyspepsia. So-called alarm symptoms (e.g., prominent weight loss, recurrent vomiting, bleeding, anemia, dysphagia, jaundice, or palpable mass) should be looked for with great care and if present, require immediate action. If there are no sinister symptoms and the patient is young (less than 45 to 50 years) and does not take nonsteroidal anti-inflammatory drugs, upper endoscopy is rarely needed as the first line. Early endoscopy is the gold standard in the diagnostic work-up of dyspeptic patients with more severe symptoms, however, and is associated with greater patient satisfaction.

Other investigations that might be considered in the work-up are upper abdominal ultrasonography or CT to evaluate for pancreaticobiliary disease, small-bowel radiography to evaluate for Crohn's disease, partial small bowel obstruction or tumors, 24-hour esophageal pH monitoring, and manometric studies of the upper gastrointestinal tract to exclude occult gastroesophageal reflux and generalized severe motor disorders. These investigations should not be performed in all patients, but based on the clinical picture, the severity of symptoms, and the refractoriness of the patient.

TREATMENT

Reassurance and education are of primary importance. It seems logical to have patients eat more frequent, smaller meals, and avoiding meals with a high fat content might be advisable. At the moment, empirical treatment with acid-suppressive agents and prokinetics is the recommended therapeutic approach in the management of these patients, despite limited efficacy. Identification and treatment of H.pylori infection has been recommended for uninvestigated dyspepsia, because it may cure underlying peptic ulcer disease, but is unlikely to provide symptomatic benefit to patients with functional dyspepsia. Refractory patients may respond to antidepressants or to psychologic treatments, but proof of efficacy is limited. New and more effective approaches are badly needed for functional dyspepsia.

Functional Constipation

Diagnostic criteria for functional constipation include presence of two or more of: (1) Straining in >1/4 defecations; (2) Lumpy or hard stools in >1/4 defecations; (3) Sensation of incomplete evacuation in >1/4 defecations; (4) Sensation of anorectal obstruction/blockade in >1/4 defecations (5) Manual maneuvers to facilitate >1/4 defecations (e.g., digital evacuation, support of the pelvic floor); and/or (6) <3 defecations/week for at least for 12 weeks, in the preceding 12 months. Loose stools are not present, and there are insufficient criteria for IBS.

Functional Diarrhea

Functional diarrhea is continuous or recurrent passage of loose (mushy) or watery stools without abdominal pain of at least 12 weeks, which need not be consecutive, in the preceding 12 months of: (1) Liquid (mushy) or watery stools; (2) Present >3/4 of the time; and (3) No abdominal pain. Restriction of foods, which seem provocative, may help. Empiric anti-diarrheal therapy (e.g., diphenoxylate or loperamide) is usually effective, especially if taken prophylactically, before meals. The occasional patient responds to cholestyramine.

Functional Vomiting

Identified as frequent episodes of vomiting, occurring on at least three separate days in a week, absence of criteria for an eating disorder, rumination, or major psychiatric disease according to DSM-IV, absence of self-induced and medication-induced vomiting and absence of abnormalities in the gut or central nervous system, and metabolic diseases to explain the recurrent vomiting. Assessment of nutritional status is vital and appropriate intervention should be provided. Anti-nauseants are worth a trial but are not of established value. Antidepressants can be helpful in full doses. Psychosocial support is important. Behavioral and psychotherapy have not been adequately tested but may be considered.

Functional Abdominal Bloating

Functional abdominal bloating comprises a group of functional bowel disorders, which are dominated by a feeling of abdominal fullness or bloating or visible distension for at least 12 weeks, which need not be consecutive, in the preceding 12 months and without diagnostic criteria for another functional gastrointestinal disorder like functional dyspepsia, IBS, or other functional disorder. Functional bloating is usually absent on awakening and worsens throughout the day. It may be intermittent and related to ingestion of specific foods. Excessive burping or farting may be present. There is no proved effective therapy for functional bloating, and its cause is unknown, so only education and reassurance are recommended.

Functional Abdominal Pain Syndrome (FAPS)

FAPS describes pain for at least six months that is poorly related to gut function and is associated with some loss of daily activities. The pain is not malingering and there are insufficient criteria for other functional gastrointestinal disorders that would explain the abdominal pain. Management depends on an effective doctor–patient relationship. Analgesics are ineffective, and narcotics should be avoided. Concurrent depression should be treated. Low doses of antidepressants can reduce pain as well as insomnia. Anxiolytic therapy, if used at all, should be limited in duration. Various types of psychotherapy have been tried without critical evaluation. A multidisciplinary pain management program may be the most promising approach.

Aerophagia

Refers to air swallowing that is objectively observed along with troublesome and repetitive belching. It is usually an unconscious act unrelated to meals, and is presumably a learned habit. A positive diagnosis is based on a careful history and observation of air swallowing. In typical cases no investigation is required. Explanation of the symptoms and reassurance are important. Treatment of associated psychiatric disease or use of stress reduction techniques may be worth considering. Dietary modification, avoiding sucking hard candies or chewing gum, eating slowly and encouraging small swallows at mealtime, and avoiding carbonated beverages are often recommended. Although tranquillizers may occasionally be useful in severe cases, drug therapy is not generally recommended.

Globus

Globus is a sensation of a lump, something stuck, or tightness in the throat. Classically a lump, it may be a hair-or crumb-like (foreign body) sensation, a constriction or a choking. The symptom is considered functional when no organic explanation is detected. Clinical evaluation centres on a history that tackles psychosocial factors and a thorough examination of the neck, larynx, and pharynx. Sensations localized above the cricoid arise in areas visible by flexible laryngoscope. Reassurance is a standard but unproved mainstay. Anecdotal reports favour use of anxiolytics and antidepressants, but patient dropout was high in a small controlled trial of tricyclic antidepressants for this disorder.

Rumination syndrome: effortless regurgitation of recently swallowed food

Functional chest pain: the feeling of chest pain, presumably of esophageal origin

Functional heartburn: persistent burning sensation in the absence of gastro esophageal reflux disease, a motility disorder, or a structural explanation

Functional dysphagia: the sensation of difficulty in swallowing

Gallbladder dysfunction: characterized by episodes of severe steady pain accompanied by decreased gall bladder emptying.

Sphincter of Oddi dysfunction: a motility disorder characterized by severe steady pain with no structural abnormalities that explain the symptoms. It sometimes occurs following gallbladder removal, but also may occur with an intact gallbladder.

Functional fecal incontinence: recurrent uncontrolled passage of fecal material where no structural or neurological cause is evident

Functional anorectal pain: Levator syndrome is a dull ache in the rectum that lasts for hours to days. Proctalgia fugax is an infrequent sudden, severe pain in the anal area of short duration.

Irritable bowel syndrome (IBS): See chapter on IBS

SUGGESTED READING

1. Hyams JS. Irritable bowel syndrome, functional dyspepsia, and functional abdominal pain syndrome. Adolesc Med Clin 2004; 15: 1-15.
2. Clouse RE. Psychotropic medications for the treatment of functional gastrointestinal disorders. Clin Perspect Gastroenterol 1999; 2:348-56.
3. Simrén M. Functional dyspepsia: evaluation and treatment. Gastroenterol Clin North Am 2003; 32: 577-99.
4. Smith DS. Diagnosis and treatment of chronic gastroparesis and chronic intestinal pseudo-obstruction. Gastroenterol Clin North Am 2003; 32: 619-58.
5. Budavari AI. Psychosocial aspects of functional gastrointestinal disorders. Gastroenterol Clin North Am 2003; 32: 477-506.

19

Narayanan VA

Intestinal Gas Syndromes

INTRODUCTION

Excessive "gas" production is one of the most common gastro intestinal symptoms. The patients complaining of "gas" fervently believe that the gas travels to all parts and that a variety of symptoms like bloating, belching, chest pain, abdominal cramps and anorexia are due to gas. Managing these patients represents a challenge to the physician. There are no simple tests that can objectively document gaseous abnormality. The gaps in our understanding in the pathogenesis of these symptoms make treatment unsatisfactory and the disorder is often dumped as functional. This review outlines the current knowledge on the physiology of intestinal gas, clinical approach to gas syndromes, investigation technique available and patient management.

PHYSIOLOGY OF INTESTINAL GAS

During intrauterine life, the intestine of fetus has no gas. As soon as the child is born gas enters the GI tract with the first cry and plain X-rays can show fundal gas shadow. After the child is fed and the digestion process starts and meconium is passed, gas shadows appear in small and large intestines.

VOLUME OF GASTROINTESTINAL GAS

The total volume of gas in intestinal tract is less than 200 ml. Volume of gas in gastrointestinal tract is measured by a body plethysmograph or by argon washout technique. Levitt demonstrated that the volume of gas is not different in patients who complain of excessive gas from that of controls. He also demonstrated that infusion of gas caused discomfort and severe pain in patients whereas normal healthy patients tolerated the same amount of infusion without difficulty.. All the patients had abnormal motility and visceral hypersensitivity as evidenced by reflux of gas from small intestine to stomach, prolonged transit time and hypersensitivity to balloon inflation. Balloon distension of the rectum in patients caused pain and discomfort at smaller volumes of air distension than in healthy controls. Thus patients with excessive gaseousness are a variant of the irritable bowel syndrome. Altered perception of gaseous distension (visceral hypersensitivity) and exaggerated motor response to normal amount of gas can explain their symptoms.

COMPOSITION AND SOURCE OF GAS

Intestinal gas consists of 64% nitrogen, 0.96% oxygen, 10% to 19% hydrogen, 8.8% methane and 14% CO_2 (Table 19.1). Nitrogen is the major component arising from swallowed air. Smokers, people who chew pan or chewing gum, rapid eaters and excessive worriers swallow more air. However, from healthy intestines with normal motility and normal sensitivity, the air is passed out. Normally 1000-1500cc of flatus is passed out in a 24-hour period (See Table 19.1)

Mean + ISD	MI	%
Volume	90+ 54	
Nitrogen (N$_2$)	64+ 52	64+21
Oxygen (O$_2$)	58+ 43	0.69+0.49
Hydrogen (H$_2$)	14.0+ 9.9	19+16
Methane (CH$_4$)	5.6+2.6	8.8+ 9.0
Carbon dioxide (CO$_2$)	9.7+ 2.4	14.0+ 7.0

Table 19.1: Composition of intestinal gas

From M.D. Levitt New Eng. J. Med 284: 1397:1971

Gut contains little oxygen as the oxygen is utilized by bacterial flora. Hydrogen, CO_2 and CH_4 are endogenously produced; CO_2 by the neutralization of hydrochloric acid by alkali in the small intestine and also by the fermentation of lactose; H_2 and CH_4 by colonic flora. However if there is bacterial overgrowth in small intestine, hydrogen is produced in the small intestine also. Breath excretion test is used as a measure of hydrogen production.

Clinical Syndromes

Table 19.2: Clinical gas syndromes

1. Chronic belching or eructations
2. Abdominal bloating and distension
3. Hepatic and splenic flexure syndromes
4. Flatulence
5. Carbohydrate malabsorption

Belching is expulsion of gas from stomach through mouth. Flatulence is excessive passage of gas from rectum, and abdominal bloating refers to the feeling of distension of abdomen. Often patients say that passage of flatus or belching relieves the discomfort (Table 19.2).

CLINICAL ASSESSMENT

History: Dietary history regarding consumption of legumes, beans, potatoes.

Medication: Sedatives, anti cholinergics, calcium-channel blockers.

Surgery: Any previous abdominal surgery.

Psychiatric disturbances: Anxiety, depression.

Systemic Diseases

Diabetes, hypothyroidism, systemic sclerosis, neurological disorders, meal related excessive bloating. Malodorous gas and nocturnal gas are likely to be due to excessive bacterial fermentation. Milk causing bloating, abdominal cramps and borborygmi may be due to lactase deficiency.

INVESTIGATIONS

Routine urine, CBC, blood sugar to exclude diabetes, upper GI endoscopy and USG abdomen to exclude peptic ulcer or gallstone.

SPECIAL INVESTIGATIONS

Radiography

Plain X-ray abdomen may show gas trapped in splenic flexure and hepatic flexure.

Radionuclide Scintigraphy

Solid or liquid, labelled with radioisotope, 99Tc is given orally. Gamma camera is used to monitor the emission. Esophageal clearance, gastric emptying and transit to colon can be quantified and compared with normal ranges. This is the most practical and useful method and is simple, non-invasive and subjects the patients to very little radiation exposure.

Real Time Ultrasound Imaging (dynamic study)

This method correlates well with scintigraphic measurements. Advantage is that it is non-invasive.

Manometry

Pressure sensitive transducers are placed in different levels in the gut and pressures at different levels are recorded. Disadvantage is that it is time consuming.

Myoelectric Techniques

Electrogastrogram (EGG): Measures electrical potentials. Cutaneous electrodes are placed overlying stomach. This is a non-invasive method that measures contractile activity. Clinical applications are emerging.

Colonic myoelectric rhythm: Colonic myoelectric rhythm can be studied by placing mucosal electrodes in colon through sigmoidoscope. This is an invasive procedure and is more of a research tool at present.

Hydrogen Breath Tests

The test is used to measure orocecal transit time and to detect bacterial overgrowth. A solution of 10 gm of lactose is ingested orally. This is not absorbed in the gut and is fermented by colonic bacteria to release hydrogen. Breath samples are taken at 15 minute intervals and are analysed for hydrogen using hydrogen electrode. Transit time is defined as a sustained plateau of breath hydrogen exceeding 20 ppm while small intestinal overgrowth is identified by a transient peak of > 20 ppm preceding the sustained plateau.

Anorectal Manometry

Records the basal anorectal sphincter pressure and anorectal pressure both in resting phase and after stimulation. Also the rectal sensation is recorded. This is a very useful study in cases of constipation associated with flatulence.

Management

Patients complaining of chronic eructation should be counselled and advised to eat slowly. Smoking, chewing gums and chewing pans, should be avoided. Stress management is helpful.

If bloating and abdominal distention are the major problem, comorbid conditions like diabetes mellitus and neurological disorders should be looked into. Diet low in carbohydrate and lactose free diet may be of help in some patients.

Simethicone, a compound that reduces surface tension has shown efficacy is some controlled trials but not in others. Activated charcoal has been claimed to absorb gas. However controlled trials have not shown much benefit. Alteration of bacterial flora using saccharomyces boullardii (Econorm/Stibs powder) or lactobacilli may be helpful in some patients. Constipation associated with splenic or hepatic flexure syndromes should be treated with regular exercise, high fiber diet and osmotic laxatives. If associated obesity is present weight reduction will be helpful. Newer prokinetic drugs like tegaserod (now available in India) and prucalopride may be useful. Treatment should be directed towards abnormal motility and visceral hypersensitivity considering these patients as variants of irritable bowel syndrome. The treatment of gastric dysfunction causing bloating and distension is summerised in Table 19.3)

Table 19.3: Treatment of gastric dysfunction causing bloating and distension		
Impaired gastric emptying	*Impaired fundal relaxation*	*Visceral hyper sensitivity*
Prokinetic agent	Fundal relaxants	Visceral afferent inhibitors
a. Cisapride	a. α2 agonist	a. Fedotozine
b. Domperidone	b. 5HT agonist	b. 5H3 antagonist
c. Metaclopramide		c. Tricyclic antidepressant (low dose)

CONCLUSION

With a good understanding of pathophysiology of intestinal gas and a modern motility lab, recent advances in investigation and therapy in this field could be utilized for the benefit of patients.

SUGGESTED READING

1. Roth J.L.A, Gaseousness In: Berk JE. Ed Gastroenterology Philadelphia W.B. Sunnders 1985;142.
2. Danhoff E, The clinical gas syndromes—a pathophysiologic approach Ann. NY Acad. Sc. 1968; 150: 127.
3. Levitt M.D. Bond JH Flatulence Ann Rev Med 1980; 31:127.
4. Levitt M.D, Furne J, Acolus M.R, et al. Evaluation of an extremely flatulent patient case report and proposed diagnostic and therapeutic approach. Am J. Gastroenterol 1998; 93:2276-81.
5. Serra, J, Azpinz F, Malagelada J.R. Intestinal gas dynamics and tolerance in humans. Gastroenterology 1998;115:42-550.
6. Levitt M.D. Volume and composition of intestinal gas determined by means of intestinal washout technique N. Eng. J. Med. 1971;284-1396.
7. Montes R, Gottal R.F, Bayless J.M. Breath hydrogen testing as a physiology lab exercise for medical students. Am. J. Physiology 1992;2622:525.
8. Kerlin P, Wong L Breath hydrogen testing in bacterial overgrowth of small intestine. Gastroenterolgy 1988; 95:1982-1984.
9. Cheni TN, Schruder M.M., Bohmaaaf ME. A simple radiological method to estimate the quantity of bowel gas. Am J. Gastroenterology 1991; 86: 599.
10. Potter, Tellif C Levitt MD. Activated charcoal in vivo and invitro studies on effect of gas formation. Gastroenterology 1985;88:620.
11. Geshon MD. Role played by 5 hydroxy tryptamine in the physiology of bowel. Alimentary pharmacology therapeutics. 199: 13 (suppl 2) 15-30.
12. Camilleri M,Chei M. Potential new pharmacological therapy in treatment of irritable bowel syndrome both in experimental studies in healthy subjects and in patients with this syndrome. Alimentary pharmacology therapeutics 1997; 11:3-15.

20

Shine Sadasivan

How to Investigate a Patient with Jaundice?

DEFINITION

Jaundice is defined as yellowish pigmentation of sclera and skin due to bilirubin deposition when the serum bilirubin is above 2 mg/dl.

A carefully elicited history, physical examination and review of the standard laboratory tests should allow the physician to make an accurate diagnosis in 85% of cases.

BILIRUBIN METABOLISM

Bilirubin is derived mainly from breakdown of senescent red blood cells. Hemoglobin is broken down into heme and globin. Heme is oxidized and converted to biliverdin by the enzyme heme oxygenase and then to bilirubin by biliverdin reductase in extrahepatic tissues mainly in the spleen and bone marrow. Unconjugated bilirubin binds tightly but reversibly with albumin and is taken up by the hepatocytes and converted into bilirubin monoglucuronide (BMG) and di-glucuronide (BDG) by the glucuronyl transferase enzyme. BMG and BDG are transported into the plasma and bind with albumin, but less tightly than unconjugated bilirubin. As they are less tightly bound to albumin, both BMG and BDG will be filtered at the glomerulus and appear in urine. Approximately 80% of human bile is in the form of BDG. The rest is formed mainly by BMG and only trace amounts are the unconjugated fraction. Conjugated bilirubin is converted into urobilinogen in the intestine by bacterial action. Urobilinogen is absorbed from the small intestine, via the entero hepatic circulation but minimally from the colon. Liver and kidneys re-excrete absorbed urobilinogen.

HISTORY

Onset of illness with preceding nausea, anorexia and arthralgia (prodromal symptoms) prior to jaundice suggests viral hepatitis. Anorexia with significant weight loss can also occur in malignancy of liver, pancreas, biliary tree and colon. Chills and fever with right upper quadrant pain suggest cholangitis. Previous history of dyspepsia, fat intolerance and biliary colic suggest cholelithiasis with or without choledocholithiasis. Jaundice with continuous severe epigastric pain radiating to the back with marked weight loss indicates pancreatic malignancy. In patients with jaundice, the constellation of symptoms of fever, arthralgia, rash and eosinophilia should raise the possibility of drug induced liver disease. Presence of pruritus and clay-colored stools suggests cholestasis. Quantification of alcohol intake is also very important in the evaluation of a patient with jaundice.

Past history of blood transfusion, parenteral injections, drug abuse, sexual history, tattoos and acupuncture are also important. Contact with jaundiced patients particularly in nurseries, camps, hospitals or schools should also be noted. Post biliary surgery jaundice indicates retained common bile duct stones, biliary stricture or viral hepatitis. Family history of jaundice is also relevant with respect to viral hepatitis, Wilson's disease and congenital non-hemolytic hyperbilirubinemia.

PHYSICAL EXAMINATION

The general examination includes nutritional status evaluation. Temporal and proximal muscle wasting suggests long-standing disease like cirrhosis. Stigmata of chronic liver disease include spider nevi, palmar erythema, gynecomastia, Dupuytren contracture, parotid gland enlargement and testicular atrophy. An enlarged left supraclavicular lymph node or para-umbilical node suggests abdominal malignancy. Elevated jugular venous pressure suggests right heart failure causing hepatic congestion.

Abdominal examination should include the size and consistency of the liver. A firm nodular liver and a palpable left lobe of the liver suggest cirrhosis of the liver. Enlarged hard liver indicates hepatocellular carcinoma or liver metastasis. Causes of tender hepatomegaly with jaundice include viral hepatitis, alcoholic hepatitis, congestive cardiac failure, etc. Jaundice with palpable gall bladder is mostly due to pancreatic head malignancy or distal cholangio carcinoma. Ascites in the presence of jaundice suggests either cirrhosis or peritoneal spread of malignancy.

CAUSES OF JAUNDICE

Most common causes

- Viral hepatitis
- Alcoholic liver disease
- Cholecystitis
- Choledocholithiasis
- Carcinoma of the pancreas

Common causes
- Drug or toxin-induced liver disease
- Chronic hepatitis
- Gilbert's syndrome
- Post-operative state
- Sepsis

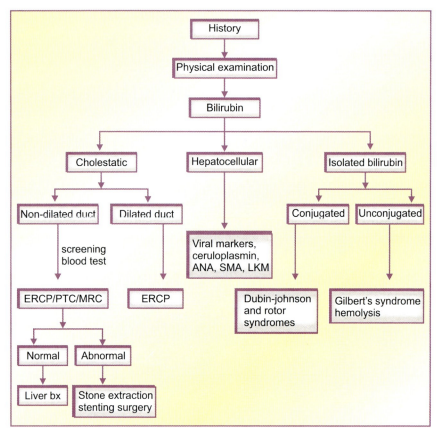

Fig. 20.1: Algorithm in the evaluation of patients with jaundice

Less common causes
- Metastatic liver disease
- Hepatocellular carcinoma
- Lymphoma

INVESTIGATIONS

Urine Examination

Bilirubin in urine is an early sign of viral hepatitis or drug induced jaundice. Persistent absence of urobilinogen suggests total common bile duct obstruction. Excess of urobilinogen with negative bilirubin in urine supports hemolytic jaundice.

Stool Examination

Positive fecal occult blood favours periampullary, pancreatic, or alimentary malignancy or it can also be due to portal hypertension.

Liver Function Test

Serum bilirubin level helps to confirm jaundice and to assess the depth and progression of jaundice. In hepatocellular jaundice there will be disproportionate elevation of transaminases than alkaline phosphatase. A very high liver enzyme in thousands of units occurs in viral hepatitis, drug induced liver disease and ischemic hepatitis. High values of transaminases can also be seen in acute biliary obstruction due to bile duct stones. AST (SGOT) more than two times the ALT (SGPT) occurs in alcoholic liver disease and Wilson's disease. In alcoholic hepatitis enzyme levels usually will not go above 300 international units.

In cholestatic jaundice, elevation of alkaline phosphatase will be more than transaminases. Gamma glutamyl transferase (GGT) will also be elevated in cholestatic jaundice. Serum albumin levels will be low in chronic hepatocellular jaundice, with increased globulin levels. Parenteral administration of vitamin K usually normalizes the prolonged prothrombin time in patients with obstructive jaundice but not in hepatocellular jaundice.

Viral Markers

Anti HAV IgM, Anti HEV IgM and anti HBc IgM are the markers of acute hepatitis A, acute hepatitis E and acute hepatitis B respectively. Hepatitis C rarely presents as acute hepatitis. For chronic hepatitis, HBsAg and anti HCV are tested usually.

Liver Biopsy

Is most useful in undiagnosed persistent jaundice. Helps in the diagnosis of conditions like alcoholic hepatitis, granulomatous hepatitis, primary biliary cirrhosis and in neoplasm of the liver like hepatocellular carcinoma or liver secondaries. Special histologic stains and quantification of iron and copper content help in the diagnosis of hemochromatosis and Wilson's disease respectively. In case of chronic viral hepatitis, the necroinflammatory scores assess the disease activity and if the score is more than three, antiviral therapy may have to be considered.

IMAGING STUDIES

Ultrasonography (USG)

USG abdomen helps to assess the calibre of the intra and extrahepatic biliary tree and reveals intrahepatic or extrahepatic mass lesions. USG is superior to CT in the detection of cholelithiasis. It is noninvasive, portable and less expensive. Disadvantages of USG are that presence of bowel gas may obscure common bile duct and the pancreas, and also cause difficulty in visualisation in obese patients (See Fig. 20.1)

CT Abdomen

Contrast enhanced CT scan of abdomen is another non-invasive means of evaluating biliary obstruction. Spiral CT increases the diagnostic accuracy. It picks up space-occupying lesions as small as 5 mm and helps to assess the resectability of malignant lesions of the pancreas, stomach or liver. CT is not operator-dependent, but is expensive, lacks portability and needs intravenous contrast.

Magnetic Resonance Cholangiopancreatography

MRCP is a technical refinement of MRI that permits rapid clear-cut delineation of biliary tract without the need of intravenous contrast. MRCP is non invasive. Use of MRCP is limited in non-dilated biliary tree. MR-angio is the investigation of choice for cholangiocarcinoma in assessing its operability.

Endoscopic Retrograde Cholangiopancreatography (ERCP)

ERCP permits direct visualization of the biliary tree as well as pancreatic ducts. It is highly accurate in the diagnosis of biliary obstruction. It also helps to take brushings for cytology and biopsies from the periampullary lesion. If a focal cause for biliary obstruction like choledocholithiasis is detected, maneuvers to relieve the obstruction such as sphincterotomy, stone extraction, dilatation and stent placement can be performed. In inoperable cases of pancreatic malignancy, cholangiocarcinoma or periampullary carcinoma, palliative stenting can be done.

Percutaneous Transhepatic Cholangiography (PTC)

Here a needle is passed through the skin and subcutaneous tissue into the hepatic parenchyma and into the peripheral bile duct. A catheter is introduced and contrast is injected through the needle. PTC is advantageous when the level of obstruction is proximal to common hepatic duct or in cases when altered anatomy precludes ERCP. It has an important role in the management of patients with cholangitis, where ERCP has failed or is not possible.

Differential Diagnosis of Jaundice

Causes and presumed sites of intrahepatic cholestasis

Hepatocellular
- Viral hepatitis
- Alcoholic liver disease
- Cirrhosis of liver

Hepatocanalicular
- Drugs (androgens, phenothiazines)
- Sepsis
- Post-operative state
- Total parenteral nutrition
- Hodgkin's and non-Hodgkin's lymphoma
- Amyloidosis

Ductular
- Primary biliary cirrhosis

Bile ducts
- Intrahepatic biliary atresia
- Choledocholithiasis
- Cholangiocarcinoma
- Primary sclerosing cholangitis

Recurrent cholestasis
- Benign recurrent intrahepatic cholestasis (BRIC)
- Recurrent jaundice of pregnancy
- Dubin-Johnson syndrome

SUMMARY OF APPROACH TO A PATIENT WITH JAUNDICE

Once jaundice is recognized clinically or biochemically, next step is to determine whether it is predominantly conjugated or unconjugated hyperbilirubinemia. Presence of bilirubin in urine indicates conjugated hyperbilirubinemia. Isolated elevation of unconjugated bilirubin indicates overproduction as in case of hemolysis or impaired uptake caused by drugs or Gilbert's syndrome. Impaired

Table 20.1: Differentiating points between intra and extra hepatic cholestasis

	Intrahepatic cholestasis	Extrahepatic cholestasis
History	Viral prodrome Blood transfusion Intravenous drugs Exposure to hepatotoxins Family history of jaundice	Abdominal pain Fever, rigor and chills Prior biliary surgeries
Physical examination	Stigmata of chronic liver disease Asterixis Encephalopathy	High fever Palpable abdominal mass Abdominal scar
Lab studies	Predominant elevation of serum aminotransferases Prothrombin time does not normalize with vitamin K	Predominant alkaline phosphatase elevation Prothrombin time normalizes with Vitamin K

glucuronide conjugation is another cause of unconjugated hyperbilirubinemia. When there is mild decrease in glucuronyl transferase it causes Gilbert's syndrome, whereas moderate deficiency causes Type 2 Crigler-Najjar syndrome and the enzyme is totally absent in Type 1 Crigler-Najjar syndrome. In jaundice with predominantly isolated conjugated hyperbilirubinemia two familial conditions are to be considered, namely, Dubin Johnson syndrome and Rotor syndrome.

If the bilirubin elevation is associated with transaminases elevation out of proportion to alkaline phosphatase, it indicates hepatocellular type of jaundice, which includes conditions like viral hepatitis, drug or alcohol-induced hepatitis, autoimmune hepatitis, Wilson's disease and cirrhosis. In hepatitis and cirrhosis there is usually interference in hepatic uptake, conjugation and excretion. But excretion is the rate-limiting step in the metabolism of bilirubin; hence conjugated bilirubinemia predominates in these conditions.

If bilirubin elevation is associated with alkaline phosphatase elevation out of proportion to transaminases, it suggests cholestatic jaundice. Cholestatic jaundice can be intrahepatic or extrahepatic. USG abdomen helps to differentiate between the two. If intrahepatic biliary radical dilatation or CBD dilatation is present, it indicates extrahepatic biliary obstruction. Next investigation is CT abdomen, which helps to assess the resectability, if there is a malignant lesion. If inoperable, patient can be taken up for ERCP and therapeutic stenting. ERCP also helps in the clearance of stone and stenting of CBD in case of biliary stricture. Cholestasis with non-dilated intrahepatic ducts has to undergo liver biopsy to find out the etiology (See Table 20.1).

SUGGESTED READING

1. Berg C.L., et al, Bilirubin metabolism and pathophysiology of jaundice in Schiff's Diseases of the liver 9th edition ER Schiff et al, Philadelphia, Lippencott, 2002.
2. Greenberger N.J, Hinlhorn D.H, History taking and physical examination essentials and clinical correlates. St Louis: Mosby year book 1992;220-61
3. Bilirubin metabolism and hereditary hyperbilirubinemia, Seminars in liver disease 1994;14:321,.
4. Roche SP; Kobos R Am Fam Physician 2004 Jan 15;69(2):299-304
5. Current concepts in diagnosis. Approach to the patient with cholestats. Jaundice. Scharschmidt B. F., Goldberg H. I., Schmid R.N Engl J Med 1983; 308:1515-19, Jun 23, 1983.
6. Pathophysiology and current concepts in the diagnosis of obstructive jaundice. Lucas WB, Chuttani R. Gastroenterologist 1995 Jun;3(2):105-18.

21

Anil John

Hepatitis A

INTRODUCTION

Hepatitis A is a major cause of acute hepatitis worldwide. It is highly prevalent in virtually all areas of suboptimal hygiene of water supply and food production and is spread by feco-oral route.

VIRUS STRUCTURE AND ASSEMBLING

Belongs to hepatoviridae; consists of a spherical protein shell (capsid) and encapsidates a single stranded RNA.

STABILITY AND SURVIVAL

Viral survival strategy imparts resistance to adverse environmental conditions. The virions survive acidic pH, which favour gastric passage. The particle can withstand dryness and heat, which explains their survival in the environment. HAV is however sensitive to strong oxidants like chlorine and is inactivated at 85°C for one minute. It survives lower heat exposure at 60°C. It can survive in sea water, dried faeces at room temperature and in live oysters.

EPIDEMIOLOGY

HAV seroprevalence declines in the population with improved socioeconomic conditions. As a result, a population of adults emerge, who having escaped HAV infection in childhood, remain non-immune and susceptible to infection in adulthood. As infection becomes less frequent in the population, cases are shifted from younger to older segments. Infection in adults leads to clinically more severe disease. So in developed countries, cases of acute hepatitis A requiring admission to hospitals are more common than a decade ago. Several developing countries are showing similar patterns of changing HAV seroepidemiology.

ROUTES OF TRANSMISSION

The primary route of transmission is feco-oral, person to person contact or ingestion of contaminated food or water.

BIOLOGY AND PATHOGENESIS

Humans are the only host in nature. When hepatitis A virus is ingested by feco-oral route, it survives gastric pH. The precise mechanism of hepatic uptake is unknown. HAV antigens can be detected in the enterocyte of the upper jejunum and ileum. HAV antigen has been shown as fine granular pattern in the heptocyte cytoplasm. The virus is distributed throughout the liver. The virus replicates exclusively in the liver cells and induces immunologically mediated hepatic necrosis. From the liver cells, the virus is released into the biliary tree. The presence of HAV in bile during acute infection explains the presence of virus in stools.

CLINICAL MANIFESTATIONS

The incubation period of the infection is about four weeks. About 10 days after the uptake of HAV, virus can be found in the stool and titres as high as 10^9 viral particles / gm stool may be seen. HAV shedding in stool decreases by the time of onset of hepatitis.

Infection may be asymptomatic or may result in acute hepatitis of variable severity. HAV does not cause carrier state or chronic hepatitis.

After the incubation period, patient experiences prodromal symptoms like fatigue, headache, myalgia, arthralgia, nausea and vomiting followed by jaundice. Physical examination reveals mild tender hepatomegaly and scleral icterus.

Hepatitis A infection may present in one of the following clinical patterns:
1. Asymptomatic and non-icteric: Seen mostly in young children.
2. Symptomatic and icteric (the usual presentation in adults): Self-limited to approximately eight weeks or less
3. Cholestatic, which lasts an average 10 weeks or more with feature of intrahepatic cholestasis
4. Relapsing, consisting of two or more bouts of acute HAV infection occuring over 6-10 weeks' period
5. Fulminant hepatitis, which is a rare clinical manifestation in around 1% infected patients

Rare complications like thrombocytopenia, renal failure, aplastic anemia and neurological sequelae have been reported with non-fulminant hepatitis A.

Acute hepatitis A, unlike hepatitis E, has not been shown to have an increased mortality in pregnancy.

LAB FEATURES

Biochemical hallmark is elevation in AST and ALT levels. Elevation in the AST and ALT precedes elevation in bilirubin, which may continue to climb even as AST and ALT levels decline. Transient neutropenia and an atypical lymphocytosis can occur.

Presence of IgM anti HAV establishes the diagnosis of acute hepatitis A with 100% sensitivity and specificity. IgM anti HAV decline in three months. Beginning with convalescence and persisting indefinitely, IgG anti HAV is associated with life-long immunity to the infection (Fig. 21.1)

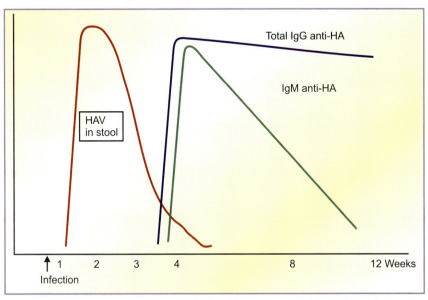

Fig. 21.1: Figure showing the time relationship between HAV shedding in the stool and appearance of IgG anti HAV antibodies

Determinant of the Severity of Acute Hepatitis A

Age of infection is a determinant of the severity of acute hepatitis A. Young children only rarely have clinical icteric hepatitis.

Management

The disease is self-limiting with no chronic sequelae. Only general supportive and symptomatic measures are required. Symptomatic therapy for nausea and bed rest as needed are recommended. No anti-viral agent has been shown to be effective clinically. Hospital admissions are usually not required except in patients with prolonged prodromal symptoms, impending encephalopathy, prolonged cholestasis or in the event of unusual complications. Corticosteroids are not helpful except in situations of intrahepatic cholestasis.

Prevention

Clean and safe water supply and environmental hygiene is important in preventing HAV infection.

PRE EXPOSURE PROPHYLAXIS

Active Immunization

Inactivated hepatitis A virus has been shown to be safe and immunogenic, and provides high protection to non-immune contacts of hepatitis A infection. Protective levels of anti HAV antibody appear within 2 weeks of vaccination and are detected for approximately 20 years following immunization.

The high risk group that must be targeted for immunization include travelers from regions of low endemicity to high endemic regions and patients with chronic liver disease who are non-immune against hepatitis A.

Dose and Schedule of Hepatitis A vaccine (Havrix)

Group	Primary immunization	Booster
Adults ≥ 19 years	1 ml IM (1440 ELISA units)	1 ml IM at 6 months
Children 2-18 years	0.5 ml IM (720 ELISA units)	0.5 ml IM at 6 months

(Adolescents)

Now, combined vaccines for both hepatitis A and B for use in adults and children at dual risk of exposure to HAV and HBV are available. The adult preparation of the combination vaccine (Twinrix by Glaxo Smithkline) is a 1 ml formulation containing 720 ELISA units of hepatitis A virus and 20 mg of recombinant yeast derived HBsAg. The paediatric formulation contains 360 ELISA units of HAV antigen and 10 mg of HBsAg in a 0.5 ml dose. The recommended primary course of vaccination consists of 3 doses administered at 0, 1 and 6 months by IM injection in the deltoid region in adults and children and antero-lateral thigh in infants.

POSTEXPOSURE PROPHYLAXIS

Human pooled immunoglobulin (Immune serum globulin – ISG) is administered in doses of 0.02 ml/kg within 2 weeks of exposure, which has an 85% efficacy in preventing acute hepatitis A. Post exposure prophylaxis can be combined with active immunization against hepatitis A.

The changing Epidemiology of Hepatitis A Infection in India and Relevance of Hepatitis A Vaccination

The reported seroprevalence of anti HAV antibodies in the general population has been 80-90%, which is reached by 10 years as per earlier reports. However, there are recent reports of decline in HAV seroprevalence especially in the higher socio-economic class. The decreased seroprevalence can result in symptomatic acute hepatitis in adults. Though there is no role for universal hepatitis A vaccination, there is definitely a relevance in providing vaccination for the susceptible non-immune population, especially if they have possible risk of exposure to hepatitis A virus.

SUGGESTED READING

1. Lemon SM, Martin a. Hepatitis a. In: Schiff e, Sorrel eds. Schiff's diseases of the liver; Lippincott Williams and Wilkins, 2003; 9th edition; 745-62.
2. John TJ, George GM. What priority for prevention of hepatitis A in India? – Editorial; Indian Journal of Gastroenterology 1998; 17:2-3.
3. Dhawan PS, Shah SS, alwares JF, Khen A, Sankaran K, Kandoth PW, et al. Seroprevalence of hepatitis A virus in Mumbai and immunogenicity and safety of hepatitis a vaccine. Indian Journal of Gastroenterology 1998; 17:16-18.
4. Asian perspectives on viral hepatitis A. Lee SDJ Gastroenterol Hepatol (Australia), Oct 2000; 15 Suppl pG94-9
5. Regev A, Schiff ER.Viral hepatitis A, B, and C. Clin Liver Dis (United States), Feb 2000; 4(1):p47-71, vi
6. Kemmer NM, Miskovsky EP. Hepatitis A. Infect Dis Clin North Am (United States), Sep 2000; 14(3):p605-15

22

Philip Augustine
Jose V Francis

Hepatitis E

INTRODUCTION

Acute viral hepatitis is a systemic infection affecting the liver predominantly. In the earlier days only two types of hepatitis were classified: infectious hepatitis and serum hepatitis. This classification was decided upon when no serological markers were available. The identification of Australia antigen in 1965, which was a landmark discovery, opened the floodgates for further identification for other causes of jaundice. The advances in molecular biology helped the medical fraternity in diagnosing the different viruses that cause hepatitis. Epidemiologic, serologic and clinical differentiation from other viruses can now be accomplished.

The various hepatitis viruses identified are hepatitis A, B, C, D, E and G. Although these agents can be distinguished by their molecular and antigenic properties, all types of viral hepatitis produce clinically similar illnesses. These range from asymptomatic and inapparent to fulminant and fatal acute infections common to all types.

Viral hepatitis remains a major public health problem and is the most common cause of liver disease worldwide. Despite advances in diagnosis and treatment, enterically transmitted viral hepatitis in the developing world continues to be highly prevalent, in fact in epidemic forms, due to the non-availability of clean drinking water and poor sanitary and hygienic conditions.

Hepatitis E virus spreads through contaminated drinking water, i.e. fecal-oral route as mentioned earlier wherever there are unhygienic living conditions. Hepatitis E was initially known as enterically transmitted non-A, non-B hepatitis. This distinct clinical entity was first considered when during episodes of epidemic jaundice the serological markers of A and B, which were the only ones available then were found to be negative. Balayan, et al obtained the proof of existence of this virus in 1983 and the genome of the virus was finally cloned in 1990.

VIROLOGY

Hepatitis E virus (HEV) is a non – enveloped single stranded RNA virus and has been found to have properties similar to those of calciviruses. At present a genus is not named; till this is determined the virus is designated in the group as the hepatitis E like viruses. Electron microscopy of the stool samples has identified a 32–34 nm virus like particle. Scientists have been able to transmit this virus to cynomolgus monkeys. This virus is approximately 7600 nucleotides in length with 5′ and 3′ noncoding regions, has at least three open reading frames (ORF) and a 3′ terminal poly A sequence. Each of the open reading frames is responsible for the replication of the viral genome, capsid protein and cytoskeletal proteins respectively.

There are two main strains of the virus, Burmese (Asian) and Mexican. Some variations have been noted and different types were detected in the USA, Taiwan, China, Italy and Greece. However no difference in the clinical presentation has been noted among the various strains.

Epidemiology

Before the identification of hepatitis E virus, epidemics of apparent water – borne, NANB (non A non B) hepatitis have been described in India, Asia, Africa, and Central America. Serology testing of the preserved sera proved that these epidemics were of hepatitis E etiology. It has been found that it resembles hepatitis A in many respects. The commonly recognized cases occur after contamination of water supplies such as after monsoon flooding, but sporadic isolated cases do occur. The other reason epidemics do occur is because the drinking water pipes run along with the sewage pipes and leakage results in contamination. An epidemiological feature that distinguishes HEV from other enteric agents is the rarity of secondary person-to-person spread from infected persons to their close contacts.

Large outbreaks in epidemic form occur in developing countries. Sporadic cases have been known to occur. Other than fecal-oral route no other transmission routes have been identified. Vertical transmission has been reported. The reservoir of infection is mainly contaminated water by sewage. This contamination is continued by the numerous cases of sub-clinical infection of HEV with the subsequent fecal shedding which follows it. Another reservoir considered is zoonotic as anti HEV is detected in cattle and swine. Thus it is easy for HEV to cause large epidemics from an environmental, human or animal reservoir.

CLINICAL FEATURES

Clinical manifestations are as follows:
- Anicteric hepatitis
- Acute hepatitis
- Cholestatic hepatitis
- Fulminant hepatic failure.

Hepatitis E cannot be distinguished from the other forms of viral hepatitis on clinical grounds alone. However, certain features may occur more or less frequently. More than 50% of patients with hepatitis E have fever. Upto one third of patients may have arthralgias. Although the disease is usually mild among individuals who survive, severe hepatitis with a high mortality can occur.

The disease is insidious in onset with a prodrome of fever, anorexia, vomiting, weakness, arthralgias and a transient macular rash. This is followed by appearance of jaundice. The prodromal symptoms subside once the jaundice appears. Physical examination is unremarkable except for icterus, tender hepatomegaly and in a few cases splenomegaly is seen. The liver function tests are consistent with acute hepatitis and it takes about one and half months to return to normal. The disease is self-limiting and usually takes a benign course and lasts for about one to four weeks. The clinical presentation can be varied. The presentation could vary from the usual jaundice, to cholesteric jaundice and even fulminant hepatic failure. An average incubation period of 35 to 40 days is observed. It is usually the young adults of the age group 15-40 years who are commonly affected. It usually has a mild clinical presentation in children. The difference in age distribution of hepatitis A and epidemic hepatitis E appears to be a significant epidemiological difference, possibly related to a difference in the intensity of exposure to the two agents in childhood, or to a failure of infection with HEV to produce long lasting protective immunity, as does infection with HAV.

Hepatitis E infection, unlike other viral hepatitis, does not produce any chronic hepatitis. Fulminant hepatic failure is seen in about 0.07-0.6%. In a few cases an entity in the form of cholestatic hepatitis occurs where there is persistent jaundice and severe intractable itching. The prognosis is good and after a prolonged course it resolves in 2–6 months.

HEPATITIS E AND PREGNANCY

Severe hepatitis has consistently been observed in pregnant women with development of fulminant hepatic failure in 22.2% of patients and mortality rates are reported to be 20–39%. The mortality was highest when the attack occurs during the second and third trimesters. Fetal wastage in the form of abortion, stillbirth and neonatal death has been reported to be common. The pathology of such a high mortality in pregnant women is unknown.

Pathology

The virus has been detected in stool, bile, and liver from infected patients as well as from experimentally infected non-human primates. Studies in humans and experimental animals have shown that HEV is excreted in the stool during the late incubation period and the immune responses to the viral antigens occur very early during the course of acute infection. Both IgM anti – HEV and IgG anti – HEV can be detected, but both fall rapidly after acute infection reaching low levels within 9-12 months. The histological features of HEV infection differ from other hepatitis in some respects. More than 50% have features of cholestatic hepatitis characterized by canalicular bile stasis and gland like transformation of the hepatocytes. In other cases the usual findings of hepatitis are found in the form of ballooned hepatocytes, acidophilic bodies and focal/confluent hepatic necrosis. No particular zone of the liver is involved. In patients with severe liver injury massive necrosis and collapse of reticulin and liver parenchyma occur.

Diagnosis

The diagnosis is based on detection of antibodies to HEV, IgM anti-HEV or HEV RNA in the patient's serum. IgM anti-HEV is the common test done for the diagnosis. Viral excretion occurs about one week prior to the onset of the illness and persists for a period of two weeks. Immunoglobulin M appears early and disappears by a few months. The immunoglobulin G levels last for four and half years only. The viral particles can be checked in the stool using immune electron microscopy.

Treatment

There is no specific treatment for hepatitis E virus infection. The usual supportive and conservative measures are the mainstay of treatment. Restricted activity, steroids and dietary modification do not alter the course of the disease. Non-specific treatments in the hospital set up, include anti-emetics, intra-venous fluids, and anti-histamines if there is severe pruritus. Fulminant hepatic failure (FHF) needs aggressive measures especially anti-cerebral edema treatment. If all else fails, then an orthotopic liver transplant may be the only answer. Pregnant patients need close monitoring, as they are likely to go into FHF. Termination of pregnancy is not considered, as it is fraught with dangers because of coagulation problems.

Prevention

Hepatitis E infection is almost non-existent in developed countries and is in epidemic form in developing countries. The sporadic cases seen in developed countries are mainly imported ones. Proper drinking water supply is essential and should be the priority. Next should be the proper disposal of human wastes and garbage. Finally, separation of drinking water supply lines from the sewage lines to prevent contamination as was the case of Hepatitis E epidemic in Delhi is essential. Boiling of water and proper chlorination of the water should be considered in the strictest possible way. Isolation of the patient is not necessary as person-to-person transmission is uncommon. The best protection for travellers from low endemic areas to highly endemic or epidemic areas is the same as for preventing all enteric diseases, namely avoiding potentially contaminated water and uncooked food. Eating from roadside stalls and contaminated food handlers may increase the risk to an extent.

Vaccines are still in the experimental stage and once this breakthrough is achieved, as in hepatitis A, this scourge can hopefully be banished from the earth. Till then, basic hygiene, clean drinking water and proper disposal of waste are the only measures, which can be undertaken. The occurrence of epidemics in endemic areas suggests, that either the anti HEV antibodies are not protective, or that there is a rapid decline in the protective antibody levels. The role of immunoglobulins has been tried and no benefit was found. Recombinant vaccines have been tried and have demonstrated protection. However, further trials are required before definite inclusion in vaccination strategies is considered. These vaccines may benefit travellers and pregnant women so that short-term protection is conferred.

CONCLUSION

Not much has changed in the scenario of various forms of viral hepatitis including hepatitis E, and all of them are preventable in many ways, which should be the main theme, and thus measures are to be taken on a war footing. Development of a vaccine in the future will be of great help in controlling the illness, even though provision of clean drinking water has to be given top priority.

SUGGESTED READING

1. Wang L, Zhuang H. Hepatitis E. An overview and recent advances in vaccine research.
2. World J Gastroenterol (China), Aug 1 2004; 10(15):p2157-62.
3. Krawczynski K, Aggarwal R, Kamili S. Hepatitis E. Infect Dis Clin North Am (United States), Sep 2000; 14(3):p669-87
4. Acharya SK, Panda SK, Saxena A, et al. 3. Acute hepatic failure in India: a perspective from the East. J Gastroenterol Hepatol (Australia), May 2000; 15(5): p473-9.
5. Aggarwal R, Krawczynski K. 4 Hepatitis E: an overview and recent advances in clinical and laboratory research. J Gastroenterol Hepatol (Australia), Jan 2000; 15(1):p9-20
6. Khuroo MS. Hepatitis E: the enterically transmitted non-A, non-B hepatitis.
7. Indian J Gastroenterol. 1991 Jul;10(3):96-100.

23

Narendranathan M

Hepatitis B and Hepatitis C: Magnitude of the Problem and Prevention

HEPATITIS B

Hepatitis B virus (HBV) infection is the tenth leading cause of death in the world. About two billion people – one third of the population of the world—are infected with the virus and among them 350 million are carriers. Fifteen to forty percent of the infected individuals develop cirrhosis, liver failure or hepatocellular carcinoma. Primary hepatocellular carcinoma (HCC) is one of the ten most common cancers in the world, and HBV is responsible for up to 80% of these cancers. Among the known human carcinogens, HBV is only second in importance to tobacco. India is categorized under the intermediate prevalence zone for HBV carrier state. The projected figure for HBsAg positive individuals in India is 47 million. There is considerable geographical variation in the prevalence of chronic HBV infection in India. The carrier rate varies from 1 to 12%. It is difficult to divide India into high prevalence and low prevalence zones because of inadequate uniformly collected data. From the available figures the mean HBsAg positivity in India is 3.34%.

Transmission

Hepatitis B is highly infectious. Every individual who is HBsAg positive, irrespective of the HBV DNA status, should be considered infective. HBV spreads through blood, blood products and body fluids. Transmission occurs when the virus from these sources comes into contact with the tissues of an individual without adequate immunity. The minimum volume of blood needed to transmit HBV infection is 0.00004 ml whereas it is 0.1 ml for HIV. The major modes of transmission are: 1. Perinatal (mother to baby during birth), 2. Person to person, 3. Sexual contact, 4. Unsafe transfusions, injections or improperly sterilized instruments and 5. Vectors like insects.

Worldwide, most infections occur from infected mother to child, from child to child contact in household settings, and from reuse of unsterilized or improperly sterilized medical tools. The commonest risk factor for acute hepatitis B infection in India appears to be reusable needles. The transmission can occur from one individual to another in the same family. Vector borne transmission is a distinct possibility as the virus persists outside the human body in insects. Sexual contact and transmission from mother-to-baby are two other ways by which hepatitis B and C can be spread. HBV does not cross the placenta, but it can be transmitted from a pregnant carrier mother to her foetus when invasive procedures, such as amniocentesis, are carried out. This mode of vertical transmission is estimated to be responsible for less than 5% of hepatitis B cases in newborns. Infants who are infected prior to birth cannot be protected by vaccination. Hepatitis B can be transmitted from a carrier mother to her child when the newborn infant comes into contact with the mother's infected blood, often during delivery.

The mode of transmission makes some groups of individuals at higher risk of acquiring HBV infection. These high-risk groups are:

1. Health care providers
2. Those requiring frequent dialysis or blood or blood products
3. Infants borne to mothers with HBV infection
4. Individuals with multiple sex partners.
5. Men having sex with men and commercial sex workers
6. Residents and staff of correctional facilities and group homes
7. Persons living in close household contact with an infected person
8. Illicit drug users
9. Immunosuppressed individuals– e.g., those receiving cancer chemotherapy
10. Individuals who get tattoos or body piercing.

Sharing any kind of needles—those used for tattooing, body piercing, acupuncture, shots for health reasons, or illegal drugs can transmit hepatitis B and C. The risk of developing HBV infection following needle stick injury is 7 to 30% with HBV where as it is 0.5% with HIV. Straws for inhaling cocaine appears to be another major means of infection—small amounts of blood from inside the nose stick to the straw, which is then passed to the next person. This is a common way that hepatitis is spread.

Prevention

Hepatitis B is a preventable disease. Preventive strategies save considerable health related costs especially in developing countries.

Screening of blood and blood products is an important prerequisite for preventing transmission of Hepatitis B and C virus infection. Using disposable needles, avoiding needle sharing among injecting drug users and safe sex practices are other measures that prevent the infection.

Prevention in Special Settings

Medical professionals should adopt a series of steps called universal precautions, which include strict cleaning procedures for all tools, using disposable needles, and wearing gloves when coming into contact with patients.

Preventing vertical transmission: Hepatitis B vaccine and hepatitis B immunoglobulin (0.13 ml/Kg) should be given to newborns of HBsAg and HBeAg positive mothers.

Postexposure prophylaxis: Immunoprophylaxis of hepatitis B is also indicated after a needle stick or sexual exposure. The recommended dose of HBIG is 0.06 ml/Kg. This should be given within 48 hours of exposure. For inadvertent percutaneous exposure, a regimen of two doses of HBIG, one given after exposure and one a month later is about 75% effective in preventing hepatitis B. For sexual exposure to a person with acute hepatitis B, a single dose of HBIG is 75% effective if administered within two weeks of sexual exposure.

HEPATITIS B VACCINE

Hepatitis B vaccine is highly effective, giving protection to 95% of individuals. Use of the hepatitis B vaccine has been monitored for 15 years, and it has not been proven to be the cause of any deaths and is only rarely linked to serious side effects. Hepatitis B vaccination is indicated for all infants, irrespective of the endemicity of the region. High-risk groups should receive the vaccination. Three doses of the vaccine given at 0, 1 and 6 months give adequate protection. Half the adult dose is given for children and young adults. Immunocompromised individuals require 40 micrograms per dose. The vaccine is given by the intramuscular route into upper thigh of infant and deltoid muscle of adult. There is evidence that booster doses are not necessary to persons who are not in the high-risk group. Recombinant DNA vaccines are available now and these should be preferred to plasma derived vaccines. There are very few contraindications for Hepatitis B vaccine. Severe allergic reaction to previous doses and fever >38.5°C are absolute contraindications. Persons with severe allergic reaction to baker's yeast should receive plasma-derived vaccines. Respiratory tract infection or diarrhea and temperature below 38.5°C, allergy, asthma, breast-feeding and pregnancy are not contraindications for the vaccine.

Types of Chronic HBV Infections

Chronic HBV infection may be HBeAg positive or HBeAg negative. Inactive HBsAg carrier state is the term given to persistent HBV infection without significant evidence of ongoing necroinflammatory disease. *Acute exacerbation or flare* can occur when the transaminase levels increase to 10 times the upper limit of normal. Reappearance of necroinflammatory disease in inactive disease is called *reactivation* of hepatitis B. Reappearance of HBeAg is called *HBeAg reversion*.

Management

The diagnosis of chronic hepatitis B can be made in the presence of histologic or ultrasound evidence of chronic liver disease in a person with positive viral markers. In the absence of the above the diagnosis of chronic hepatitis can be made when there is evidence that the infection was present for more than six months.

Initial Evaluation of a Patient with Chronic Hepatitis B Virus Infection

1. History and physical examination—Specifically look for symptoms and signs of portal hypertension and liver failure (jaundice, hematemesis, ascites, encephalopathy, etc.)
2. Laboratory tests—Liver function tests, complete blood counts, renal function tests
3. Screen for esophageal varices (upper gastrointestinal endoscopy)
4. Screen for hepatocellular carcinoma (ultrasonography and alpha-fetoprotein levels)
5. Tests for viral replication status (HBeAg, anti-HBe, hepatitis B virus DNA)
6. Screen for coinfection with other parenterally transmitted viruses (anti-hepatitis C virus antibodies, HIV serology)
7. Liver biopsy (optional)

Inactive HBsAg carriers have normal alanine aminotransferase activity. These patients should be followed up with 6 monthly ALT estimations. They should also be screened for the presence of hepatocellular carcinoma. No antiviral treatment is indicated in these patients.

Hepatitis C, D or HIV coinfection, renal failure, immunosuppressive treatment or decompensated cirrhosis makes treatment difficult.

Some cases of chronic hepatitis respond to therapy. As antiviral therapy is expensive and potentially toxic it is essential to identify those who would respond to the treatment. Patients who respond are those with histologic evidence of active hepatitis, presence of HBeAg or HBV DNA and elevated transaminases.

It has to be emphasized that many persons seeking employment in Gulf are found to be HBsAg positive during medical check up. The reason why they seek medical help is to get rid of the HBsAg. Interferon therapy or lamivudine rarely if ever clears the HBsAg from the blood. This should be explained to the patient before embarking on treatment. The aim of treatment in chronic infection is to stop HBV replication. This is evidenced by sustained clearance from the blood of HBeAg and HBV DNA and appearance of anti-HBeAg. Anti viral treatment should be given to those with high ALT (more than twice the upper limit of normal) and presence of HBV DNA in the blood. The recommended dose of alpha interferon is 5 million units thrice weekly for 16 weeks. Higher dosage schedules are less tolerated by our patients. Patients with hepatic decompensation should not be given interferon for treatment for HBV.

Lamivudine in a dose of 100 mg per day is another drug effective in chronic HBV infection. The indication for treatment is evidence of HBV replication – HbeAg positivity or HBV DNA positivity. Lamivudine is the preferred drug in those with hepatic decompensation. The dose should be reduced in those with renal failure. Lamivudine can be stopped two months after HBeAg seroconversion. Adefovir is another drug that is effective in chronic HBV infection. This is recommended for those who do not respond to lamivudine.

HEPATITIS C

The global prevalence of Hepatitis C ranges from 0.1 to 5% with a mean of 3%. About 170 million people are infected with HCV worldwide. There are eleven genotypes (1 to 11) and twenty-two subtypes of the virus. In India the prevalence is around 1%. The prevalence increases with age. In India about 30% of HCV positive individuals had elevated transaminase levels. HCV genotype one and three are the major genotypes in India.

The routes of transmission are like HBV. Blood and blood products that have not been screened for HCV are a major source of HCV transmission. This mode of transmission is coming down in many countries with strict guidelines for testing blood and blood products. The risk of HCV transmission through sexual contact or through ordinary household contact is very low. This is a definite risk and should not be ignored. Mother-to-child transmission is known to occur.

Transmission of HCV in health care settings is an important mode of transmission. Well-documented outbreaks of nosocomial transmission have occurred among patients with immunosuppressive conditions who have frequent venepuncture or access to veins. Dialysis units may also be responsible for transmission of HCV. The need for proper cleaning and sterilization of all instruments entering sterile body sites is obvious and the exhortation to health care workers to regularly and thoroughly wash their hands needs constant reemphasis. The risk of occupational transmission of HCV has been investigated. The data suggest that the risk of transmission of HCV through percutaneous injury is higher than for HIV but lower than for HBV. Predictably, risk of acquiring HCV occupationally is related to frequency of blood contact, volume of blood involved, prevalence of HCV in the patient population and probably the level of viremia. Injecting drugs is the commonest mode of acquiring HCV in some countries. Open wounds in patients may be a source of transmission to household contacts. In about 30% of patients no known risk factor or exposure can be identified.

Acute HCV infection is generally anicteric and relatively asymptomatic, making it difficult to determine when infection occurred. Of people infected with HCV, most will fail to eliminate it, and estimates of those who develop chronic HCV infection vary between 50 and 90%. Follow-up of transfusion-associated cases of HCV infection indicate that the average time taken to develop cirrhosis is about 20 years, but the time range over which liver disease develops is wide. HCV disease is often slowly progressive and potentially results in severe liver disease. Alcoholism, acquiring disease later in life and coinfection with HBV or HIV adversely affects the outcome of cases with chronic HCV infection. HCV infection can progress through CLD and ultimately result in hepatocellular carcinoma.

Treatment for chronic HCV is recommended only for those with histologic evidence of activity or raised ALT. IFN-ribavirin combination is the first line treatment. Pegylated IFN 180 microgram weekly for 48 weeks plus ribavirin is superior to the IFN-ribavirin combination. For genotypes two and theee, duration of therapy is six months. Genotypes one and four require longer treatment. Persistently elevated ALT, positive HCV RNA by PCR and liver biopsy evidence of septal fibrosis or necro-inflammation are necessary to start treatment.

SUGGESTED READING

1. Hepatitis B in India, Prevention and Management. Editors: SK. Sarin and AK. Singal, CBS Publishers and Distributors, New Delhi. First Edition. 2004.
2. Lauer G. M., Walker B. D. Hepatitis C Virus Infection. N Engl J Med 2001; 345:41-52
3. Lee W. M. Hepatitis B virus infection. N Engl J Med 1997; 337:1733-45.
4. Ganem D., Prince A. M. Hepatitis B Virus Infection — Natural History and Clinical Consequences. N Engl J Med 2004; 350:1118-29.
5. Lok AS, McMahon BJ; Practice Guidelines Committee, American Association for the Study of Liver Diseases (AASLD). Chronic hepatitis B: update of recommendations. Hepatology. 2004; 39:857-61.
6. Lok AS, McMahon BJ; Practice Guidelines Committee, American Association for the Study of Liver Diseases. Chronic hepatitis B. Hepatology 2001; 34:1225-41

7. E B Keeffe and others. A Treatment Algorithm for the Management of Chronic Hepatitis B Virus Infection in the United States. Clinical Gastroenterology and Hepatology 2004; 2: 87-106.

8. Pawlotsky JM. Use and interpretation of hepatitis C virus diagnostic assays. Clin Liver Dis 2003; 7: 127-37.

9. Pawlotsky JM. Hepatitis C virus genetic variability: pathogenic and clinical implications. Clin Liver Dis 2003; 7: 45-66.

10. Geller SA. Hepatitis B and hepatitis C. Clin Liver Dis 2002; 6: 317-34.

24

Rajesh G

Management of Cholestasis

INTRODUCTION

'Cholestasis' is a clinical and biochemical syndrome characterized by pruritus, jaundice, and elevated serum alkaline phosphatase. It results from a generalized impairment in the secretion of bile.

EXTRAHEPATIC CHOLESTASIS

Extra-hepatic biliary obstruction usually results in acute cholestasis. Common benign causes include choledocholithiasis, biliary strictures, and biliary ascariasis. Malignant conditions leading to extra-hepatic biliary obstruction include periampullary carcinoma, hilar cholangiocarcinoma, gallbladder malignancy, metastatic deposits in liver, and metastases in porta hepatis. Secondary consequences of chronic cholestasis like malabsorption are rare in this subgroup whereas they are a hallmark of intrahepatic cholestasis. Most of these conditions will need endoscopic or surgical interventions.

INTRAHEPATIC CHOLESTASIS

These are cholestatic disorders that impair bile secretion within the liver. Jaundice and pruritus are often present whereas signs and symptoms of severe parenchymal injury e.g., ascites, coagulation defects, and encephalopathy, are typically absent. Common conditions, which present with intrahepatic cholestasis include viral hepatitis, alcoholic hepatitis, drug induced hepatitis, infiltrative disorders of the liver, cholestasis of pregnancy, primary biliary cirrhosis (PBC), primary sclerosing cholangitis (PSC), and various familial and metabolic conditions.

Physiology of Bile Formation and Flow

The functional unit of the liver is the lobule in which hepatocytes are arranged in plates along which blood flows from portal to central veins. Within these plates the small apical domains of adjacent hepatocytes form a tubular lumen, the canaliculus, which is the site of primary bile formation. From the canalicular network, bile flows to small ductules and subsequently to the larger ducts.

Mechanisms of bile formation are still incompletely understood. Hepatic bile is formed by the active transport of bile acids and other organic anions and electrolytes from the blood into the hepatocyte. In contrast with urine formation, bile flow is not dependent on hydrostatic forces, but driven by osmotic pressure of solutes secreted across the apical membrane of hepatocytes and bile duct epithelial cells. The main constituents of primary biliary fluid are bile salts; hence flow mainly depends on the extent of bile salt secretion.

Enterohepatic Circulation of Bile Salts

There occurs an enterohepatic circulation of bile, which conserves the endogenous bile acid pool.

Pathology

In intrahepatic cholestasis, bile may accumulate in hepatocytes, Kupffer cells, and bile canaliculi. Typically, retention of bile is most marked in centrilobular regions, probably because of the lobular gradient that determines bile flow. In severe cholestasis, bile infarcts may be seen. In later stages, bile ductular cells may proliferate and mononuclear cells may infiltrate the portal tracts. In chronic cholestasis, peri-portal fibrosis develops ultimately leading to portal-portal bridging and biliary cirrhosis.

Features favoring extra-hepatic cholestasis include bile plugging of interlobular bile ducts, bile stained infarcts, marked ductular proliferation, edema, and predominant polymorphonuclear infiltration of portal tracts.

Clinical Features of Cholestatic Syndrome

Feature	Clinical consequence
A. Primary: accummulation of biliary constituents	
Bilirubin	jaundice
Bile acids	pruritus
Pruritogenic substances	
Lipids	xanthoma, xanthelasmata
	hypercholesterolemia
	abnormal RBC morphology (echinocytes)
Copper	Kayser-Fleischer rings(rare)
Liver enzymes	alkaline phosphatase
	gamma-glutamyl transferase
	5' nucleotidase
B. Secondary: decreased intestinal content of bile acids, causing malabsorption of	
Dietary fat	steatorrhea
	weight loss
	? finger clubbing

Vitamin A	night blindness
Vitamin D	osteomalacia
Vitamin E	neuromyelopathy
Vitamin K	bleeding tendency

Primary Features

Jaundice is a common feature and typically follows the onset of symptoms such as pruritus and raised alkaline phosphatase by weeks, or even years, as with primary biliary cirrhosis.

Pruritus is a major but not invariable feature, occurring in 20-50% patients with jaundice and in most patients with primary biliary cirrhosis. It can have marked negative impact on the patient's quality of life and lead to significant sleep deprivation and depression and even suicidal ideation and actions. Severe intractable pruritus is an indication for liver transplantation. The pathogenesis of pruritus of cholestasis remains unclear. It is believed to result from accumulation of unidentified pruritogenic agents normally excreted in bile. A causative role for bile acids has been postulated. Bile acid binding agent cholestyramine often relieves the pruritus of cholestasis but may also relieve the pruritus of uremia and polycythemia rubra vera, where bile acids are not elevated. Histaminergic pathways may be involved, and the role of increased central opiate activity seems much more important than has previously been recognized. *Elevation of alkaline phosphatase (ALP)* is the most characteristic liver function abnormality in cholestasis and often the first clinical sign. This may be related in part to increased hepatic bile acid concentration. Gamma glutamyl transferase (GGT) is raised in most forms of cholestasis, exceptions being progressive familial intrahepatic cholestasis (PFIC) types1 and 2 and benign recurrent intrahepatic cholestasis (BRIC), where levels are usually normal.

Hyperlipidemia is a common feature with elevation in serum cholesterol and phospholipids; serum triglycerides may also be raised. Some of this cholesterol is incorporated into abnormal serum low-density lipoprotein (lipoprotein X). Lipoprotein X levels are usually higher in extra hepatic as compared to intrahepatic cholestasis; however this has little discriminatory value. Chronic hyperlipidemia results in cholesterol deposits in periorbital skin folds (xanthelasma) and in tendon sheaths, bony prominences, and peripheral nerves (xanthomas). Cholesterol also accumulates in RBC membranes, resulting in decreased membrane fluidity and deformed cells (echinocytes).

Copper accummulation may be a feature of cholestatic disorders like primary biliary cirrhosis and primary sclerosing cholangitis as bile is the major route of copper excretion. Although the copper concentration in liver may be elevated, serum copper and serum ceruloplasmin levels may be normal or high. Rarely in chronic cholestasis, corneal deposits with Kayser-Fleischer rings may be seen. Copper deposits in kidneys may lead to renal tubular acidosis, which is often a feature of PBC.

Secondary Complications

Fat malabsorption: Steatorrhea is common in advanced stages of chronic cholestatic liver disease and is primarily due to an inability to digest dietary lipids. Fat malabsorption often results in profound weight loss in advanced cholestasis. Patients with idiopathic cholestasis of pregnancy may have biochemical evidence of steatorrhea, which can result in failure to gain weight normally in pregnancy. Steatorrhea also results in decreased absorption of fat-soluble vitamins, and impaired calcium absorption due to the formation of insoluble calcium-fatty acid complexes (soaps).

Bone disease: The major bone disease in chronic cholestasis is osteoporosis. Between 10 and 40% of the patients have vertebral thinning and/or crush fractures on radiography. Bone mineral density correlates inversely with severity and duration of cholestasis.

Investigations

Ultrasound abdomen is the first investigation of choice to differentiate intra and extrahepatic cholestasis. Spiral CT scan of abdomen, magnetic resonance cholangiopancreatography (MRCP) and endoscopic ultrasound (EUS), are other imaging procedures employed in the work up of extrahepatic cholestasis. Endoscopic retrograde cholangiopancreatography (ERCP) has both diagnostic as well as therapeutic potential. Liver biopsy might be needed in many cases of intrahepatic cholestasis where the diagnosis remains elusive after appropriate laboratory and imaging procedures.

Disorders of Intrahepatic Bile Ducts

Several cholestatic disorders are associated with progressive damage to interlobular bile ducts. The diseases leading to obliteration of bile ducts are collectively known as *'vanishing bile duct syndrome'* or 'duct paucity' or 'ductopenia'. Histologically it can be diagnosed by presence of <0.5 bile ducts per portal triad when associated with normal numbers of hepatic arterioles and portal venules. Important causes of chronic cholestasis and bile duct paucity are PBC, PSC, autoimmune cholangiopathy, drugs and hepatic sarcoidosis.

Infiltrative and Metabolic Diseases of the Liver

Hodgkin's disease, non-Hodgkin's lymphoma, tuberculosis, histiocytosis-X, systemic mastocytosis, amyloidosis, cystic fibrosis, and alpha-1 anti-trypsin deficiency can all present as cholestatic syndrome.

Drug Induced Cholestasis

Cholestatic liver injury typically occurs one week to three months after initial exposure. The latency period may be as short as 24 hours if patient had previous exposure to the drug. Amiadarone, diclofenac, sulindac, and thiabendazole are known to have longer latency periods. Usual LFT pattern is of a near normal ALT, with a $>=2$ fold rise in ALP and an ALT/ALP ratio $\leq =2$. Skin rashes may be a feature with allopurinol or sulindac. Peripheral blood eosinophilia is seen in 10% cases. On withdrawal of offending drug, biochemical improvement is seen in about four weeks.

Cholestasis of Pregnancy

Idiopathic cholestasis of pregnancy (ICP) usually presents with pruritus as the first symptom in third trimester, but may be as early as six week. Jaundice usually follows 2-3 weeks later. Jaundice and pruritus are usually relieved within two weeks following delivery, although occasionally it can take several months. No medical therapy is needed if cholestasis is mild. UDCA can be tried. The mother should be monitored for signs of fetal distress and early delivery induced if this occurs. ICP should be differentiated from other causes of cholestasis in pregnancy like viral hepatitis, pre-eclampsia and HELLP syndrome, and fatty liver of pregnancy.

Cholestasis of Sepsis

In sepsis, bilirubin excretion may be affected by various mechanisms. There may often be deep jaundice (usually 75-80% is conjugated hyperbilirubinemia). Serum ALP is usually <3 times upper limit of normal. However pruritus is not a feature. Weil's disease may present with conjugated hyperbilirubinemia and mild elevation of liver enzymes. Brucellosis, malaria, typhoid and toxoplasmosis may also present with marked cholestasis but usually there is marked elevation in transaminases.

Benign Recurrent Intrahepatic Cholestasis (BRIC)

This is a rare condition with recurrent episodes of cholestasis lasting from 2-24 months (usually three months), interspersed with long asymptomatic periods with normal liver histology (even reported upto 30 years).

Miscellaneous Conditions

Total parenteral nutrition may be associated with cholestasis. Cholestasis develops in 10% of patients 1-2 weeks after coronary artery bypass surgery and is also seen occasionally after major abdominal surgery. Usually the picture is one of 'pure' intrahepatic cholestasis with normal serum aminotransferases.

Cholestasis in Infants and Children

Common causes include extrahepatic biliary atresia, neonatal hepatitis, progressive familial intrahepatic cholestasis (PFIC), galactosemia, and choledochal cyst.

Treatment of Pruritus of Cholestasis

The management of pruritus remains a challenge. Resins such as cholestyramine are the first line of therapy. In cases where cholestyramine has failed, rifampicin and antihistamines may be beneficial. Opiate antagonists hold great potential if opioid withdrawal-like syndromes can be avoided. Ursodeoxycholic acid has an advantage in not only relieving pruritus but also potentially retarding disease progression in PBC. Other agents such as propofol and S-adenosylmethionine remain experimental. The therapeutic options for relief of cholestatic pruritus are summarized below:

Medication	Dose/Mode of administration/Frequency
Cholestyramine	3.3-12 g/PO/day
Rifampicin	150 mg/PO/BD if serum bilirubin>3 mg/dL
	150 mg/PO/TDS if serum bilirubin<3 mg/dL
Naloxone	0.2 mcg/kg/min/IV infusion preceded by 0.4 mg IV bolus
Naltrexone	25 mg PO/BD day 1 followed by 50 mg PO daily
Ondansetron	8 mg IV followed by 8 mg PO/BD daily

A clear rationale for therapeutic interventions used to treat the cholestasis is not always apparent. The available modes of therapy, based on apparent effect expected, can be classified as:

a. *Removal of pruritogens from the body:* The most common medication used is the non-absorbable anion exchange resin, **cholestyramine. Colestipol**, and more recently **colesevalam** are also non-absorbable anion exchange resins that have been used for this purpose. These compounds bind anions, including bile acids in the small intestine, and decrease their enterohepatic circulation. The aim of resin treatment is to increase the fecal excretion of pruritogens. Cholestyramine powder (4 g/dose) in solution is administered before and after breakfast in patients who have gallbladders, based on the inference that pruritogens are stored in the gallbladder during overnight fast. The dose should not exceed 16 g/day. The most common side effects are bloating and constipation. Prothrombin time and serum vitamin concentrations should be monitored during prolonged administration of these agents, because treatment may result in malabsorption of fat-soluble vitamins. There should be sufficient time interval between resin administration and other medications to avoid interference with their absorption. Other measures which have been used to remove pruritogens from the circulation in patients with cholestasis include plasmapheresis, charcoal hemoperfusion, and extra corporeal albumin hemodialysis. Surgical approaches include **partial external diversion** of bile and **ileal diversion** in children with chronic cholestasis and pruritus.

b. *Antihistaminics:* Sedation seems to be the therapeutic value of anti-histaminics in the pruritus of cholestasis. This action is important if it enables the patient to sleep. Hence their use without some clear benefit does not seem justified.

c. *Hepatic enzyme inducers:* **Rifampicin** at doses of 300-450 mg/day or 10 mg/kg has been reported to improve the pruritus of cholestasis secondary to primary biliary cirrhosis. Rifampicin can be hepatotoxic at doses used to manage pruritus; hence follow-up liver function tests are necessary when this drug is used. Phenobarbitol and flumezenil are other enzyme inducers, which have been used.

d. *Opiate antagonists:* **Naloxone** as continuous infusion 0.2 mcg/kg/hr. preceded by 0.4 mg IV bolus results in significant relief of pruritus. It can be used in emergency cases such as those associated with self-injury in desperately pruritic patients. **Naltrexone**, an orally bioavailable opiate antagonist is used at doses of 50 mg/day. Naltrexone can be hepatotoxic and its metabolites can accumulate in decompensated liver disease; thus, in these patients it should be used with caution. However in the clinical context, generally pruritus is seen to cease as hepatocellular function deteriorates. To minimize the potential occurrence of opiate withdrawal-like reaction in patients with cholestasis, these agents should be introduced at a low dose. Continuous infusions of naloxone can be started at dose of 0.002 mcg/kg/min and gradually increased to 0.8 mcg/kg/min according to response of the patient. Subsequently, treatment with oral naltrexone can be started in low dose (e.g. one fourth tablet, 12.5mg) and naloxone can be discontinued.

e. *Serotonin antagonists:* Ondansetron has been used to treat the pruritus of cholestasis.

f. *Corticosteroids:* They are indicated in viral hepatitis with prolonged cholestasis and can cause rapid fall in serum bilirubin and relieve pruritus in about 70% cases. However use of steroids in chronic hepatitis B may lead to increased viral replication.

g. *Miscellaneous treatments:* Propofol, at subhypnotic doses is effective in ameliorating the pruritus of cholestasis. S-adenosylmethionine has been reported to reverse the cholestatic effects of several experimental agents and to ameliorate the pruritus of cholestasis. It has anti-depressant properties and possibly central specific or non-specific anti-pruritic effects. Lignocaine, antioxidants, androgens and phototherapy have been found to be useful. Lignocaine may provide relief by its anesthetic properties because pruritus is a nociceptive stimulus.

Ursodeoxycholic Acid (UDCA)

It is a hydrophilic bile acid useful in several cholestatic disease like primary biliary cirrhosis, primary sclerosing cholangitis, cystic fibrosis, idiopathic cholestasis of pregnancy, drug induced cholestasis, benign recurrent intrahepatic cholestasis, progressive familial cholestasis, etc. The dose of UDCA is 13-15mg/kg/day in 2-3 divided doses. It has many postulated actions including choleresis, displacement of hydrophobic hepatotoxic bile acids from endogenous bile acid pool, immunomodulation, cytoprotection and membrane stabilization.

Treatment of Secondary Consequences

The steatorrhoea of cholestasis can usually be corrected by a low fat diet (<40 g/day), and medium chain triglyceride supplementation. In patients who do not respond, the possibilities of pancreatic dysfunction and jejunal villous atrophy should be considered, because pancreatic enzyme replacement or withdrawal of gluten may then be of benefit.

The role of routine vitamin A supplementation is controversial. Periodic assessment for night blindness should be performed if cholestasis is severe. In such patients, oral vitamin A (25000 to 50000 units/day) will return vitamin A levels to normal and may improve vision.

Not all patients with cholestasis need vitamin D supplementation because serum levels of 1,25-hydroxyvitamin D are usually normal, and osteomalacia is uncommon. However, patients with long-standing cholestasis who have a poor diet, and get little exposure to sunlight, should receive at least 100000 units of vitamin D_2 or D_3 IM every month, or 40000 units (1 mg) of oral vitamin D_2 or D_3 daily. The dose should be adjusted so as to keep the serum 25-hydroxyvitamin D level in the normal range. An alternative approach is to administer 50-100 mcg of 25-hydroxyvitamin D daily.

Osteoporosis associated with cholestasis does not respond to vitamin D. However, patients with cholestasis and osteoporosis, even with normal serum levels of vitamin D, tend to have impaired calcium absorption, possibly from fat malabsorption. In these patients, a low fat diet containing at least 1.5 g of calcium per day is recommended. Other agents include bisphosphonates, hormonal replacement therapy, and raloxifene.

In children with cholestasis and established neurological deficit due to vitamin E deficiency, clinical improvement following repletion is modest, and routine supplementation after the age of three years is recommended. In adults with cholestasis, routine vitamin E replacement is probably not necessary, but patients should be monitored for development of neurological signs and symptoms. If the cholestasis is moderate, deficiency may be corrected by parenteral vitamin E (20 mg IM twice monthly) or by large doses of oral vitamin E.

When the coagulopathy of vitamin K deficiency is mild, it is seldom a clinical problem and only requires correction by parenteral vitamin K (10 mg) when liver biopsy or surgery is contemplated.

SUGGESTED READING

1. Gleeson D, Boyen J. Intrahepatic cholestasis. In BircherJ, Benhamou JP, Mc Intyre N, Rizzelto M, Rodes J (eds). Oxford textbook of Clinical Hepatology, 2nd ed., Oxford University Press, 1999; Oxford.
2. Cholestasis. In: Sherlock S and Dooley J (eds). Disease of the liver and biliary system. 11th ed, Blackwell, Oxford.
3. Bergasa NV. An Approach to the management of pruritus of cholestasis. Clin Liver Dis. 2004; 8:55-66.
4. Trauner M., Meier P. J., Boyer J. L. N Mechanisms of Disease: Molecular Pathogenesis of cholestasis. Engl J Med 1998; 339:1217-1227, Oct 22, 1998
5. The pathology of cholestasis. Semin Liver Dis 2004 Feb; 24(1): 21-42
6. Elferink RO. Cholestasis. Gut 2003 May;52 Suppl 2:ii42-8

25

Thomas Alexander

Cirrhosis Liver: Management and Prevention of Complications

INTRODUCTION

Cirrhosis liver is a distinct pathological entity that has diffuse fibrosis and regenerative nodule formation as its hallmarks. Generally considered irreversible, early stages are often silent and may be diagnosed only by a liver biopsy. Cirrhosis is the end result of a variety of insults to the liver, some of which are preventable. With complications like ascites, GI bleed, hepatic encephalopathy and hepatocellular carcinoma, it is a major cause of morbidity and mortality.

ETIOLOGY

Alcohol and chronic viral hepatitis are undoubtedly the major causes of cirrhosis, worldwide. However as mentioned above any chronic injury to the liver can lead to cirrhosis. Multiple etiologic factors (e.g., HCV + alcohol) may occur in a patient; when the effect is additive.

The common causes include:

- Alcohol
- Chronic hepatitis B
- Chronic hepatitis C
- Chronic hepatitis D
- Autoimmune hepatitis
- Wilson's disease
- Hemochromatosis
- Alpha 1 antitrypsin deficiency
- Budd Chiari syndrome
- Drug induced
- Biliary obstruction
- Cardiac failure

PATHOLOGY

Fibrosis and nodule formation are the essential components.

CLASSIFICATION

Morphological: Micronodular (nodules < 3 mm), macronodular (nodules > 3 mm), mixed.

Etiological: Alcoholic, posthepatitic, metabolic, biliary, drug induced, cardiac.

CLINICAL FEATURES

A patient with early cirrhosis may be completely asymptomatic with no abnormalities on clinical examination. Later on *jaundice, edema,* and *coagulopathy* often occur. These are due to a decrease in the quantum of functioning hepatocyte mass. *Splenomegaly* and *gastroesophageal varices* are other common manifestations and these are due to fibrosis and distortion in the vasculature causing portal hypertension. *Ascites* and *encephalopathy* are due to both factors.

GENERAL EXAMINATION

Poor nutritional status, clubbing, white nails, pedal edema, spider naevii, palmar erythema, gynecomastia, testicular atrophy, Dupuytren's contracture and parotid enlargement are found in alcoholics.

Neurological: Altered mental status, flaps. (asterixis) in hepatic encephalopathy.

ABDOMEN

The liver may be normal, increased (particularly left lobe) or decreased in size. Splenomegaly, ascites, umbilical hernia and abdominal wall collaterals are other physical findings.

The term decompensated cirrhosis is used when jaundice, pedal edema, ascites or variceal bleed develop. Gallstones, peptic ulcer disease and infections are more common among cirrhotics. Due to changes in intrarenal circulation, there is a predisposition for renal failure.

Diagnosis

After a thorough history and physical examination, the minimum work up for a patient with cirrhosis would include the following:
a. Imaging: A good ultrasound study of the abdomen – size of the liver, coarse echotexture, SOL, splenomegaly, free fluid
b. Liver function test and prothrombin time – PT elevated, low albumin and increased globulin
c. Blood routine, platelet count, renal functions – anemia, low platelets, abnormal renal functions (in advanced cirrhosis)
d. Viral markers for hepatitis B and C
e. Upper GI endoscopy: to assess varices (esophageal and gastric)
Additional imaging like CT scan abdomen or liver / spleen radionuclide scan; etiological tests like se.ceruloplasmin and copper studies (Wilson's); iron studies (hemochromatosis); autoantibodies (autoimmune), etc. would depend on the clinical scenario. A liver biopsy is the definitive test, but may not be required in many cases, as the diagnosis will be obvious.

Prognosis: Depends on child's grading, being best in child's A and worst in C.

Child-Pugh grading: A clinico-laboratory score is compiled as follows

Parameter	Score 1	Score 2	Score 3
S. Bilirubin (mg/dl)	< 2.0	2.0 – 3.0	> 3.0
S. Albumin (g/dl)	> 3.5	2.8 – 3.5	< 2.8

Prothrombin time (difference in seconds)	< 3	3 – 6	> 6
Ascites	None	Mild–moderate	Gross
Encephalopathy	None	Mild	Severe
Child's A	Total score 5 or 6		
Child's B	Total score 7, 8 or 9		
Child's C	Total score 10 or greater		

General Management of Cirrhosis

- Prevent ongoing insult e.g., stop alcohol, eradicate or suppress hepatitis B / C activity
- Adequate balanced diet with at least 1 gm of protein/day
- Correction of vitamin deficiencies
- Primary prophylaxis of variceal bleed (pharmacological agents e.g., beta blockers)
- Vaccination against hepatitis B (in the non infected, nonimmune)
- Sodium restriction if pedal edema, ascites present
- Remember that surgery in patients with cirrhosis carries high morbidity and mortality (particularly in Child's C)

Complications

1. Ascites
2. Portal hypertensive hemorrhage
3. Hepatic encephalopathy
4. Hepatorenal syndrome
5. Hepatocellular cancer.

Ascites

Accumulation of peritoneal fluid is due to a combination of increased pressure in the portal system along with decreased oncotic pressure, secondary to decreased se.albumin concentration.

Detection: A fluid thrill will be present if the ascites is tense. Shifting dullness requires about 1500 ml of fluid. An ultrasound study of the abdomen is the most sensitive test and can pick up as little as 100 ml of fluid.

Prognostic significance of ascites in cirrhosis: Fifty percent of cirrhotics will develop ascites within 10 years and there is a 50% mortality within two years of onset of ascites.

An ascitic tap to analyze the fluid and exclude infection is of paramount importance.

Paracentesis–Practical Aspects

a. Choose either of the lower quadrants
b. Avoid surgical scars
c. Use sterile precautions
d. 22G needle for diagnostic tap and 18G for therapeutic tap
e. Use long needle (LP needle) in obese patients
f. Use Z tract technique in tense ascites to prevent leak from aspiration site
g. Insert the needle slowly with intermittent aspiration

Ascitic Fluid Analysis

Albumin, WBC total and differential count should be done in all patients.

Ascitic fluid culture, protein, cytology and adenosine deaminase (for tuberculosis) should be done where appropriate.

Ascitic Fluid Culture

Directly innoculate 5 ml of fluid into bottles of glucose broth and bile broth, just like sending a blood culture. The positivity rate by this method in infected specimens is over 90%.

SAAG (Serum Ascites Albumin Gradient)

This is obtained by subtracting ascitic fluid albumin from se. albumin.

A value > 1.1 indicates the presence of portal hypertension with 97% accuracy.

SAAG Classification of Ascites

High Gradient (>1.1 g/dl)	Low Gradient (<1.1 g/dl)
Cirrhosis	Peritoneal carcinomatosis
Alcoholic hepatitis	Tuberculous peritonitis
Budd Chiari syndrome	Nephrotic syndrome
Massive liver metastasis	Pancreatic ascites
Fulminant hepatic failure	Biliary ascites
"Mixed" ascites	Post-op lymphatic leak
Cardiac ascites	Ischemic bowel
	Serositis

Pitfalls in SAAG estimation

1. Serum and ascitic fluid samples ideally should be taken within the same hour; or at least on the same day.
2. Systemic hypotension and hyperglobulinemia can lead to a narrow gradient.

General Dietary Principles

Renal sodium retention is the fundamental pathogenetic factor in the development of cirrhotic ascites. Hence sodium restriction is the key to its control. Every gram of sodium retains 200 ml of fluid. One gram of salt contains 0.4 g of sodium.

a. All food to be cooked without salt
b. Allow 2 g salt / day
c. Omit pickles, salted, canned food
d. Omit items with baking powder or baking soda (e.g., bread, papad).
e. Predominantly vegetarian diet since most animal proteins have high sodium content
f. Allow 1 to 1.5 l of fluids/day (do not encourage excessive intake of barley water, etc.)

Diuretics

Initiate with spironolactone and frusemide. The usual dose is spironolactone 100 mg + frusemide 40 mg. This can be progressively increased if required, while monitoring se. electrolytes till a maximum dose of 400 mg spironolactone + 160 mg. frusemide is achieved.

Side Effects of Diuretics

a. Gynecomastia—switch to amiloride (10 mg amiloride = 100 mg spironolactone)
b. Electrolyte imbalance
c. Renal failure
d. Hepatic encephalopathy
e. Hepatorenal syndrome

Refractory Ascites

Definition: Uncontrolled Ascites despite adequate sodium restriction and maximum dose of diuretics (as above). Inadequate compliance with sodium restriction is often the cause.

Treatment Options

a. Large volume paracentesis
- This is the most practical method.
- Remove 5 litres or more at one sitting
- Safe procedure when there is associated pedal edema
- When there is no pedal edema colloid replacement is essential: 125 ml Hemaccel for every litre of fluid removed or 6 grams of albumin per litre of fluid
- Contraindications: Child's C status; se. creatinine >3 mg

b. Peritoneo-venous shunt (Le Veen shunt): of historical interest

c. TIPS (Transjuglar Intrahepatic Portosystemic Shunt): an expensive short term modality, as a bridge to transplantation

d. Liver transplantation (See Fig. 25.1).

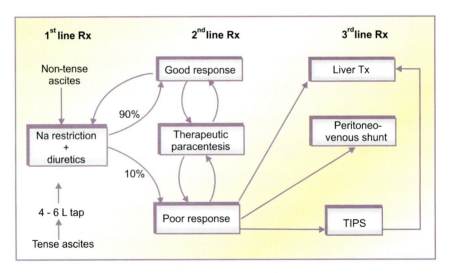

Fig. 25.1: Algorithm for treatment of cirrhotic ascites

Complications of Ascites

a. Infection
b. Pleural effusion (hepatic hydrothorax)
c. Abdominal wall hernias
d. Tense ascites with consequent respiratory embarrassment

Ascitic Fluid Infections

a. Spontaneous bacterial peritonitis
b. Monomicrobial non neutrocytic ascites
c. Culture negative neutrocytic ascites

Spontaneous Bacterial Peritonitis (SBP)

This can quickly kill a patient, and the clinician should always be on the lookout for this complication. A single episode of SBP in a patient is sufficient indication for a liver transplant listing, irrespective of the Child Pugh grade.

Definition: a. Ascitic fluid neutrophil count > 250/cmm
b. Ascitic fluid culture positive
c. No intra abdominal sepsis

Clinical features: May be very subtle with altered mental status only. Abdominal pain, tenderness and fever are not as prominent as in secondary bacterial peritonitis. A high index of suspicion is necessary, and ascitic fluid should be routinely examined in any cirrhotic who suddenly worsens. Injection cefotaxime 2 gm intravenously q 8 h for 5 days is the standard treatment.

Primary prophylaxis with norfloxacin (400 mg bd) is offered to all hospitalized patients, whose ascitic fluid protein (not albumin) is less than 1 gm.

Portal Hypertension Associated GI Bleed

The most common site of acute bleed is from esophageal varices followed by gastric varices. Colorectal and ectopic varices are other sites. Portal hypertensive gastropathy is a cause for chronic blood loss, rather than acute.

Variceal bleed usually presents as hematemesis and/or melena, depending on the site and rapidity of bleed. Prompt hemodynamic resuscitation is the all—important first step. Pharmacological agents like octreotide (100 mcg IV bolus, followed by 50 mcg/hr) or somatostatin (250 mcg IV bolus followed by 250 mcg/hr) are useful in reducing portal pressures. Vasopressin, a much older drug, is also effective in reducing portal pressures, but has a potential for significant toxicity. Precipitation of coronary ischemia is its most dreaded complication.

The diagnosis of the bleeding site is determined by endoscopy, and definitive endoscopic therapy (variceal ligation, sclerotherapy, glue injection) is delivered at the same time. (See chapter on management of upper GI bleed). A Sengstaken-Blakemore tube (or one of its variants like the Minnesota tube) is used for mechanical tamponade if bleeding persists despite pharmacological agents.

Transjugular Intrahepatic Portosystemic Shunt (TIPS) or emergency surgery (esophageal transection or shunt surgery) are kept as rescue measures.

The prognosis of variceal bleed is grave. Though earlier mortality rates were reported to be about 35%, with the increased use of pharmacological agents to acutely reduce portal hypertension and better endoscopic treatment modalities, the mortality rate has decreased to about 10%. Any patient with a variceal bleed should be given parenteral antibiotic prophylaxis with ciprofloxacin on admission itself, as there is a high risk for sepsis.

It is important to realize that a major problem is that of rebleed and hence endoscopic therapy should continue until all varices are fully obliterated. Concomitantly, secondary prophylaxis with propranolol (in those without contraindications to the drug) should also be given. Propranolol should be given in a dose, such that the resting pulse rate is 60/minute.

The primary prophylaxis of a variceal bleed is important, and at present propranolol or endoscopic variceal ligation (where the drug is contraindicated or poorly tolerated) are the recommended modalities.

Hepatic Encephalopathy

Hepatic encephalopathy, also known as portosystemic encephalopathy, is a reversible neurologic dysfunction that occurs in liver disease.

The changes are graded as follows

Clinical stage	Intellectual function	Neuromuscular function
Subclinical	Normal examination; work or driving may be impaired	Slight changes on psychometric or number connection tests
Stage 1	Impaired attention, irritability, depression or personality change	Tremor, inco-ordination, apraxia
Stage 2	Drowsiness, behavioral change, poor memory, sleep disorders	Flap, ataxia, slowing or slurring of speech
Stage 3	Confusion, disorientation, somnolence, amnesia	Hyperreflexia, rigidity, clonus, nystagmus
Stage 4	Stupor and coma	Dilated pupils, decerebrate posturing, oculocephalic reflex, no response to stimuli

Putative pathogenetic mechanisms in hepatic encephalopathy include toxins like ammonia and mercaptans, alteration in gamma amino butyric acid (GABA) related neuronal transmission, and false neurotransmitters.

Common precipitating factors include azotemia, use of sedatives, GI bleed, electrolyte imbalance (particularly hypokalemia), infection (especially SBP), constipation and increased dietary protein.

The clinical diagnosis is based on the table above. It is important to realize that unilateral or focal signs are not a feature of hepatic encephalopathy. Arterial ammonia levels and EEG changes, though described, are not generally routinely done and the diagnosis is often made clinically.

Management of hepatic encephalopathy is dealt with in a separate chapter.

The prognosis depends on whether there is a remediable precipitating factor. Absence of such a factor(s) indicates a poor prognosis, because it implies a grossly deficient functioning hepatocellular mass.

Hepatorenal Syndrome

This is functional kidney failure, without structural damage, in advanced cirrhosis liver. The condition is progressive. The pathogenesis is thought to be altered hemodynamics of renal circulation with vasoconstriction of the arterioles of renal cortex. The result is decreased glomerular filtration and renal flow.

The onset may be precipitated by hyponatremia, hypokalemia or by hepatic encephalopathy. There will be oliguria (< 500 ml/day), serum creatinine >2.5 mg/dL, urinary sodium concentration < 10mEq/l, and a concentrated urine. The condition is often irreversible and carries a very high mortality. Infusions of albumin and terlipressin bring about temporary improvement. The only definitive treatment is liver transplantation.

Hepatocellular Carcinoma (HCC)

This is a dreaded complication of cirrhosis, which is often diagnosed only at a late stage. Cirrhosis per se can be considered to be a preneoplastic lesion. Chronic hepatitis B and C, and hemochromatosis associated cirrhosis carry an exceptionally high risk. Chronic hepatitis B can cause hepatocellular carcinoma without the development of cirrhosis.

Manifestations: Early stages are often asymptomatic and the clinician should always suspect the development of an HCC when there is a sudden change in a cirrhotic's condition. Upper abdominal pain, asthenia, anorexia, weight loss, increasing ascites and jaundice indicate advanced stages of the disease. Sometimes the patient may present with paraneoplastic manifestations like hypoglycemia, polycythemia, hypercalcemia, watery diarrhea, polymyositis or neuropathy.

Clinical examination might reveal a firm to hard tender liver. A bruit is a useful clinical clue. Jaundice and ascites may be present.

The diagnosis is generally made by an imaging study and presence of tumor markers (usually elevated se. alpha feto-protein—AFP). A fine needle aspiration cytology or biopsy may be required at times.

Management options include resection (if small tumor with good liver status), percutaneous chemical ablation with absolute alcohol or 50% acetic acid, chemoembolization, other ablative methods like radiofrequency heating, microwave cooking, etc. A small HCC in a cirrhotic would be an indication for a liver transplant. (see chapter on GI tumors also).

The management of a cirrhotic with all attendant potentially fatal complications can be a daunting challenge. Newer and better drugs and other tools to manage these, are the focus of constant research. However it is imperative that the preventable causes, particularly alcohol and hepatitis B, be eliminated by effective public information campaigns.

SUGGESTED READING

1. Benvegnu L, Gios M, Boccato S and Alberti A. Natural history of compensated viral cirrhosis: A prospective study on the incidence and hierarchy of major complications. Gut 2004; 53:744.
2. Runyon BA: Care of patients with ascites. N Engl J Med 1994; 330:337.
3. Jalan R and Hayes PC. UK guidelines on the management of variceal hemorrhage in cirrhotic patients. Gut 2000;46 (Suppl 3) 46:1.
4. North Italian Endoscopic Club for the Study and Treatment of Esophageal varices. Prediction of the first variceal hemorrhage in patients with cirrhosis of the liver and Esophageal varices
5. N Engl J Med 1988; 319:983.
6. Kudo M: Imaging diagnosis of hepatocellular carcinoma and premalignant/ borderline lesions. Semin Liver Dis 1999; 19:291.
7. Gines P, Cardenas A, Arroyo V, Rodes J. Management of cirrhosis and ascites N Engl J Med. 2004 15; 350: 1646-54.
8. Bosch J, Garcia-Pagan JC. Complications of cirrhosis. I. Portal hypertension. J Hepatol. 2000; 32(1 Suppl): 141-56.
9. Arroyo V, Jimenez W. Complications of cirrhosis. II. Renal and circulatory dysfunction. Lights and shadows in an important clinical problem. J Hepatol 2000; 32 (1 Suppl): 157-70.
10. Garcia-Tsao G. Current management of the complications of cirrhosis and portal hypertension: variceal hemorrhage, ascites, and spontaneous bacterial peritonitis. Gastroenterology, 2001; 120:726-48.

26

Narayanan VA

Alcohol and the Liver

INTRODUCTION

Alcohol induced liver disease (ALD) is a major cause of illness and death in India. Alcohol consumption in India is increasing to alarming levels and there is a direct correlation between liver related mortality and per capita ethanol consumption. Fatty liver is the most common form of alcoholic liver disease and it is reversible with abstinence. More serious forms of alcoholic liver disease are alcoholic hepatitis, characterized by inflammation of liver, and cirrhosis liver characterized by progressive scarring of liver tissue. Both conditions are fatal and treatment options are limited. During the past five years, research has significantly increased our understanding of the mechanism of alcoholic liver damage.

PREVALENCE OF ALCOHOLIC LIVER DISEASE

Approximately 10-35% of heavy drinkers develop alcoholic hepatitis and 10 to 20% cirrhosis liver.

Alcohol equivalent

Whisky	30 ml	10 gm
Wine	100 ml	10 gm
Beer	250 ml	10 gm

Less than 40 gm ethanol daily is perhaps a safe limit and more than that for long time carries risk for occurrence of liver disease. Susceptibility to ALD differs considerably among individuals and only a small proportion of heavy drinkers develop liver disease. Genetic polymorphism of the cell types may be a factor influencing the susceptibility. Nutritional factors like high fat, low calorie diet promote liver damage in alcohol fed rats and high amounts of PUFA (Poly unsaivraied fatty acids) promote the development of cirrhosis in animals. Women develop alcoholic liver disease after consuming lower levels of alcohol for a shorter period of time compared to males. The mechanism that underlies the gender related difference is not known. Co-infection with hepatitis C virus accentuates liver injury. Alcohol consumption can increase the adverse effects of drugs. For example, acetaminophen has been associated with severe liver damage in alcohol drinkers.

MECHANISM OF LIVER DAMAGE

Fatty Liver

Alcohol related steatosis can occur as microvesicular steatosis (small fat globules inside liver cells) or macrovesicular, mostly in zone three, surrounding the central vein. The mechanism by which fat accumulates in hepatocytes has been unraveled by recent research. Ethanol alters intramitochondrial redox potential via generation of NADH by alcohol dehydrogenase. In addition, ethanol metabolism causes oxidative stress. This impairs B-oxidation of fatty acids and tricarboxylic acid cycle activity resulting in elevated intrahepatocellular free fatty acids and fat globules accumulate in hepatocytes. Also ethanol upregulates lipogenic enzymes and inhibits the endogenous fatty acid receptor, which plays a role in fatty acid degradation. Oxidative stress causes increased lipid peroxidation and by a combination of all these factors accumulation of fat occurs.

Alcoholic Hepatitis

If ethanol consumption continues the steatosis may progress to steatohepatitis. Persistence of alcohol consumption can cause acute hepatitis by numerous mechanisms. ATP depletion occurs due to oxidative stress and leads to inflammation. Alcohol also causes increase in gut permeability leading to raised endotoxin levels. Endotoxemia has been consistently shown in alcoholic liver disease. This activates hepatic stellate cells to produce pro-inflammatory cytokines and liver cell necrosis occurs.

Alcoholic Cirrhosis

The Figure 26.1 summarizes the mechanism of fibrosis leading to cirrhosis of liver.

PATHOLOGY

Fatty change can be quantitated by histopathology—less than 25% of liver cells containing fat in stage I, 25-50% in stage II, 50-75% in stage III and more than 75% liver cells containing fat is stage IV. Fat mostly appears in centrizonal and midzonal areas.

Balloon degeneration, acidophilic bodies, mallory bodies, giant mitochondria, fat globules, sclerosing hyaline necrosis and polymorphonuclear infiltration are the characteristic features of histopathology of alcoholic hepatitis. Mallory bodies are purplish red intracytoplasmic inclusions. Varying degrees of fibrosis also may be present in alcoholic hepatitis. Fibrosis progresses and regenerating nodules appear. Then it becomes alcoholic cirrhosis liver.

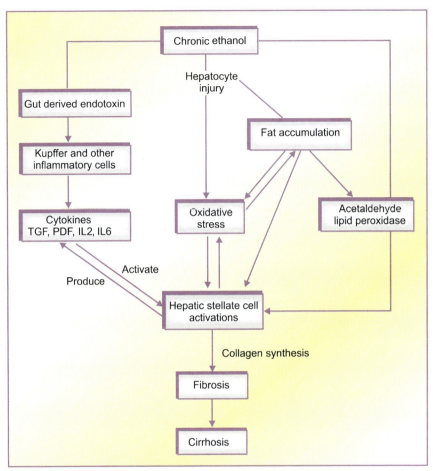

Fig. 26.1: Algorithm showing the pathogenesis of alcoholic liver cirrhosis

CLINICAL FEATURES

Fatty liver is often asymptomatic. Some patients have vague right upper quadrant heaviness and easy fatiguability. Ultrasound scan or CT scan shows fatty changes in liver and by ultrasound it can be quantitated. The only biochemical abnormality in fatty liver is raised GGT (gamma glutamyl transferase), which is specific for alcoholic disease. If alcohol is stopped, these changes may reverse.

Alcoholic hepatitis presents with easy fatiguability, nutritional deficiency features and jaundice. Abdominal pain may be present. Some patients may have cholestatic features.

Cirrhosis liver presents with features of hepatic dysfunction and portal hypertension. GI bleed, ascites and jaundice are the features. Spleen may be palpable. Veins may be present on the anterior abdominal wall. The stigmata of liver insufficiency such as palmar erythema, parotid enlargement, gynecomastia Dupuytren's contracture are all often seen. The liver is moderately enlarged and firm. Spleen is usually small compared to post hepatitis cirrhosis. Ten to 15% of patients develop hepatocellular carcinoma.

INVESTIGATIONS

Urinalysis, hemogram, platelet count, INR, electrolytes, LFT, renal function tests, USG abdomen, AFP (alpha feto-protein), CT scan and upper GI endoscopy for varices are the usual investigations ordered. The investigations help to establish the diagnosis and exclude other etiologies. Serological markers are done to exclude co-existing viral B, or C infection. Elevated GGT is an early feature even in the absence of other liver function abnormalities. Low albumin, prolonged INR, grossly raised serum bilirubin all indicate severe disease. Refractory ascites, which rapidly re-accumulates, serum albumin persistently low despite albumin infusions, hyponatremia, renal involvement and INR more than three, all indicate end-stage liver disease. USG/ CT scan and AFP estimation help to monitor development of superadded malignancy. Endoscopy is done to grade varices and in early stage, there may be only portopathy.

TREATMENT

Cessation of alcohol intake and nutritious balanced diet are the most important aspects in the treatment. Vitamin and mineral supplements should be given to make up deficiencies. Without these any other therapy will not be effective. Early fatty liver may reverse and cure can be achieved by complete abstinence.

In alcoholic hepatitis the treatment options are limited. Ursodeoxycholic acid 300 mg twice daily or silimarin 140 mg daily are conventionally given. The role of steroids is controversial. In severe alcoholic hepatitis, when no co-existing infection exists and renal functions are normal with no ascites, steroids may be tried in conventional dosage. Other drugs tried are pentoxyphylline in dosage of 1200 mg daily and colchicine in 1 gm dosage. Albumin dialysis (MARS) also has been tried in severe cases.

Variceal bleeding is treated in the conventional way. Ascites is treated with salt restriction, aldactone and frusemide. Hyponatremia in end-stage is common and difficult to correct. End-stage liver disease will require liver transplantation.

CONCLUSION

The single most important prognostic factor is the patient's ability to stop drinking alcohol. Once ascites develops, only 50% of patients survive five years.

SUGGESTED READING

1. Tig H, Diehl AM. Cytokines in alcoholic and non-alcoholic steatohepatitis. N Engl J Med 2000; 343: 1467-76.
2. Arfeel GE, Marsano L, Mendez C, Bentley F, Meclan CJ. Advances in alcoholic liver disease. Best Pract Res Clinicar Gastroenterology 2003; 17: 625-47.
3. Blendis LM. The treatment of alcoholic liver disease. Alimentary pharmacology and therapeutics 1992; 6:541-8.
4. Brunt EM. Alcoholic and non-alcoholic steatohepatitis. Clin Liver Dis 2002; 6: 399-420
5. Grove J, Daly AK, Bassendine MF, Day CP. Association of a tumor necrosis factor promoter polymorphism with susceptibility to alcoholic steatohepatitis. Hepatology 1997; 26:143-6.
6. French SW. Rationale for therapy for alcoholic liver disease. Gastroenterology 1995; 109:617-20.
7. Leevy CM, Leevy CB.Liver disease in the alcoholic. Gastroenterology 1993; 105:294-6.

27

Anil John

Non-Alcoholic Steatohepatitis

INTRODUCTION

In 1980, Ludwig and colleagues gave the name non-alcoholic steatohepatitis (NASH) to a clinico pathological syndrome that occurred in diabetic females who denied alcohol use but in whom the hepatic histology was consistent with alcoholic hepatitis. The liver biopsy specimens were characterized by the presence of macrovesicular fatty changes and evidence of focal lobular necrosis with mixed inflammatory infiltrates and mallory bodies. Fibrosis was present in most specimens and some patients had cirrhosis. The authors concluded that the cause of NASH was unknown and no effective therapy existed. However progress had been made in our understanding to the extent that it is not an entirely benign clinical entity but rather a common disease with potentially serious clinical sequelae.

Non-alcoholic steatohepatitis (NASH) represents only a stage within the wide spectrum of non-alcoholic fatty liver disease (NAFLD). The spectrum could range from simple steatosis to steatohepatitis, advanced fibrosis and cirrhosis.

DEFINITION

Non-alcoholic steatohepatitis (NASH) is defined as the presence of macro vesicular fatty changes with lobular inflammation in the absence of significant alcohol abuse in amounts likely to cause liver damage (usually less than 20 g/day).

EPIDEMIOLOGY

Both fatty liver and NASH have been reported in all age groups including children. The highest prevalence is between 40 and 49 years of age. Though studies published before 1990 emphasized that NASH occurs mostly in women, most recent studies have shown that NASH occurs with equal frequency in men as well.

Using the presence of hyperechoic liver on ultrasound as a diagnostic criteria, 14% of 2574 randomly selected Japanese subjects had fatty liver. Since ultrasound can detect only fat, not all of these patients had documented inflammation to make a diagnosis of NASH. Autopsy studies demonstrate NASH in 18.5% of obese subjects and 2.7% of normal weight people. In US 20% of apparently normal people evaluated as donors for living related liver transplantation had fatty liver and 7.5% had NASH. The above figures do suggest that NASH is not an uncommon clinical entity.

Obesity defined as body mass index (more than 30 kg/m^2) is associated with NASH. Type II diabetes mellitus is associated with both obesity and NASH.

There is evidence that NASH often represents the hepatic component of a metabolic syndrome characterized by obesity, type II diabetes mellitus, insulin resistance, hyperinsulinemia, hypertriglyceridemia and hypertension. Hypertriglyceridemia rather than hypercholesterolemia may increase the risk of non-alcoholic fatty liver disease.

Secondary Causes for Fatty Liver

Non-alcoholic fatty liver with or without hepatitis should be differentiated from secondary causes because these conditions have distinctly different pathogenesis and out comes. NASH should be a diagnosis of exclusion, i.e. all secondary causes for fatty liver should be excluded. Some examples of secondary causes for fatty liver are given below.

Nutritional	Protein calorie malnutrition Total parenteral nutrition Rapid weight loss GI surgery for obesity
Drugs	Glucocorticoids Amiodarone Tetracycline
Metabolic causes	Acute fatty liver of pregnancy Lipodystrophy Dyseta lipoproteinemia Wilson's disease
Miscellaneous causes	Inflammatory bowel disease HIV Infection HCV Infection Environmental hepatotoxins like petrochemicals and phosphorus

CLINICAL MANIFESTATIONS

Most patients have no symptoms or signs of liver disease at the time of diagnosis. However some patients report fatigue or malaise and a sensation of fullness or discomfort in the right side of the upper abdomen. Hepatomegaly is the only physical finding in most patients. Acanthosis nigricans may be found in children with fatty liver.

LABORATORY ABNORMALITIES

Mild to moderately elevated serum ALT/AST or both are common and is the only lab abnormality most often seen in patients with NASH. The ratio of AST to ALT is usually less than one but the ratio increases as fibrosis advances leading to the loss of its diagnostic accuracy. Serum alkaline phosphatase and gamma glutamyl transferase or both are usually normal but mild elevations can be consistent with diagnosis of NASH. Features like hypoalbuminemia, prolonged PT and increased bilirubin would signify the progression of NASH to fibrosis and cirrhosis. Elevated serum ferritin and transferrin saturation levels can be seen in some patients. However hepatic iron index and hepatic iron levels are usually in the normal range.

IMAGING STUDIES

On ultrasound, fatty infiltrations of liver produce a diffuse increase in echogenicity as compared to kidneys. Ultrasound has a sensitivity of 90% and specificity of 93% in detecting steatosis and is an excellent screening test. Fatty infiltrations of liver produce low-density hepatic parenchyma on CT scan. Steatosis is diffuse in most patients with non-alcoholic fatty liver disease (NAFLD) but occasionally is focal. Consequently ultrasound or CT scan can be misinterpreted as liver masses. In such cases MRI can distinguish a space-occupying lesion from focal fatty infiltrations or focal fat sparing.

HISTOLOGICAL FINDINGS

Non-alcoholic fatty liver disease is indistinguishable from liver damage due to alcohol abuse. Liver biopsy features include steatosis, mixed inflammatory infiltrate, hepatocyte ballooning and necrosis, Mallory hyaline and fibrosis. The presence of these features alone or in combination accounts for a wide spectrum of non-alcoholic fatty liver disease. Portal tracts are relatively spared from inflammation, unlike chronic viral hepatitis. A finding of fibrosis in non-alcoholic fatty liver disease suggests more advanced and severe liver injury. According to a cross sectional study of 673 liver biopsies some degree of fibrosis is seen in up to 66% of patients at the time of diagnosis in NASH whereas severe fibrosis was found in 25% and cirrhosis in 14% patients.

The combination of steatosis, infiltration by inflammatory cells with hepatocyte ballooning and spotty necrosis is known as **non-alcoholic steato-hepatitis (NASH),** which is a subset of **non-alcoholic fatty liver disease (NAFLD).** Most patients with this type of non-alcoholic fatty liver disease will have some degree of fibrosis whereas Mallory's hyaline may or may not be present. The severity of steatosis can be graded on the basis of the extent of involved hepatic parenchyma (Table 7.1). A system that combines the lesions of steatosis and necro inflammation into grades and those of the type of fibrosis into a stage has been proposed (Table 27.2).

Table 27.1: Grading for Steatosis
Grade 1 <33% of hepatocytes affected
Grade 2 33% to 66% of hepatocytes affected
Grade 3 >66% of hepatocytes affected

Table 27.2: Grading of Steatohepatitis

Grade 1: mild

Steatosis: macrovesicular, up to 66% of lobules

Ballooning: occasionally in zone 3 hepatocytes

Lobular inflammation: scattered mild acute inflammatory response and occasionally chronic inflammatory cells

Portal inflammation: none

Grade 2: moderate

Steatosis: any degree, mixed macrovesicular and microvesicular

Ballooning: obvious in zone 3

Lobular inflammation: polymorphonuclear cells in association with ballooned hepatocytes and pericellular fibrosis

Portal inflammation: mild

Grade 3: severe

Steatosis: more than 66% of lobules, mixed steatosis

Ballooning: marked zone 3

Lobular inflammation: scattered, acute and chronic inflammation. Polymorphonuclear cells are concentrated in zone three areas of ballooning and peri sinusoidal fibrosis

Portal inflammation: mild to moderate

Staging of Fibrosis

Stage 1   Zone three perivenular, perisinusoidal or pericellular fibrosis: focal or extensive
Stage 2   As above, with focal or extensive peri-portal fibrosis
Stage 3   Bridging fibrosis, focal or extensive
Stage 4   Cirrhosis

PATHOGENESIS

Pathogenesis still remains poorly understood. It is not yet known why simple steatosis develops in some patients whereas steatosis and progressive liver disease in others. Difference in body fat distribution or antioxidant systems in the context of genetic predisposition may be a possible explanation. A net retention of lipids within the hepatocytes in the form of triglycerides is a pre requisite for the development of NASH. The primary metabolic abnormalities leading to lipid accumulation are not well understood but they could consist of alterations of pathway in the uptake, synthesis, degradation or secretion in hepatic lipid metabolism resulting from insulin resistance. Insulin resistance is the most reproducible factor in the development of NASH. The molecular pathogenesis of insulin resistance is multi factorial and several molecular targets involved in insulin inhibition have been identified. Insulin resistance leads to fat accumulation in the hepatocyte by two mechanisms, i.e. lipolysis and hyperinsulinemia. Increased intrahepatic levels of fatty acids provide a source of oxidative stress, which may in large part be responsible for progression of steatosis to NASH and cirrhosis. Mitochondria are the main cellular source of reactive oxygen species, which may trigger steatohepatitis and fibrosis by mechanisms of cytokine induction and lipid peroxidation. Patients with NASH have ultra structural mitochondrial lesions including crystalline inclusions in mega mitochondria. This mitochondrial injury is remarkably absent in most patients with simple steatosis.

Thus although the symptoms of liver disease rarely develop in patients with fatty liver who are obese, have diabetes mellitus or hyperlipidemia, a steatotic liver may be vulnerable to fibrotic injury when challenged by additional insults. This led to the presumption that progression from simple steatosis to NASH and advanced fibrosis results from two distinct events. First insulin resistance leads to accumulation of fat within hepatocytes and second, mitochondrial reactive oxygen species causes lipid peroxidation and cytokine induction inciting further injury and necro inflammatory process leading to NASH.

DIAGNOSIS

The diagnosis of NASH is usually suspected in persons with asymptomatic elevation in AST/ALT, radiological findings of fatty liver and unexplained persistent hepatomegaly. Clinical diagnosis and liver tests do not predict histological involvement. Imaging studies, although helpful in detecting the presence of fatty infiltration, cannot be used to accurately determine the severity of the liver damage. The clinical suspicion of non-alcoholic fatty liver disease and its severity can only be confirmed by liver biopsy.

Diagnosis of NASH mandates exclusion of alcohol and secondary causes of fatty liver, which is very vital. The daily intake of alcohol should be less than 20 g (300 mL of beer, 120 mL of wine and 45 mL of hard liquor each contain 10 g of alcohol). Other causes like hepatitis C virus infection, metabolic and hereditary factors and drugs/toxins should be ruled out. The extent of serological work up should be individualized. Specific lab tests and histological features of other liver diseases help in the process of exclusion.

ROLE OF LIVER BIOPSY

Liver biopsy is the best diagnostic tool in confirming NASH and in prognosticating. It also helps in detecting response to treatment measures since liver function tests and imaging studies correlate poorly with histology in NASH. Argument against a liver biopsy includes generally good prognosis of most patients with non-alcoholic fatty liver disease and lack of effective therapy. In addition the risks of liver biopsy have also to be considered. Although it is essential to include only biopsy proven cases of NASH in clinical trials, the decision to perform a liver biopsy in routine clinical practice should take into account the specific clinical questions that are relevant in each case. The issues that may further prompt a liver biopsy are exclusion of alternate causes of liver disease and ascertainment of the degree of fibrosis. Thus the decision to perform a liver biopsy in a case of suspected NASH and timing of biopsy should be individualized and the patient should be included in the decision making process.

NATURAL HISTORY AND RISK OF PROGRESSION TO CIRRHOSIS

Only limited data is available on the natural history of the spectrum of the histological lesions in non-alcoholic fatty liver disease. There are several distinct histological states within the spectrum of NAFLD that denote prognosis. These include fatty liver, steatohepatitis, steatohepatitis with fibrosis and eventually cirrhosis. Cross-sectional studies have shown that fatty liver without inflammatory response is essentially benign and they have the best prognosis. The risks of progression are determined by severity of histological damage. In a series 54 of the 257 patients with NAFLD who underwent liver biopsy, 28% had progression to liver damage, 59% had no change and 13% had improvement or resolution of liver lesions, over a follow up period of 3.5 to 11 years. Hence in some cases progression of steatohepatitis to more advanced fibrosis and eventually cirrhosis is a possibility. However the natural history of cirrhosis resulting from NASH has not been clearly defined.

MANAGEMENT

General Recommendations

Gradual weight loss with appropriate metabolic control of glucose and lipids is the first step. Reducing fat and calorie intake with regular exercises to ensure a weight loss of 500 g to 1 kg/week has been advocated. However the most effective rate and degree of weight loss has not been established. There are some reports that very rapid weight loss though reduces fatty infiltration can some times increase necroinflammatory activity. The degree of fatty infiltration usually decreases with weight loss in most patients.

In patients with diabetes mellitus or hyperlipidemia, good metabolic control results in improvement in liver functions. But this does not always ensure reversal of fat accumulation in the liver.

Drug Therapy

No medicine has been proven to reverse liver damage independent of weight loss. The drug trials have been small pilot studies so far. Gemfibrozil, vitamin E (alpha tocopherol) and metformin have been shown to improve liver functions in small studies. Ursodeoxycholic acid and betaine have shown to improve liver functions as well as histological findings in NASH. However these observations require confirmation in larger trials.

SUMMARY

Non-alcoholic fatty liver disease is a major cause of liver-related morbidity and its spectrum ranges from simple steatosis to steatosis with inflammation and fibrosis. There is increasing evidence that this can progress to cirrhosis and liver failure. Physicians have to actively check for the presence of liver disease especially in those who are overweight and diabetic. There is no established treatment for NAFLD. Treatment is directed at optimizing body weight and achieving metabolic control of lipids and glucose. The role of pharmacological agents is still evolving.

SUGGESTED READING

1. Non alcoholic fatty liver disease: Seminars in liver disease: Volume 2001;21:1.
2. AGA technical review on Non-alcoholic fatty liver disease: Gastroenterology 2002:123:1705-25.
3. Angulo P. Medical progress: Non-alcoholic fatty liver disease. N Engl J Med 2002; 346:1221-31.

4. Tilg H., Diehl A. Cytokines in alcoholic and non-alcoholic steatohepatitis. M. N Engl J Med 2000; 343:1467-76.
5. McCullough AJ. The clinical features, diagnosis and natural history of non-alcoholic fatty liver disease Clin Liver Dis-2004; 8: 521-33.
6. Harrison SA. Pharmacologic management of non-alcoholic fatty liver disease. Clin Liver Dis 2004; 8: 715-28.
7. Neuschwander-Tetri BA, Caldwell SH. Non-alcoholic steatohepatitis: summary of an AASLD Single Topic Conference. Hepatology 2003; 37:1202-19.

28

Musthafa CP

Management of Ascites

INTRODUCTION

Ascites is the pathologic accumulation of fluid in the peritoneal cavity. Approximately 80% of patients with ascites have cirrhosis. Peritoneal carcinomatosis, tuberculosis, heart failure, nephrotic syndrome and pancreatic diseases are other causes of ascites. Patients with fulminant hepatic failure, alcoholic hepatitis and hepatocellular carcinoma can develop ascites without cirrhosis. The development of ascites in chronic liver disease is a poor prognostic sign. Treatment of ascites depends on the cause of the fluid retention.

PATHOGENESIS OF ASCITES

Three theories of ascites formation have been proposed in cirrhotic patients. The underfill theory postulates that an alteration in hydrostatic oncotic balance leads to leakage of intravascular fluid into the peritoneal cavity leading to contraction of intravascular space and triggers neurohormonal excitation, activation of the renin angiotensin aldosterone system and sympathetic system. The overfill theory suggests that overflow of fluid into the peritoneal cavity occurs due to primary sodium retention. A more recent concept is that underfill theory operates in the early phase and later, overflow theory takes over.

Exudation of proteinaceous fluid from the peritoneal lining occurs in peritoneal carcinomatosis and tuberculous peritonitis. Peripheral vasodilatation applies in nephrotic syndrome, congestive cardiac failure and Budd-Chiari syndrome.

EVALUATION OF ASCITES

The initial evaluation of a patient with ascites should include directed history, focused physical examination and a diagnostic paracentesis with ascitic fluid analysis.

Directed history related to cirrhosis, tuberculosis, congestive heart failure, and cancer is important. Physical examination is done to make the diagnosis of ascites by flank dullness and shifting dullness, and to determine the causes of ascites. Overall accuracy of physical examination to detect ascites is 58%, hence abdominal ultrasound examination is recommended to confirm the presence of ascites and to help in determining the etiology of ascites.

PARACENTESIS

Paracentesis with ascitic fluid analysis is the most rapid and cost effective way to determine the cause of ascites and this should be done routinely in all patients with new onset, clinically apparent ascites. Initial routine screening tests consist of cell count, albumin, total protein and culture. In a cirrhotic patient diagnostic paracentesis should be repeated if patient develops fever, abdominal pain or tenderness, hypotension, encephalopathy, renal failure, peripheral leukocytosis or acidosis. Coagulopathy is not a contraindication for paracentesis unless clinically apparent disseminated intravascular coagulation or primary fibrinolysis is present.

ASCITIC FLUID CELL COUNT

The white cell count is the single most important test. The cell count provides immediate information about possible bacterial infection. A sample with an absolute polymorphonuclear leukocyte count of 250 cells/mm^3 is treated as having ascitic fluid infection until proven otherwise. Patients with tuberculous peritonitis, and peritoneal carcinomatosis have elevated ascitic fluid WBC counts, predominantly lymphocytic.

ALBUMIN CONCENTRATION AND SAAG

The SAAG is widely used to categorize ascites (Table 28.1). Portal hypertension results in an abnormally high hydrostatic pressure gradient between hepatic sinusoids and peritoneal fluid, similar in gradient to oncotic pressure gradient between serum and ascitic fluid. Albumin concentration of ascitic fluid allows calculation of the serum ascites albumin gradient (SAAG) to classify specimens into high or low gradient categories. SAAG is calculated by subtracting the albumin concentration of ascites from the albumin concentration of serum. Obtained on the same day. Patients with significant portal hypertension have SAAG equal to or greater than 1.1 g/dl, whereas those without portal hypertension have SAAG less than 1.1 g/dl. SAAG predicts the presence of portal hypertension with 97% accuracy.

ASCITIC FLUID TOTAL PROTEIN

Ascitic fluid total protein concentration (AFTP) greater than 2.5 g/dl is called exudate. High AFTP in an appropriate clinical scenario should raise the suspicion of peritoneal carcinomatosis, tuberculous peritonitis, cardiac ascites, Budd-Chiari syndrome and myxedema. This is also seen in lymphatic rupture, intestinal perforation, biliary ascites and pancreatic ascites. The AFTP level depends on serum total protein concentration and portal pressure. Around 20% of cirrhotic patients and all patients with cardiac ascites have high AFTP and most of the SBP patients have low AFTP. SAAG is superior to AFTP estimation in the analysis of ascites. But AFTP may alert the clinician about other potential causes of ascites.

CULTURE IN BLOOD CULTURE BOTTLES

The most common bacterial infection of ascitic fluid is monomicrobial with a very low concentration of organism. Bed-side innoculation of 10-20 cc of ascitic fluid to blood culture bottle has high detection rate (85%).

OPTIONAL TESTS

Additional ascitic fluid tests include glucose, LDH, amylase, triglyceride, bilirubin levels and cytology. In late stages of spontaneous bacterial peritonitis (SBP) and gut perforation ascitic fluid glucose can drop to 0 mg/dl. The LDH level in the ascitic fluid may rise above that in the serum during SBP and may become very high in the presence of gut perforation. The ascitic-fluid amylase concentration helps detect pancreatic ascites and perforation of the gut into the peritoneal cavity. In pancreatic ascites, the amylase level averages 2000 IU/L and becomes six fold the magnitude of serum amylase. Chylous ascites has a triglyceride level of at least 200 mg/dl and usually above 1000 mg/dl. Gram staining of ascitic fluid may be helpful to identify gut perforation. Cytologic examination is expected to be positive only in peritoneal carcinomatosis. Positive cytology is not expected in hepatocellular carcinoma, massive liver metastases and lymphoma without peritoneal metastases. Send 50 cc of ascitic fluid for cytologic evaluation.

LAPAROSCOPY

Suspected tuberculosis, which cannot be proven by other tests, is an indication for laparoscopy. Sensitivity for tuberculosis reaches 100% when both peritoneal biopsy and histologic study are performed. If analysis of ascitic fluid does not provide pathologic diagnosis, laparoscopy can be used to obtain tissue diagnosis in carcinomatosis peritonitis.

MIXED ASCITES

Approximately 5% of the patients have mixed ascites. Mixed ascites results from two causes of fluid retention (e.g., cirrhosis and tuberculosis or peritoneal carcinomatosis).

Table 28.1: Relationship of SAAG (Serum Ascites Albumin Gradient) to the etiology of ascites	
Causes of high (>1.1gm/dl) serum ascitic albumin gradient	*Causes of low (<1.1gm/dl) serum ascitic albumin gradient*
• Cirrhosis • Alcoholic hepatitis • Cardiac ascites • Massive liver metastases • Fulminant hepatic failure • Budd-Chiari syndrome • Portal vein thrombosis • Veno-occlusive disease • Myxedema • Fatty liver of pregnancy • *Mixed ascites*	• Peritoneal carcinomatosis • Tuberculous peritonitis • Pancreatic disease • Biliary ascites • Nephrotic syndrome • Serositis • Bowel obstruction or infarction

Treatment of Ascites

The treatment of ascites depends on the cause of fluid retention. The SAAG is useful for guiding treatment. High SAAG ascites (>1.1 gm/dl) usually respond to salt restriction and diuretics. The most important treatments are the restriction of dietary sodium intake and the use of oral diuretics. Treatment can be attempted in an outpatient setting. Patients with a low SAAG usually do not respond to conservative measures.

Treatment of High SAAG Ascites

Patients with small volume ascites can be managed initially as outpatients. Hospitalization is indicated for large volume ascites, unsuccessful outpatient management, or intensive inpatient education. Sodium restriction to 2 g/day (88 mmol/day) and diuretics are the mainstay of treatment in cirrhotic ascites. Fluid restriction is not necessary for most patients and should be advised only in patients with serum sodium <120 mmol/L. These measures will achieve successful diuresis in 90% of the cases. Spontaneous diuresis with salt restriction alone is possible only in 10-15% of cirrhotic patients.

The combination of spironolactone and furosemide is the most effective oral diuretic. This is given as a single morning dose. A typical starting daily dose is 100 mg of spironolactone and 40 mg of furosemide. If there is no decrease in body weight or increase in urinary sodium excretion after two or three days, the doses of both drugs can be titrated up to maximum doses of 400 mg of spironolactone and 160 mg of furosemide per day. Once pedal edema disappears, dose of diuretic should be reduced to maintain diuresis of 750 ml/day to avoid azotemia and electrolyte disturbances. Physician should reduce the diuretic dose to maintain a stable weight.

Amiloride (starting dose, 10 mg per day; maximal dose, 40 mg per day, 1:10 ratio with furosemide) can be substituted for spironolactone if patients develop side effects of spironolactone like painful gynecomastia or hyperkalemia. However, amiloride is more expensive and less effective.

Serial monitoring of urinary sodium excretion may help to determine the optimal diuretic dose. If the urinary sodium concentration is less than 10 mmol per liter and the urine volume is less than 1 liter per day despite diuretic treatment, the diuretic dose must be increased to achieve natriuresis.

Contraindications for diuretics include hepatic encephalopathy, serum sodium >120 nmol/L, and renal insufficiency.

Large Volume Paracentesis (LVP)

Large volume paracentesis (five or more liters of fluid) is indicated when the patient has tense ascites to relieve shortness of breath, to decrease early satiety, and prevent pressure-related leakage of fluid from the site of the paracentesis. Therapeutic paracentesis may improve cardiac function. A simple 16 to 18 gauge disposable metal needle is connected by phlebotomy tubing to vacuum bottles for therapeutic paracentesis. A single 5 liter paracentesis can be done safely without colloid infusion. Since paracentesis doesn't address the underlying disease, ascitic fluid usually re-accumulates requiring repeated paracentesis. Therapeutic paracentesis should not be routinely recommended in diuretic sensitive patients.

Refractory Ascites

There are two subgroups for refractory ascites: diuretic resistant and diuretic intractable ascites. In diuretic resistant ascites, ascites cannot be mobilized with maximum dose of diuretic and intensive salt restriction. In diuretic intractable ascites, diuretic induced complications prevent from using effective diuretic dose. Therapeutic paracentesis, peritoneo-venous shunting, transjugular intrahepatic portosystemic stent shunts (TIPS), and liver transplantation are available treatment options for these patients.

In large-volume paracentesis, four to six liters of fluid are removed daily and 10 gm of albumin given for each liter of ascitic fluid removed. Albumin infusion is given because of concern for rapid re-accumulation of ascites, acute intravascular fluid shift, and renal failure and electrolyte disturbances. The role of albumin infusion is still debated. The American Association for the study of Liver Diseases suggests that albumin infusion as optional for LVP of more than five liters but is not recommended for paracentesis of lesser volume.

TIPS is a side to side porta-caval shunt. TIPS allows the blood to flow form portal circulation to systemic circulation. TIPS may be reserved for patients with refractory ascites that recurs despite multiple LVP attempts. In patients whose predicted survival is short, TIPS is offered as bridge to liver transplantation. If the predicted survival is prolonged, then TIPS may be a preferred therapeutic option.

Peritoneovenous (e.g., LeVeen or Denver) **shunt** is a subcutaneously tunneled plastic tubing that returns the ascitic fluid by a unidirectional valve system into the jugular vein. Although survival is not prolonged, shunting may improve patient's comfort by reducing the volume of ascitic fluid and by better response to diuretics. Peritoneovenous shunt is rarely used nowadays.

Liver transplantation: Two year survival is 50% once ascites develops and drops to 25% with refractory ascites and 20% after an episode of SBP. Overall one-year survival after liver transplantation exceeds 75%. Patients with diuretic-resistant ascites who are otherwise good candidates for transplantation should be offered liver transplantation.

Ascitic Fluid Infection

Ascitic fluid infection can be spontaneous or secondary to an intra abdominal or surgically treatable source of infection. More than 90% of ascitic fluid infections in cirrhotic patients are spontaneous.

SBP (spontaneous bacterial peritonitis) is defined as ascitic fluid with polymorphonuclear cell (PMN) counts 250/mm^3 or more and positive culture; and absence of surgically treatable cause. Culture negative neutrocytic ascites is defined as an ascitic fluid PMN count of more than 250 mm^3 with a negative culture. Monomicrobial non-neutrocytic bacterascites is defined as an ascitic fluid PMN count of < 250 cells/mm^3 with a positive culture for a single organism. Secondary bacterial peritonitis is elevated PMN leucocytes with a positive ascitic fluid culture and presence of intra abdominal infection.

Ascitic fluid infection is treated with cefotaxime or a similar third generation cephalosporin. Cefotaxime 2 gm given 8th hourly for 5 days is effective. Empirical treatment for SBP is started as soon as possible, when hospitalized patient with ascites develops clinical signs of possible infection (fever, abdominal pain, encephalopathy) or shows deterioration in clinical or laboratory parameters, after initiating cultures and ascitic fluid analysis.

Secondary bacterial peritonitis is treated surgically. Antibiotics should be given to cover both aerobic and anaerobic infections.

Short-term prophylaxis of SBP is indicated in cirrhotic patients with gastrointestinal hemorrhage and low ascitic fluid protein (<1 gm/dl) and long term prophylaxis in patients with a prior episode of SBP. Norfloxacin, trimethoprim-sulfamethoxazole and ciprofloxacin are used for prophylaxis.

Peritoneal Carcinomatosis

Peritoneal carcinomatosis is the most common form of low albumin gradient ascites. Except in breast and ovarian cancer, the presence of malignant ascites in patients with neoplastic diseases frequently heralds the terminal phase of cancer. It is a poor prognostic indicator, with a median survival time ranging from 1 to 4 months. In general, malignant ascites remains refractory to medical treatment. Peripheral edema in these patients responds to diuretics. Mainstay of treatment for non-ovarian peritoneal carcinomatosis is outpatient therapeutic paracentesis. Paracentesis will improve quality of life and will provide acceptable palliation in symptomatic ascites.

Intra-peritoneal chemotherapy along with systemic chemotherapy is an effective way to palliate malignant ascites. Mitomycin C with or without cisplatin, or cisplatin and etoposide with hyperthermia in patients with gastric, colon, and ovarian cancer-induced ascites have produced encouraging results. In addition to controlling malignant ascites, patient survival is improved in selected cases.

Tuberculous peritonitis: Ascites caused by tuberculous peritonitis is cured by anti-tuberculous treatment. Diuretics do not speed weight loss unless the patient has underlying portal hypertension from cirrhosis.

Pancreatic ascites: Pancreatic ascites may resolve spontaneously, may require endoscopic stenting or operative intervention, or may respond to somatostatin therapy.

Other causes: Other causes are rare and are treated on individual case basis.

SUGGESTED READING

1. Gines P, Arroyo V, Rodes J. Pathophysiology, complications, and treatment of ascites. Clin Liver Dis 1997; 1: 129-55.
2. Bataller R, Gines P, Arroyo V. Practical recommendations for the treatment of ascites and its complications Drugs 1997 Oct; 54(4): 571-80.
3. Chutaputti A. Management of refractory ascites and hepatorenal syndrome. J Gastroenterol Hepatol. 2002; 17: 456-61.
4. Roberts LR, Kamath PS. Ascites and hepatorenal syndrome: pathophysiology and management. Mayo Clin Proc 1996; 71: 874-81.
5. Habeeb KS, Herrera JL. Management of ascites. Paracentesis as a guide. Postgrad Med 1997; 101: 191-2, 195-200.

29

Viswanath N

Hepatic Encephalopathy— Testing Clinical Talents

INTRODUCTION

Hepatic encephalopathy (HE) can be defined as a reversible change in neurologic function caused by liver disease. This vague definition reflects the varied neurologic manifestations that develop as a consequence of a spectrum of liver diseases (Figure 29.1). The cardinal feature is the reversibility of the neurological syndrome with improvement of the status of the liver.

Though no prevalence data are available, fulminant hepatic failure (FHF) is likely to be more common in India than in the West, largely due to the greater incidence of viral and toxic hepatitis. Chronic liver disease is probably no less frequent than what it is in the west; the etiology however may differ. A sizeable percentage of all cirrhotics in later stages develop hepatic encephalopathy.

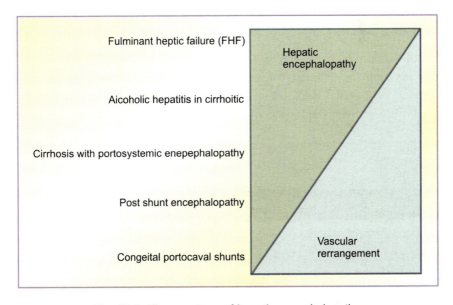

Fig. 29.1: The spectrum of hepatic encephalopathy

CLASSIFICATION

This has been confusing. The following is based on the recommendations of the Working Party of World Congress of Gastroenterology (2002) (Table 29.1).

Minimal (earlier called subclinical) encephalopathy denotes the group of patients with chronic liver disease who are clinically normal but have mild impairment of higher mental functions as assessed by psychometric analysis.

Table 29.1: Proposed nomenclature for hepatic encephalopathy

HE Type	Nomenclature	Subcategory	Subdivisions
AHE	Associated with acute liver disease		
BHE	Associated with porto-systemic bypass and no intrinsic liver disease		
CHE	Associated with cirrhosis and portal hypertension or portosystemic shunts	Episodic HE	Precipitated Spontaneous Recurrent
		Persistent HE	Mild Severe Tt dependent
		Minimal HE	

PATHOPHYSIOLOGY

In theory, hepatic encephalopathy could occur as a consequence of a) synthesis of encephalopathogenic substances by liver, b) reduced synthesis of substances essential for normal function of the brain and c) impaired extraction and metabolism of encephalopathogenic substances or their precursors by the failing liver.

Many events have been noted to precipitate encephalopathy in cirrhotics (Table 29.2).

Table 29.2: Factors that may precipitate hepatic encephalopathy

Oral protein load Upper GI bleed Constipation	Act via the gut – portal vein
Diuretic therapy Diarrhea and vomiting Abdominal paracentesis	Dehydration, electrolyte, acid/ base imbalance (e.g., alkalosis)
Hypotension, hypoxia anemia, hypoglycemia	Adverse effect on brain and liver
Sedatives, hypnotics infection, surgery Azotemia Creation of a porto systemic shunt	

Historically hypotheses have ranged from single unifying theories to the notion that hepatic encephalopathy is a multifactorial process caused by several toxins affecting brain function at different levels. The latter is the more favoured view.

Table 29.3: Circulating factors implicated in the pathogenesis of encephalopathy	
1	Ammonia
2	Synergistic toxins ; mercaptans, phenols, short chain fatty acids
3	False neurotransmitter hypothesis; more of aromatic amino acids enter brain which may lead to formation of neurotransmitters
4	GABA / endogenous benzodiazepines-GABA and substances (endozepines) that interact with GABA A receptor. Recently peripheral benzodiazepine receptor activation has been stressed
5	Cytokines TNFa, IL-1b and IL-6 recently postulated to play a role

Ammonia is the most studied toxin causing hepatic encephalopathy, but not the only one (Table 29.3).

The gastrointestinal tract is the primary site of production of ammonia from the ingested proteins and secreted urea. The portal vein ammonia levels are 5 to 10 fold greater than mixed venous blood. The first pass clearance of ammonia by liver is very high; little enters the systemic circulation. In healthy persons 50% of ammonia is taken up by muscle explaining why a wasted cirrhotic slips into encephalopathy easily.

Despite strong evidence favouring the role of ammonia in causation of hepatic encephalopathy, the precise cellular mechanisms involved remain elusive. Potential mechanisms include decrease in concentration of glycogen in cultured astrocytes, impaired glial neuronal communication and interference with synaptic transmission.

A variety of other toxins and changes in organ functions brought on by impaired hepatocellular function and/ or portosystemic shunting acting in tandem, cause the neuropsychiatric syndrome (Figure 29.1)

Diagnosis

Hepatic enceophalopathy presents as a cluster of neurological abnormalities, though the clinical features are by and large nonspecific. Subtle changes in personality, memory or consciousness are easily overlooked if the underlying liver disease is not recognized. On the other hand, the clinical presentation of florid encephalopathy in a patient with overt liver disease is unmistakable. However, the diagnosis of hepatic encephalopathy is a diagnosis of exclusion. Intracranial space occupying lesions, vascular events, infectious causes and other metabolic disorders may all need to be considered.

A precipitant needs to be diligently searched for in a cirrhotic. In fulminant hepatic failure too, a correctable precipitant may modify the outlook. These include :

- Infection—culture of body fluids especially ascites is important. Spontaneous bacterial peritonitis may present with hepatic encephalopathy.
- GI bleed—stool examination or placement of an NG tube may be needed.
- Use of psychoactive medication
- Constipation and/or ingestion of excessive protein
- Renal and electrolyte abnormalities. In uremia, urea is broken down to ammonia in the gut and absorbed. Hypokalemia and hypovolemia favour entry of ammonia into the brain.
- Worsening hepatic function. Superimposed liver injury such as portal vein thrombus, a hepatoma, alcohol abuse and so on, may need consideration.

The grade of encephalopathy: Two commonly used ones are the Glasgow coma scale and the West Haven criteria

1. Glasgow coma scale. The best score is 15, the worst is 3, with values less than 12 indicating more severe encephalopathy.
2. The gradation based on West Haven criteria includes the following:

Table 29.4: Grading system for hepatic encephalopathy

Grade	Level of consciousness	Personality and Intellect	Neurologic signs
0	Normal	Normal	None
Minimal	Normal	Normal	Abnormalities only on psychometric analysis
1	Inverted sleep pattern, restlessness	Forgetfulness, mild confusion, agitation irritability	Tremor, apraxia, incoordination, impaired writing
2	Lethargy, slow responses	Disorientation as regards time, amnesia decreased inhibitions, inappro- priate behaviour	Asterexis, dysarthria ataxia, hypoactive reflexes
3	Somnolent but rousable, confusion	Disorientation as regards place, aggressive behaviour	Asterexis, hyperactive reflexes, Babinski's sign, muscle rigidity
4	Coma	None	Decerebration

TREATMENT

General Care

A patient with altered mental status needs proper supportive care. Intravenous access may be needed to provide fluids and electrolytes; hydration is important even in presence of ascites. Diuretics are better avoided unless essential as in pulmonary edema. Urinary catheters and nasogastric feeding tubes may be needed. Care needs to be exercised to avoid line sepsis, pressure sores and aspiration pneumonia. In deeply unconscious patients tracheal intubation and ventilation may be necessary.

Adequate nutritional support is essential. It is recommended to provide 25-35 kcal/kg/d and 0.5-1.2 G/kg/d of protein to reduce endogenous protein breakdown. However, in general, during the first 2-3 days of coma, patient may better be on intravenous glucose only. Later, oral or nasogastric feeding may be started. With improvement of sensorium, protein may be raised. In patients with prolonged coma, nitrogen supplements may be given preferably enterally. BCAA (branched chain amino acids) rich feeds may be used in this setting.

Medical Treatment

Hepatic encephalopathy in acute liver failure is generally rapid in onset, progression and usually complicated by cerebral edema if it deepens to grade 4 coma. Though management with protein restriction, unabsorbable disaccharides and other supportive means as discussed is started, in severe liver failure, if liver function does not recover soon enough, cerebral edema and death are very likely. Several predictors of outcome have been assessed. In the era of orthotopic liver transplantation (OLT), it is important to identify who will need OLT and who have a better chance of survival by conservative management (Table 29.5).

Table 29.5: King's College criteria for liver transplantation

Non-acetaminophen	Acetaminophen
PT >100s (INR >6.5) (irrespective of grade of hepatic encephalopathy)	pH <7.3 (irrespective of HE grade)
Or any three of the following 1. Age <10 or >40 y 2.Etiology: negative serology for hepatitis A and B, 3. Halothane, idiosyncratic drug reaction, 4. Wilson's disease. 5. Period of jaundice to encephalopathy >7days 6. PT >50s (INR >3.5) 7. Serum bilirubin >17.5 mg/dl	Or all three of the following 1. Grade III – IV encephalopathy 2. PT >100 s (INR >6.5) 3. Serum creatinine >3.4 mg/dl

A few etiologies of fulminant hepatic failure demand specific and immediate treatment. These include acetaminophen overdosage (N-acetyl cysteine); *Amanita* mushroom poisoning (high dose penicillin and silibinin); herpes simplex infection (acyclovir) and acute fatty liver of pregnancy (rapid delivery of the infant)

Patients in acute liver failure with Grade III – IV coma are recommended elective ventilation to protect airways and to manage cerebral edema and mannitol by repeated bolus injections (0.5 G/kg over a period of 10 mts). Continuous dextrose infusion and six hourly blood sugar monitoring are essential to avoid lethal hypoglycemia. Hypokalemia and other dyselectrolytemias need to be watched for and corrected.

In hepatic encephalopathy with chronic liver disease, a precipitating event is apparent on careful search. Several factors may operate in a given patient at the same time to produce hepatic encephalopathy. For instance, septicemia or bacterial peritonitis with gram negative enteral flora develops within 48 hours in about half of patients with Child-Pugh class C cirrhosis and acute gastro intestinal bleeding. Hypokalemia and alkalemia complicating diuretic use lead in turn to increased renal production of ammonia and increased diffusion of ammonia through the blood brain barrier, respectively. Every effort should be made to identify the precipitating factor, the cofactors and correct them if possible.

Reduction of Production and Absorption of Ammonia

- The intestinal production of ammonia can be restricted by restricting protein intake. But patients need a minimum of 0.8-1.0 G / kg of protein a day to maintain nitrogen balance. After restricting to 10-20 g/d, increase intake by 10 G increments every three to five days to achieve the level of patient's tolerance or the minimum requirement. Vegetable proteins are believed to cause less of encephalopathy due to their higher fibre content. This a) increases rate of transit through intestine and b) lowers pH of colonic lumen due to fermentation by bacteria.

- The ammoniagenic substances are removed from gut by the osmotic cathartic action of nonabsorbable disaccharides such as lactulose (b-galactosidofructose) or lactisol; the daily dose has to be titrated to result in 2-4 soft acidic (pH <6) stools.

- Lactulose lowers colonic pH by production of organic acids by bacterial fermentation. The pH is hostile for urease producing intestinal bacteria and help growth of nonurease producing lactobacilli. In addition, acidification not only reduces absorption of ammonia by nonionic diffusion, but also results in the net movement of ammonia from blood to bowel lumen. Lactulose enemas may also be used.

- Antibiotics with activity against urease producing bacteria such as neomycin (4-6 g/d) or metronidazole (800 mg /d) also reduce intestinal ammonia. A small percentage of neomycin may be absorbed and could be nephrotoxic or ototoxic in the long term. Antibiotics and nonabsorbable disaccharides could interact by depletion of the bacteria fermenting the disaccharides. Trials show that in the majority there is no interaction. In some patients, stool pH has been noted to rise with use of antibiotics. In these one could discontinue antibiotics. Colonising the bowel with nonurease producing bacteria has been attractive. *Enterococcus faecium* was found to be effective alone or even after discontinuing the administration of bacilli.

- *H.pylori* is believed to contribute to blood ammonia. Although evidence is still unclear, there are many who suggest *H.pylori* eradication in patients who had hepatic encephalopathy.

To Effect Changes in Conversion of Ammonia in Tissues

- Ornithine and aspartate are critical substrates in the conversion of ammonia to urea and glutamine respectively. Controlled trials indicate that ornithine and aspartate but not ornithine and alpha ketoglutarate are of therapeutic benefit in hepatic encephalopathy.
- Benzoate and phenylacetate, which react with glycine to yield hippurate and with glutamine to form phenacetyl glutamine respectively have been found to be beneficial (10 g of sodium benzoate may be as effective as lactulose)
- Two of the five urea cycle enzymes are zinc dependent. Cirrhotics are often deficient in zinc. Zinc sulphate 600 mg/d was found to be helpful.

Neurotransmitter Mediated Mechanisms

- Formula low in aromatic amino acids and rich in branched chain amino acids have not been shown to be of benefit in trials
- Controlled trials show no benefit with levodopa and bromocriptine.

GABA –Benzodiazepine Receptor Mediated Mechanisms and Manganese

- Only incomplete improvement was seen with flumazenil, a benzodiazepine antagonist
- Manganese chelation has not been studied in patients with hepatic encephalopathy.

Liver Support Systems

The liver is critical in multiple processes; clearance of endogenous compounds, in synthesis of macromolecules and in organ specific biotransformations. The reproduction of this complexity in a device has been a daunting challenge. However the success of liver transplantation has changed expectations; A "bridge to transplantation" is the new goal.

Conceptually liver support systems are divided into three groups; artificial (nonbiologic) support, biological approaches and the hybrid devices. Molecular Adsorbent Recycling System (MARS) is a nonbiologic liver support system which has shown some promise in managing acute on chronic liver disease with encephalopathy, but still of no definite benefit in fulminant hepatic failure, save some biochemical improvement and change in level of coma. Though there have been more expectations from hybrid and biologic systems in fulminant hepatic failure, they are yet to be fulfilled. However the future of liver support looks promising.

TRANSPLANTATION

Liver transplantation has revolutionalized management of fulminant hepatic faliure. In carefully selected patients, it offers a survival between 65 and 80%. The decision should balance the likelihood of spontaneous recovery with risks of surgery and long-term immunosuppression.

Development of hepatic encephalopathy in a patient with chronic liver disease indicates severe portosystemic shunting and hepatic dysfunction. Prognosis for such a patient is grim; 80% 1-yr, 65% 2-yr and 55% 3-yr survival reported. Hence in the ideal setting, the only definitive treatment for these patients will be a transplant.

SUGGESTED READING

1. Juan Cordoba, Andres T Blei; Hepatic encephalopathy in Schiff's Diseases of the liver; 9th edition; 2004
2. David A Sass, A Obaid Shakil Fulminant hepatic failure; Gastroenterology clinics; December 2003; 32:4.
3. Andres T Blei, Diagnosis and treatment of hepatic encephalopathy. Bailliere's Clinical Gastroenterology. 2000; 14:6.
4. Liver support systems; section from Brenner and Rector. The Kidney 7th edition 2004.
5. Peter Ferenci, Alan lockwood and Members of the Working Party Hepatology; 2002; 35:3.
6. Gerber T, Schomerus H. Hepatic encephalopathy in liver cirrhosis: pathogenesis, diagnosis and management. *Drugs*. 2000; 60:1353-70.
7. Mullen KD. Newer aspects of hepatic encephalopathy.Indian J Gastroenterol. 2003; 22 Suppl 2:S17-20.
8. Blei AT, Cordoba J. Practice parameters committee of the American College of Gastroenterology. Hepatic Encephalopathy. Am J Gastroenterol. 2001; 96: 1968-76.
9. Butterworth RF. Complications of cirrhosis III. Hepatic encephalopathy. J. Hepatol. 2000; 32 (1 Suppl): 171-80.
10. Tandon BN. Hepatic encephalopathy syndromes. Indian J Gastroenterol. 2003; 22 Suppl 2:S4-6

30

Sudhindran S

Liver Transplantation: What a Physician needs to Know

INTRODUCTION

Liver failure can affect individuals of all ages and in most cases results in their death, or greatly impairs their quality of life. In India patients with chronic liver disease, along with their loved ones accept this fate as untreatable or inevitable. This is a sobering concern because most such cases are readily treatable by orthotopic liver transplantation (OLT). Thousands of children and adults who were otherwise doomed to die due to irreversible acute or chronic liver failure currently live and have an excellent quality of life after OLT. Over the last two decades, the number of liver transplants escalated exponentially along with an extension in the list of indications for transplantation. This article focuses on the current indications for referral of adult patients for liver transplantation, some surgical considerations, modern results and current dilemmas facing the transplant community.

The first attempts at OLT in humans were made at three separate institutions in 1963, each resulting in the death of the recipient. Four years later an 18-months old child with hepatoma survived OLT, however recipient died 13 months later. Factors leading to a transformation in the field of solid organ transplantation and the consequent extraordinary success of OLT include:

- Development of the ever-expanding choice of immunosuppressant drugs heralded by cyclosporine in 1978 and later followed by tacrolimus, sirolimus, mycophenolate, etc.
- Discovery of the University of Wisconsin (UW) perfusion solution
- Surgical and anesthetic refinements
- Understanding the mechanics of coagulopathy and development of blood products like fresh frozen plasma (FFP), cryoprecipitate, platelet concentrates and antifibrinolytics like aprotinin

Early referral of potential candidates can prevent avoidable deaths and facilitate better outcome after OLT. Prior to reviewing the indications for liver transplant, it may be pertinent to discuss the contraindications for OLT, which have steadily declined over the last decade.

- **Absolute contraindication**
  - Extrahepatic malignancy other than skin cancers
  - Uncontrolled sepsis
  - Advanced cardiopulmonary disease
  - AIDS
- **Relative contraindication**
  - HIV positivity
  - Active alcohol or illicit drug abuse within the previous six months

- Advanced age (>70 years)
- Cholangiocarcinoma
- Severe psychiatric disorder
- Portal vein thrombosis

Indications for Referral of Patients for Liver Transplantation

The major purpose of an evaluation for OLT is to determine if a particular patient is likely to benefit from liver transplantation. Additional goals of a complete evaluation are to predict the optimal timing of transplantation, to maximize nutritional and medical therapy during the waiting period and finally, to provide education to the patient and family.

Acute Liver Failure

The leading causes of acute liver failure in India are acute viral hepatitis, idiosyncratic drug reactions, autoimmune hepatitis and occasionally metabolic causes such as Wilson's disease. The fatality is close to 80% and liver transplantation is an important treatment option in the management of severe cases of acute liver failure. However deciding whether an individual patient requires transplantation or whether conservative therapy might suffice can be challenging. The etiology of liver failure and the interval between the onset of jaundice and encephalopathy have major prognostic significance. The King's College criteria are very commonly used for selecting patients with acute liver failure for OLT.

King's College Hospital Criteria for Transplantation in Acute Liver Failure

- Acute liver failure due to paracetamol poisoning
  - pH <7.30 (irrespective of grade of encephalopathy) or
  - Prothrombin time >100 seconds and serum creatinine >3.4 mgm/dl if in grade III or IV coma
- Non-paracetamol causes
  - Prothrombin time >100 seconds (irrespective of grade of encephalopathy) or
  - Any three of the following (irrespective of grade of encephalopathy):
    - (i) Etiology: non-A, non-B (indeterminate) hepatitis, halothane, hepatitis, idiosyncratic drug reactions
    - (ii) Age <10 or >40 years
    - (iii) Jaundice to encephalopathy interval >7 days (paradoxically!)
    - (iv) Prothrombin time >50 seconds
    - (v) Serum bilirubin >18 mgm/dl

Chronic Liver Failure

The diagnosis of cirrhosis is not an indication to straight away recommend OLT, but urges a need to anticipate potential complications, such as hepatocellular carcinoma (HCC) or the onset of decompensation, that would indicate a need for referral to a transplant program. Studies from both sides of the Atlantic have shown that the survival of patients with cirrhosis decreases significantly after clinical decompensation. *Clinical decompensation is defined as the acute or insidious onset of ascites, jaundice, variceal hemorrhage, encephalopathy, spontaneous bacterial peritonitis or hepatocellular carcinoma.* An accurate prognostic model of chronic liver disease, which in turn can be the basis for evaluating the need for OLT is still lacking. The currently existing models or recommendations can be grouped as disease specific and non-disease specific.

DISEASE SPECIFIC RECOMMENDATIONS

In India the bulk of the indication for OLT in adults would be end stage liver disease due to hepatitis C, hepatitis B or alcoholic liver disease and hepatocellular carcinoma (HCC) complicating cirrhosis.

Hepatitis B Virus (HBV) Liver Disease

Transplantation is the only option open to patients with HBV liver disease that goes on to develop end stage cirrhosis since antiviral therapy does not modify the course of disease at this stage. However, OLT perse does not prevent virological recurrence from extrahepatic reservoir sites. Accordingly recurrence of HBV related liver disease is the main determinant of outcome after transplantation in this population and is closely related to the pretransplant replication status of the virus. Measurement of HBe antigen and circulating HBV DNA is mandatory prior to transplant. Active viral replication at the time of transplantation heralds an inferior outcome. Co-infection with hepatitis delta virus (HDV) is probably advantageous for both disease recurrence and survival. The current guidelines regarding OLT for HBV associated end stage liver disease are:

- Patients with end stage chronic HBV related liver disease must be HBV DNA negative before transplantation. Most HBV DNA positive patients can be rendered HBV DNA negative with antiviral treatment and should not be excluded from assessment for OLT.

- Long-term passive immunization with hepatitis B immunoglobulin is an effective strategy to prevent re-infection. Hepatitis B immunoglobin therapy should start from the "anhepatic phase" of the transplant. Unfortunately, the major issue that deters its utilization is the prohibitive expense.
- Antiviral agents such as lamivudine and adefovir have potential use in optimising the outcome after OLT.
- Mutant HBV or HDV coinfections are not contraindications to transplantation.

Hepatitis C Liver Disease

Patients with end stage hepatitis C cirrhosis should be considered for transplantation. Genotype and viral load should not influence transplant assessment. Recurrence of the virus from reservoir sites is universal after successful OLT. High dose immunosuppression increases viraemia and may promote disease recurrence. Whether disease recurrence will affect long-term graft survival still remains a moot question. The use of interferons, ribavirin and drugs like sirolimus in reducing the recurrence of Hepatis C after OLT is under rigorous scrutiny in ongoing trials. Concomitant alcohol misuse should be actively excluded. Hemophilia is not a contraindication to transplantation .

Hepatic tumors

Hepatocellular Carcinoma

Transplantation is rarely indicated in HCC developing within a non-cirrhotic liver. The optimal management of HCC complicating cirrhosis is more problematic. An evaluation of the likelihood of decompensation from the underlying cirrhosis, and obtaining tumor-free resection margins needs to be calculated before choosing resection as the preferred treatment. The risk of mortality is increased by the presence of portal hypertension, a Child-Pugh score of B or C, and the number of liver segments resected. Recommendations for transplantation in HCC complicating cirrhosis are as follows:

- Single tumor less than 5 cm diameter or multiple tumors less than three in number each less than 3 cm in diameter are suitable for transplantation.
- Local or systemic extrahepatic malignant disease is an absolute contraindication
- The fibrolamellar variant of HCC is not constrained by the size and volume criteria for transplantation as they are slower growing, less aggressive tumors.

Cholangiocarcinoma is not an indication for transplantation unless performed in conjunction with a novel management strategy.

Epithelioid hemangioendothelioma is one malignancy where even extrahepatic spread may not be a contraindication for transplantation. Five year survival figures between 40% and 75% have been reported. Distinguishing this tumor from an angiosarcoma is essential as transplantation is followed by universal recurrence and early mortality in the latter.

Metastatic Disease

Neuroendocrine tumors are the only metastatic liver tumors suitable to be transplanted for palliation. Several reports confirm that worthwhile symptomatic relief, and on occasion cure, can result from transplantation where resection is not feasible. Extrahepatic disease from neuroendocrine tumors is a contraindication to transplantation. The overall results of transplantation for nonneuroendocrine liver metastases have been poor.

Alcohol Related Liver Disease (ALD)

There are three main issues to be addressed whilst evaluating this disorder for transplantation:

- Is there a potentially reversible element to the disease following alcohol abstinence? If so transplantation should not be done
- Is the alcoholic liver disease associated with alcohol dependence and can abstinence be achieved following transplantation? Non-abstinence or recidivism leads to a very poor prognosis after OLT. Accordingly a six-month period of supervised abstinence is desirable. Nevertheless, young patients on first presentation need not fulfil this criteria if the illness is life threatening.
- Are there other co-morbid alcohol related illnesses, which will jeopardise the outcome? Organic brain damage from chronic alcohol abuse, alcoholic cardiomyopathy, pancreatitis and protein calorie malnutrition are specific areas that require careful assessment.

Despite the apparent difficulties in selecting patients, transplant programmes are reporting that sustained and serious recidivism rates are unexpectedly low. The liver transplant registry data from the United States demonstrate that survival figures for ALD are similar to non-ALD indications. These figures have been achieved despite a generally sicker pre-transplant clinical status. Lower rejection rates may be a part of the explanation.

Primary Biliary Cirrhosis (PBC) and Primary Sclerosing Cholangitis (PSC)

The recommendations for transplantation in PBC and PSC are:

- PBC and PSC are excellent indications for transplantation.
- Transplantation can be indicated for both prognosis in end stage liver disease and for symptomatic relief of intractable pruritus or debilitating lethargy. Although recurrence of PBC and PSC in the liver graft is evident histologically in a proportion of cases, subsequent graft failure is extremely rare.
- In PBC referral should be made for transplantation once the serum bilirubin exceeds 6 mgm/dL or significant impairment of liver function ensues.
- In PSC, age, bilirubin level, splenomegaly, histological stage, and Child-Pugh score have consistently been shown to be the most important prognostic variables. Mayo Clinic model uses these parameters and assesses risk of death at the time of referral to a tertiary centre. A Mayo model score of more than five or a Child grade C score justifies referral for transplantation.
- In PSC, stringent efforts to detect superadded cholangiocarcinoma are necessary but tests are often unreliable. The risk of colonic dysplasia complicating inflammatory bowel disease is also increased by up to fivefold in these patients and demands colonoscopic surveillance.

  Other conditions where OLT is a viable option include chronic liver disease or HCC complicating autoimmune hepatitis, Wilson's disease, hemochromatosis, and Budd-Chiari syndrome.

NON-DISEASE SPECIFIC CRITERIA

In the west, the wide disparity between available livers and potential recipients has lead to a contentious debate involving how this sparsely available organ should be allocated. It has been affirmed that urgency for liver transplantation should take the highest priority so-called "sickest first" philosophy. This requires a means to assess the severity of illness. The Child-Turcotte-Pugh scoring (CTP score) is an empiric, qualitative, classification of the severity of the "hepatic functional reserve" and comprises ascites, encephalopathy, albumin, bilirubin, and prothrombin time. A CTP score of more than seven was recommended as the minimal listing criteria for entry into the transplant waiting list in USA. However CTP scoring had significant limitations, which were:

- "The ceiling effect": a patient with 3.0 mg/dL of bilirubin and another with 20 mg/dL are classified within the same degree of severity. Something similar happens with albumin levels, and INR.
- This model cannot be applied to groups of diseases such as malignancy, fulminant liver failure and cholestatic liver disease

- Ascites and encephalopathy are very subjective criteria
- CTP classification provides three strata only. As a result, to distinguish two potential candidates within the same CTP class, the waiting time on the list took an unwarranted significance.

In February 2002, CTP scoring was replaced by the MELD (Model for End Stage Liver Disease) score for adults and PELD (Pediatric End Stage Liver Disease) for children in USA to decide on allocation of cadaveric livers for potential recipients on the waiting list. MELD score is based on a complicated calculation of bilirubin, creatinine and INR. Patients with HCC were given additional points depending on the stage of HCC (HCC MELD). This new allocation system appears to have decreased the death of patients on the waiting list, although the long-term impact on survival remains to be seen.

SURGICAL CONSIDERATIONS

Liver transplantation has four major phases:
- **Donor hepatectomy:** there are two types of donors
  - Cadaveric donor
    The liver is usually implanted in its entirety with the inferior vena cava (classical liver transplantation). Sometimes, an adult cadaveric liver will be split into two such that the smaller part, usually comprising segments 2 and 3 can be used for a child whilst the larger part (segments 4,5,6,7,8) is transplanted into an adult (split liver transplantation).
  - Living donor
    The left lateral segment, the left lobe or the right lobe from the living donor can be used depending on the relative sizes of the donor and the recipient.
    The donor liver is kept viable by cold preservation using UW (University of Wisconsin) at 4 °C. This way, a liver can be kept for up to 16 hours.
- **Recipient hepatectomy** is often the most difficult part of the procedure because of complicating features such as portal hypertension, coagulopathy, and adhesions from prior surgery. In classical transplantation, the hepatectomy is performed with the accompanying inferior vena cava. In **Piggy-Back technique**, the liver is removed separately from the inferior vena cava, which will be left almost intact apart from the areas of drainage of the main hepatic veins.
- **The implantation of liver** which in turn comprises three important phases
  - **Anhepatic phase** when the patient has no functioning liver. The problems that are to be anticipated are acidosis, impaired venous return

leading to cardiovascular instability, coagulopathy, fibrinolysis and electrolyte imbalance such as hyperkalemia.

- **Implantation** when the new liver is sutured to the recipient starting with the vascular outflow anostamoses first, including the suprahepatic vena cava and infrahepatic vena cava (or the hepatic veins in piggy-back technique), followed by the vascular inflow of the portal vein and finally hepatic artery.
- **Reperfusion**, which is usually done after the portal vein anostomosis. All the problems in the anhepatic phase can be accentuatated during this period. A specialized anesthesia team that understands the metabolic complexities of a patient with end stage liver disease is crucial to the success of the procedure.

The biliary anastomosis is done after this final phase. A bile duct to bile duct anostomosis (choledochostomy) is usually preferred. A Roux-en-Y bilio-enteric anastomosis is obviously necessary for those with abnormal native biliary systems such as biliary atresia and primary sclerosing cholangitis.

Operative Complications

Early surgical complications of liver transplantation include primary non-function of the hepatic graft, bleeding, hepatic artery thrombosis, and bile leak. Primary non-function (PNF) is a catastrophic event, estimated to occur in 2% to 5% of adult liver transplant recipients and treatable only by re-transplantation. The condition is characterized by acidosis, persistent and worsening coagulopathy, rising liver enzymes, and cholestasis. Although the cause is unknown, it is likely to be due to the result of donor factors such as poor retrieval technique rather than recipient factors.

Hepatic artery thrombosis can have a disastrous outcome as well and often requires re-transplantation.

MEDICAL CONSIDERATIONS

Rejection

Rejection is the primary medical complication of liver transplantation. Standard prophylactic regimens to prevent rejection usually include a calcineurin inhibitor (cyclosporine or tacrolimus) together with azathioprine or mycophenolate and steroid therapy. There is increasing support for eventual withdrawal of steroid therapy. Despite prophylactic therapy, rejection is seen in 40-50% of recipients usually within 7 to 10 days following successful liver transplantation. Rejection is generally suspected based on laboratory findings before symptoms develop, and is characterized by rising liver enzymes. Clinical features include fever and headache, followed by cholestasis. Liver biopsy is indicated to confirm the diagnosis as other causes of liver enzyme elevation (for example viral infection) may be exacerbated by the increased immune suppression used to treat rejection. Acute rejection is generally easily controlled with pulses of steroid therapy.

Infection

Complications of immunosuppression depend on the medications used but always include increased risk for serious infection from pathogens such as cytomegalo virus, Epstein-Barr virus, various fungi and bacteria. The use of perioperative prophylactic antibiotic, antifungal, and antiviral therapy is widespread.

Non-infectious Complications of Immune-suppression

Non-infectious complications of immune-suppression vary by the agent used. Post-transplant lympho-proliferative disease (PTLD) is a complication of immune-suppression that is believed to develop in response to the cumulative degree of immune-suppression and viral exposure, usually Epstein-Barr virus. Other less serious complications include hypertension, diabetes, renal impairment, hypercholesterolemia, osteoporosis, hirsuitism, gingival hypertrophy, skin malignancies, etc.

SUMMARY

Liver transplantation is a remarkably successful therapy for acute and chronic end-stage liver disease. Major developments in medical management, donor availability and procurement, operative techniques, and post-operative management all contributed to the dramatic improvement in outcome and growth of liver transplantation from its inception in 1963. The current 1-year and 5-year survival after OLT approach 90% and 60% respectively.

Liver transplantation has now, regrettably, become a victim of its own success. The two critical issues facing the transplant community are the crisis in the cadaveric organ supply and the consequences of long-term immunosuppression and its potentially life-threatening complications. Future advances in transplant immunobiology, organ availability (by xenotransplantation and genetic bio-engineering) and infection control are likely to lead to still greater improvements in short and long-term outcome of liver transplantation.

SUGGESTED READING

1. Starzl TE. The saga of liver replacement, with particular reference to the reciprocal influence of liver and kidney transplantation (1955–1967). J Am College of Surgeons 195(5): 587–610.
2. J Devlin, J O'Grady. Indications for referral and assessment in adult liver transplantation: a clinical guideline. Gut 1999; 45(Suppl 6): VI1-VI22.
3. Samuel D, Muller R, Alexander G, et al. Liver transplantation in HBsAg positive patients; an European experience 1977–1990. N Engl J Med 1993; 329: 1842–7.
4. Grellier L, Mutimer D, Ahmend M, et al. Lamivudine prophylaxis against reinfection in liver transplantation for hepatitis B cirrhosis. Lancet 1996;348: 1212–15.
5. Bismuth H, Chiche L, Adam R, et al. Liver resection versus transplantation for hepatocellular carcinoma in cirrhotic patients. Ann Surg 1993;218: 145–51.
6. Malinchoc M, Kamath PS, Gordon FD, Peine CJ, Rank J, ter Borg PC. A model to predict poor survival in patients undergoing transjugular intrahepatic portosystemic shunts. Hepatology 2000;31:864-871.
7. Noble-Jamieson G, Barnes N. Diagnosis and management of late complications after liver transplantation. Arch Dis Child 1999; 81(5):446-51.
8. Sudan DL, Shaw BW Jr. The role of liver transplantation in the management of portal hypertension. Clin Liver Dis 1997; 1: 115-20, xii.
9. Esquivel CO. Current status and outcome of pediatric liver transplantation. Clin Liver Dis 1997; 1: 397-415, ix-x.
10. Tung BY, Kowdley KV. Liver transplantation for hemochromatosis, Wilson's disease, and other metabolic disorders. Clin Liver Dis 1997; 1: 341-60.
11. Maldonado JR. Keeffe EB. Liver transplantation for alcoholic liver disease: selection and outcome. Clin Liver Dis 1997; 1: 305-21.
12. Bzowej NH, Wright TL. Prophylaxis and treatment strategies for chronic viral hepatitis in liver transplant patients. Clin Liver Dis 1997; 1: 323-39.

31

Sudheer OV

Investigation and Management of Gallstone Disease

INTRODUCTION

The incidence of biliary calculus disease varies widely throughout the world. In India there is geographical variation with northeastern region having more incidence of gall stone disease than the rest of the country.

Even though the incidence of gallstones is high, all patients do not need treatment. Except in special situations, only symptomatic gallstones require treatment.

The management of gallstone disease depends on the clinical presentation that the patient comes to you with. This setting can vary and can be considered under three basic headings:
1. Acute cholecystitis
2. Biliary colic, dyspeptic symptoms and chronic cholecystitis
3. Complicated gallstone disease with common bile duct (CBD) stones, cholangitis, biliary pancreatitis or other complications.

The final management pathway in all theses situations will be a cholecystectomy. In the first two settings the temporal sequence of medical management and the timing of surgery will vary. In the subset of patients with complicated gallstone disease the initial management will consist of the management of complications and then the clearance of the ductal stones that are almost invariably present in these settings.

ACUTE CHOLECYSTITIS

Acute cholecystitis is the most common complication of gallstone disease. This involves an acute inflammation of the gallbladder.

The initiating event in this entity is believed to be an occlusion of the cystic duct or the infundibulum of the gallbladder. This, in combination with altered biliary lipid composition, initiates a cycle of events that finally cause release of chemical mediators of inflammation within the gallbladder mucosa. This results in inflammation. The bacterial infection that is seen in most biliary cultures in acute cholecystitis is a result of secondary invasion by bacteria into the inflamed gallbladder.

The patient with acute cholecystitis will present with right upper quadrant abdominal pain and fever. The pain in this setting differs from biliary colic in its nature, in that it is reported as being more constant and lasts days instead of the few hours that the biliary colic does.

The classical clinical examination finding for acute cholecystitis is Murphy's sign, which is an inspiratory arrest on deep palpation in the right upper quadrant. The laboratory evaluation in this setting will show elevated counts and a small percentage (10%) of patients might have a mild jaundice. The confirmation of the diagnosis is by imaging studies; the most widely used one being an ultrasonogram of the abdomen. The findings on an ultrasonogram that suggest acute cholecystitis is increased wall thickness of the gallbladder, edema within the wall of the gallbladder and the presence of pericholecystic collections. The CT scan is not better at picking up gallbladder calculi but will be valuable in this setting to rule out other causes for acute abdominal pain like pancreatitis. A CT will also be useful in complicated cases where collections or mass lesions causing biliary obstructions are being considered. Though biliary imaging by radionuclide scans are highly accurate the relative scarcity of equipment and the long time taken for acquisition of the images generally make this a less preferred imaging technique.

Treatment of Acute Cholecystitis

Unlike most of the other aspects of treatment of gallstone disease there is no controversy in the decision regarding the final treatment of a patient who has acute cholecystitis—it is a cholecystectomy. But here the controversy lies in the timing and the type of the surgery.

Immediate Versus Delayed Cholecystectomy

Initial conservative management by antibiotics followed by cholecystectomy after 4-6 weeks was the approach that was followed previously. The major problem with this approach is that a significant number of patients do develop repeat attacks of acute cholecystitis in the waiting period and they go in for septic complications. Hence most centers now follow a policy of an initial period of stabilization of the patient followed by a cholecystectomy in the index admission itself.

However, this policy should be individualized according to the patient. A good example might be the case where a patient presents to you with a tender inflammatory mass in the right upper quadrant. In such situations an early attempt at cholecystectomy is likely to encounter dense inflammatory adhesions and significant wound sepsis.

Laparoscopic versus Open Cholecystectomy

Current evidence shows that a carefully done laparoscopy in the setting of acute cholecystitis is a safe procedure. Initial reports had suggested that laparoscopy is unsafe in severe cholecystitis, gangrenous gallbladder, empyema of the gallbladder, etc. But as the expertise improved these have all become relative contraindications. One point to bear in mind is that there should be lower threshold to convert the procedure to an open cholecystectomy. This is especially true when the anatomy in the Calot's triangle is distorted by the inflammation.

Medical Management in Acute Cholecystitis

As mentioned above the medical management in the setting of acute cholecystitis is an adjunct and not the primary treatment. This includes stabilization of the patient with correction of fluid and antibiotic therapy.

Antibiotic therapy should be aimed against the common biliary pathogens *E. coli, Klebsiella* and enterococcus. Since the cystic duct is occluded during acute cholecystitis the biliary penetration of the antibiotic agent is not a decision-making parameter.

BILIARY COLIC AND CHRONIC CHOLECYSTITIS

Biliary colic is the commonest indication for a cholecystectomy. The symptomatology in this group of patients may vary from vague dyspepsia and flatulence to recurrent bouts of biliary colic requiring hospital visits or analgesics. The classical biliary colic is an epigastric or right upper quadrant pain setting in about 30-60 minutes after the ingestion of a meal. The pain can radiate to the right scapula or the right shoulder.

No biochemical abnormalities are expected in this setting. The imaging studies follow the same guidelines as was suggested for acute cholecystitis and form the key point around which the diagnosis and the treatment hinges. A CT scan is better than an ultrasound in detecting CBD stones.

Asymptomatic Gallstones—Should they be Treated?

This issue is complicated by the lack of a strict definition of gallstone symptoms. Only about 50% of patients with gallstones give history of symptoms on questioning. A large percentage of patients do not give history of the recurrent biliary colic. They might instead have post prandial fullness, dyspepsia and vague epigastric discomfort. It is seen that the patients with such symptoms are less likely to have a satisfactory outcome after surgery. However about 70% of the patients do get improvement in their symptoms. The incidentally detected gallstone in the asymptomatic patient is best left alone. The patient with symptoms other than pain should be counselled prior to surgery that he/she faces a 30% possibility of having persistence of the symptoms. The patient who suffers from pain should be offered an early cholecystectomy.

The previous belief that diabetics or patients with non-functioning gallbladders should have cholecystectomies since they are prone to have acute cholecystitis has not been confirmed in studies that longitudinally followed up patients with gallstones for long periods of time. The risk of carcinoma of the gallbladder is low and hence a prophylactic cholecystectomy is not warranted for this indication. However patients with a coexisting calcification of the gallbladder (porcelain gallbladder) are at 25-60% risk for carcinoma gallbladder and should have a prophylactic cholecystectomy.

Medical Therapy for Gallstones

Can I take medicines to dissolve the stones? Surgeons are likely to face this question as long as they treat gallstones.

One point to be borne in the mind while looking at the data on oral dissolution and contact dissolution is that the ideas were mooted and the brunt of the research work was conceived prior to the era of the laparoscopic cholecystectomy. Since laparoscopic cholecystectomy is a simple procedure with morbidity so low that it has become a day care procedure much of the total advantages of the dissolution therapy are not relevant any more.

Oral dissolution uses UDCA (urso deoxy cholic acid) or CDCA (chenodeoxy cholic acid). Both act by reducing cholesterol absorption, increasing the conversion of cholesterol to bile acids and decreasing cholesterol biosynthesis by inhibiting HMG CoA reductase. The ideal patient for dissolution therapy is a thin lady with pure cholesterol stones less than 5 mm diameter in a functioning gallbladder. Moreover the therapy needs to be continued for 6-12 months. The recurrence rates at five years reach 50% even with the use of maintenance treatment.

Thus the role of dissolution therapy in the current scenario is limited. The utility is further limited by the fact that they are effective only against the pure cholesterol stones; this makes them practically unusable in Asia.

Contact Dissolution

Contact dissolution with MTBE requires an interventional radiologic procedure for access to the gallbladder. This procedure is not in clinical use for gallbladder stones any more.

Is Lithotripsy an Option?

The studies on lithotripsy in gallstones were spurred on by the good results obtained in patients with renal stones. So far the results obtained in urology have not been carried on to the biliary tree. Only about 20% of patients remain asymptomatic at six months.

Laparoscopic versus Open Cholecystectomy

In the setting of biliary colic / chronic cholecystitis the decision is clear. The standard of care for a patient with symptomatic gallstones is laparoscopic cholecystectomy. Open cholecystectomy should be reserved for patients who have medical contraindications to laparoscopy or where there is a suspicion of a co-existing gallbladder cancer.

Complicated Gallstone Disease and Choledocholithiasis

Gallstone disease is the commonest cause of cholangitis and choledo-cholithiasis. Choledocholithiasis can be due to stones arising de-novo in the bile duct (primary) or those that pass into the bile duct from the gallbladder (secondary). Primary stones are associated with stasis and or infection in the biliary tree.

About 10-15% of patients reporting with gallbladder stones have associated ductal stones. In centers that practice routine intraoperative cholangiogram the incidence of previously unsuspected CBD stones ranges from 5 to 8%.

In addition to the symptoms of biliary colic, patients with CBD stones can present with cholangitis or pancreatitis. The laboratory tests show an obstructive jaundice pattern. The levels of serum bilirubin and alkaline phosphatase will be elevated. The rise in bilirubin is generally moderate. In cases with borderline elevations in the alkaline phosphatase and bilirubin levels, a GGT (gamma glutamyl transferase) level assessment can confirm the presence of a biliary obstruction.

Imaging in suspected CBD stones should start with an ultrasonogram of the abdomen to confirm the presence of gallbladder calculi. A sonogram will also pick up dilatation of the CBD and intra hepatic biliary radicles. But the sonogram is not as sensitive for picking up CBD stones as it is for the gallbladder calculus. CT scans are to be used selectively; these will be useful in patients who are detected to have terminal CBD obstructions.

Once a biliary dilatation is identified the patient should have a cholangiogram. In the clinical setting of stone disease the preferred technique will be to get an endoscopic retrograde cholangiogram (ERC) done. This also assesses the ampulla for any growth.

Management of Patients with CBD Stones

A CBD stone can be detected
1. Pre operatively by imaging and biochemistry
2. Intraoperatively
3. Post operatively as a retained stone.

Preoperatively Detected Stone

When a stone is suspected by biochemical evaluation or by imaging the options of treatment will be either to clear the CBD pre operatively by an ERCP and stone clearance or to do a laparoscopic CBD exploration and cholecystectomy in the same sitting.

In patients who have imaging or biochemical parameters pointing to the presence of a CBD stone only about 20-25% have stones detected on routine ERCP. Thus the large majority of patients will be subjected to unnecessary ERCP.

The expertise and instrumentation to do laparoscopic CBD exploration is still not widespread. If these are available a laparoscopic CBD exploration is a good option to complete the treatment in a single sitting. A practical approach will be to schedule patients with documented CBD stones for ERCP with stone clearance.

Intraoperatively Detected CBD Stones

Routine intraoperative cholangiogram is being practiced in many centers. Primarily this is done to identify and avoid major CBD injuries. A CBD stone could be identified in such a procedure incidentally which was not seen in previous work up. The management in such a situation is controversial. The options are an expectant management, laparoscopic CBD exploration, or conversion to open cholecystectomy with CBD exploration.

Most of the CBD stones which are less than 8 mm will pass by themselves. The morbidities and complications of CBD exploration in the setting of a nondilated CBD is significant. In such situation laparoscopic transcystic CBD exploration without incising the CBD would be a better option if expertise is available. If the cholangiogram reveals a dilated CBD, with a stone, CBD exploration and stone removal is to be undertaken. If Laparoscopic approach fails or expertise is not available, it is advisable to convert the procedure to open cholecystectomy with CBD exploration.

Postoperatively Detected CBD Stones

Retained or missed stone is one of the causes for post cholecystectomy bile leak. It can also present as post operative obstructive jaundice or cholangitis. An endoscopic removal of the stones is advocated in such cases. It would require surgical exploration of CBD if endoscopic retrieval fails or is not possible.

SUGGESTED READING

1. Palazzo L. O'Toole D. Biliary stones: including acute biliary pancreatitis. Gastrointest Endosc Clin N Am 2005; 15: 63-82.
2. Gupta SK, Shukla VK. Silent gallstones: A therapeutic dilemma. Trop Gastroenterol 2004; 25: 65-8
3. Patino JF, Quintero GA. Asymptomatic cholelithiasis revisited. World J Surg. 1998; 22: 1119-24.
4. Tham TC, Lichtenstein DR, Vandervoort J et al. Role of endoscopic retrograde cholangiopancreatography for suspected choledocholithiasis in patients undergoing laparoscopic cholecystectomy. Gastrointest Endosc. 1998; 47: 50-6
5. Medical Progress: Pathogenesis and Treatment of Gallstones Johnston D. E., Kaplan M. M. N Engl J Med 1993; 328:412-421.
6. Ko CW, Lee SP. 2 Epidemiology and natural history of common bile duct stones and prediction of disease. Gastrointest Endosc (United States), Dec 2002; 56 (6 Suppl):pS165-9
7. Agrawal S, Jonnalagadda S. Gallstones, from gallbladder to gut. Management options for diverse complications. Postgrad Med (United States), Sep 1 2000; 108(3). p143-6, 149-53.
8. Rosseland AR, Glomsaker TB Eur J Asymptomatic common bile duct stones. Gastroenterol Hepatol (England) Nov 2000; 12(11):p1171-3

32

Raj VV

How do we Manage Acute Pancreatitis?

INTRODUCTION

The terminology of acute pancreatitis and its complications are often confusing and conflicting. The definition of pancreatic inflammatory disease has been the subject of several international conferences, in Marseille 1963, Cambridge 1983, Marseille 1984, and Atlanta 1992. The 1992 Atlanta International symposium definitions of various terminologies are as follows:

Acute pancreatitis

Acute pancreatitis is an acute inflammatory process of the pancreas, with variable involvement of other regional tissues or remote organ systems.

Severe acute pancreatitis

Severe acute pancreatitis is associated with organ failure and/or local complications such as necrosis (with infection), pseudocyst or abscess. Most often this is an expression of the development of pancreatic necrosis, although patients with edematous pancreatitis may manifest clinical features of a severe attack.

Mild acute pancreatitis

Mild acute pancreatitis is associated with minimal organ dysfunction and an uneventful recovery. The predominant pathological feature is interstitial edema of the gland.

Acute fluid collections

Acute fluid collections occur early in the course of acute pancreatitis, are located in or near the pancreas, and always lack a wall of granulation or fibrous tissue.

Pancreatic necrosis and infected necrosis

Pancreatic necrosis is a diffuse or focal area(s) of non-viable pancreatic parenchyma, which is typically associated with peripancreatic fat necrosis. The onset of infection results in infected necrosis, which is associated with a trebling of the mortality risk.

Acute pseudocyst

An acute pseudocyst is a collection of pancreatic juice enclosed in a wall of fibrous or granulation tissue that arises following an attack of acute pancreatitis.

Formation of a pseudocyst requires four or more weeks from the onset of acute pancreatitis.

Pancreatic abscess

A pancreatic abscess is a circumscribed intra-abdominal collection of pus, usually in proximity to the pancreas, containing little or no pancreatic necrosis, which arises as a consequence of acute pancreatitis.

Etiology of acute pancreatitis

Toxins
Alcohol
Drugs

Structural
- Gallstones, microlithiasis
- Sphincter of oddi spasm
- Pancreas divisum
- Traumatic.

Infectious
- Viral
- Bacterial
- Parasitic.

Metabolic
- Hyperlipidemia
- Hypercalcemia.

Vascular
- Vasculitis
- Atherosclerosis.

Other specific etiologies
- Hereditary
- Coronary bypass
- Neoplasia
- Cystic fibrosis
- Post ERCP
- Idiopathic.

DIAGNOSIS

Symptoms

Pain is the most common symptom and is present in 95% of patients. This deep, visceral pain is often located in the epigastric and umbilical region and may last for hours to days. Nausea and vomiting are present in 85% of patients and may occur without ileus or gastric outlet obstruction. Respiratory failure, confusion or coma with or without abdominal pain are rare modes of presentation.

Signs

Tachycardia and hypotension are found in upto 40% of patients. Abdominal tenderness and guarding are common and bowel sounds are often decreased or absent. Occasionally, body wall ecchymoses (Cullen's sign at the umbilicus, Grey-Turner's sign in the flanks) will be evident. Pleural effusion is most often found on the left side.

The diagnosis of acute pancreatitis may be difficult to make despite the many types of investigation available. It is imperative that other life threatening conditions are excluded (for example, mesenteric ischemia, visceral perforation, leaking abdominal aortic aneurysm).

LABORATORY TESTS

Markers of Pancreatic Injury

Serum Amylase and Lipase

In the majority of instances, given the appropriate clinical setting, the diagnosis of acute pancreatitis is made by a serum amylase activity four times above normal (or by a lipase activity greater than twice the upper limit of normal). The advantages of measuring lipase are that its activity remains increased for longer than that of serum amylase and that there are no other sources of lipase to reach the serum and thus this test has a high specificity.

Other Enzymes

Trypsinogen activation peptide (TAP) is a small peptide removed during activation of trypsinogen to trypsin. TAP assays, however may be too insensitive to be used as the primary test for pancreatitis. Urinary trypsinogen–2 measurements using a rapid dipstick assay is a promising test.

Inflammatory Markers

Several serum markers have been used to quantitate the pancreatic inflammatory response. IL-6, C-reactive protein (CRP) and neutrophil-specific elastase are a few of them; however, unlike serum amylase and lipase, they have more prognostic value.

Markers of Biliary Tract Involvement

Most patients with gallstone pancreatitis have elevation of alaninine aminotransferase and elevation of serum amylase of greater than 2000 IU/L. The ratio of lipase to amylase may be greater in alcoholic than in biliary pancreatitis.

Severity Assessment

Severity assessment allows the clinician to predict the patient's course, need for hospitalization, direct investigations such as CECT (contrast enhanced CT) or ERCP and directing therapies such as antibiotics. There are three categories: specific laboratory tests, clinical and physiologic assessment and CT scan.

Laboratory Tests

CRP, IL-6 and neutrophil elastase are some of the new tests that hold promise for separating mild disease from those with severe disease.

Clinical and Physiologic Assessment Criteria

Ranson	Simplified Glasgow
On admission	
Age >55y	Age> 55y
WBC > 16,000 mm^3	WBC. 15,000 mm^3
LDH >350 IU/L	LDH > 600 IU/L
Glucose >200 mg/dL	Glucose >180 mg/dl
AST > 250 IU/L	Albumin < 3.2 g/dl
	Calcium <8 mg/dl
Within 48h	Arterial Po$_2$ < 60 mm Hg
Hematocrit decrease by >10%	Urea > 45 mg/dl
Urea nitrogen increase by > 5 mg/dl	
Serum calcium < 8 mg/dl	
Arterial PO2 < 60 mm Hg	
Base deficit > 4 mEq/L	
Estimated fluid sequestration >6L	

Ranson's criteria are most widely used for the assessment of severity of acute pancreatitis. The disadvantage of Ranson's criteria is that they include 11 variables that must be monitored over 48 hrs. Glasgow criteria can be used any time and measures only eight variables. A score of three or more indicates severe pancreatitis. The prognostic accuracy of Glasgow is similar to that of Ranson's.

The Acute physiologic and chronic health evaluation (APACHE) II uses 14 routinely measured parameters of physiologic activity and biochemical parameters. The advantage of APACHE is that it can be calculated instantaneously from routine measurements.

Computed Tomography

All patients predicted to have a severe attack by one or more of the objective criteria outlined earlier should undergo an intravenous contrast enhanced (dynamic) CT scan between three and 10 days after admission.

Grade of Acute Pancreatitis

	Points
A. Normal pancreas	0
B. Pancreatic enlargement	1
C. Inflammation confined to pancreas and peripancreatic fat	2
D. One pancreatic fluid collection	3
E. Two or more fluid collections	4

Degree of Necrosis

No necrosis	0
Necrosis of one third of pancreas	2
Necrosis of one half of pancreas	4
Necrosis of more than half	6

CT severity index (CTSI) is calculated by adding up points for grade of pancreatitis and degree of necrosis. A score of less than 3 signifies mild pancreatitis, score of 4 to 6 moderate severity and 7 to 10 severe pancreatitis. The morbidity and mortality increases with increasing CTSI scores.

Management of Mild Pancreatitis

Acute pancreatitis predicted to be mild by objective criteria usually runs an uneventful self-limiting course and this form of disease constitutes 80% of all attacks and less than 5% of deaths.

General Management

These patients can be managed in the general ward with basic monitoring of temperature, pulse, blood-pressure, and urine output. Although all patients will require a peripheral intravenous line for fluids and sometimes a nasogastric tube, few will warrant an indwelling urinary catheter.

Antibiotics

Antibiotics should not be administered routinely as there is no evidence that their use in mild cases will affect outcome or reduce the incidence of septic complications. Antibiotics are warranted when specific infections occur (chest, urine, bile, or cannula related).

Specific Treatment

A variety of pharmacological and therapeutic treatments have been used in both mild and severe acute pancreatitis. These include aprotinin, glucagon, somatostatin, fresh frozen plasma, and peritoneal lavage. None of these have proven value and therefore cannot be recommended.

CT Scanning

Routine CT scanning is unnecessary unless there are clinical or other signs of deterioration.

MANAGEMENT OF SEVERE PANCREATITIS

General Management

The initial management involves full resuscitation and a multidisciplinary approach. The cornerstone of therapy is providing supportive care. Pancreatitis often leads to intravascular volume depletion, which may in turn worsen pancreatic perfusion and exacerbate pancreatitis. Fluids and electrolytes should be adequately replaced and periodically assessed based on urine output and vitals. Nasogastric suction should be used in those patients with severe pancreatitis and ileus.

Antibiotics

There is some evidence to support the use of prophylactic antibiotics in the prevention of local and other septic complications in severe acute pancreatitis.

In this respect, intravenous cefuroxime is a reasonable balance between efficacy and cost. Imepenem and quinolones are other antibiotics, which reduce sepsis in acute severe pancreatitis. The duration of prophylactic treatment is unclear at present.

Nutrition

Early nutritional support may aid recovery. Enteral feeding has been shown to be safe, as effective as total parenteral nutrition, and well tolerated in severe acute pancreatitis. Enteral nutrition is less expensive, helps to maintain mucosal function, and limits absorption of endotoxins and cytokines from the gut. Pancreatic stimulation can be avoided by placement of feeding tube distal to the Treitz ligament. Enteral feeding has largely replaced total parenteral nutrition in the management of patients with severe acute pancreatitis.

Pharmacologic Therapy

Inhibition of pancreatic enzyme activation, secretion, inflammation and cytokines are proposed as having potential benefit in ameliorating pancreatitis. Inhibitors of pancreatic proteases and octreotide have not shown to be of benefit in severe pancreatitis. Lexipafant, inhibitor of inflammatory cascade has been reported to improve course of acute severe pancreatitis, but later studies do not support this.

Role of ERCP in Pancreatitis

Severe gallstone pancreatitis in the presence of increasingly deranged liver function tests and signs of cholangitis (fever, rigors, positive blood cultures) requires an immediate therapeutic ERCP. Failure of the patient's condition to improve within 48 hours despite intensive initial resuscitation is an indication for urgent ERCP and sphincterotomy in gallstone pancreatitis. Available evidence from clinical trials suggests that this intervention may reduce overall morbidity from severe attacks in this subset of patients.

Complications

Immediate Complications

- Acute respiratory distress syndrome
- Acute renal failure, hypotension
- Disseminated intravascular coagulation
- Metabolic encephalopathy.

Late Complications

- Pseudocyst
- Pancreatic abscess
- Pancreatic fistulae – internal / external
- Vascular complications.

Surgery in Acute Pancreatitis

Necrotising Pancreatitis

Lack of improvement with full supportive intensive care therapy over 72 h is an indication for surgical intervention to remove pus and adjacent peripancreatic or pancreatic necrosis.

Pancreatic Abscess

Abscess tends to be circumscribed and may be much better treated than infected pancreatic necrosis. External drainage is the favored modality of treatment.

Acute Fluid Collection and Pseudocyst

Most of these complications resolve spontaneously. Failure of resolution can lead to the formation of circumscribed or multilocular sterile pseudocyst. This usually takes four weeks to develop and may cause pressure effects on duodenum, CBD or stomach causing symptoms. Persisting pseudocyst that is symptomatic has to be drained which can be achieved endoscopically, radiologically or surgically.

SUGGESTED READING

1. Guidelines for the management of acute pancreatitis. Journal of Gastroenterology and hepatology 2002 17 (suppl) s15-39
2. United Kingdom Guidelines for management of acute pancreatitis Gut 1998; 42 (Suppl 2): S1-S13 (June)
3. Chapter on acute pancreatitis; Sleisenger 7th edition, 2002, Sandess.
4. Recurrent acute pancreatitis: An algorithmic approach to identification and elimination of inciting factors Lehel Somogyi[*,‡], Stephen P. Martin[*], Thangham Venkatesan[*,‡], Charles D. Ulrich, IIGastroenterology 2001;120(3):708-17.
5. Management of acute pancreatitis: from surgery to interventional intensive care. Werner J, Feuerbach S, Uhl S, and Büchler M W. Gut, Mar 2005; 54: 426-36.
6. United Kingdom guidelines for the management of acute pancreatitis. Gut, Jun 1998; 42: 1-13.
7. Initial management of acute pancreatitis: critical issues during the first 72 hours. Tenner S Am J Gastroenterol (United States), 2004, 99(12):2489-94.
8. Medical treatment of acute pancreatitis. Mayerle J, Simon P, Lerch MM Gastroenterol Clin North Am (United States), 2004, 33(4):855-69.

33

Balakrishnan V

Experience with Chronic Pancreatitis

INTRODUCTION

Chronic pancreatitis is a world-wide disease. The disease is very much prevalent in India, although there are variations in the pattern and causes of the disease as observed in different parts of India.

Definition

Chronic pancreatitis is inflammatory damage of the pancreas with resultant morphological and functional changes of a permanent nature involving the exocrine and endocrine tissues.

ETIOLOGY

The commonest cause of chronic pancreatitis in the western world and in Japan is abuse of alcohol. Usually, drinking for several years is necessary to produce pancreatitis; however, there is no cut-off level beyond which alcoholic pancreatitis occurs. There is no direct correlation between the amount and duration of drinking and development of the disease. Moreover, only a percentage of alcoholics develop pancreatitis. This is possibly related genetic factors.

In many comparatively poor tropical countries, chronic pancreatitis is observed in younger patients who are non-alcoholic and who have no other known etiological factors. Nutritional deficiency, especially of micronutrients and antioxidants or/and dietary toxins such as cyanogenic glycosides (from cassava or tapioca, maize and other food stuffs) have been implicated in the causation. However, final proof for this hypothesis is yet to come.

Gallstones usually produce acute pancreatitis. Acute recurrent pancreatitis has been described to lead to chronic pancreatitis.Other causes of pancreatitis are hypercalcemia, hypertriglyceridemia, hyperparathyroidism, drugs and trauma, even though these factors usually cause acute pancreatitis. A hereditary form of pancreatitis has been found to be due to a mutation in the cationic trypsinogen gene (PRSSgene). Other rarer causes of pancreatitis include hemochromatosis, primary sclerosing cholangitis and primary biliary cirrhosis. A congenital anomaly of the pancreatic duct, "pancreas divisum", where there is an incomplete fusion between the fetal ventral and dorsal ducts of the pancreas, has been found to be associated with acute recurrent pancreatitis, even though a causal association has not been proven.Genetic mutations, especially of the SPINK-1 (PSTI) gene have come to the forefront over the past few years as an important etiological association in chronic pancreatitis. This may possibly have a facilitatory role, along with other etiological factors. There are many reports from different parts of our country about this association.

Recently, an autoimmune form of pancreatitis has been described, particularly from Japan. This form of the disease may be accompanied by other autoimmune manifestations.

PATHOGENESIS

There are several theories about the pathogenesis of chronic pancreatitis. These are the toxic metabolic theory, the small duct hypothesis, necrosis-fibrosis events, and the antioxidant deficiency theory. According to the toxic metabolic theory, it is the acinar tissue that is damaged first, followed by ductal changes, and later, the islets are destroyed.The small duct theory propounded by Prof. Sarles and colleagues lays emphasis on early damage to the small pancreatic ducts. Protein plugs formed from a hyperviscous pancreatic juice block the ducts causing stasis and the plug acts as a nidus for calculus formation, abetted by supersaturation of the juice with calcium. The necrosis fibrosis theory implicates acute recurrent attacks progressively leading to chronic pancreatitis.Relative deficiency of antioxidants and micronutrients, facilitating pancreatic damage by unquenched free oxygen radicals, is the core of the antioxidant theory.

It is possible that many of these pathogenetic mechanisms operate concurrently. Oxidant stress, ischemia and immunological factors, all may play different roles in the progression of the disease. Genetic defects, such as SPINK I mutations, predispose the individual to injury caused by environmental factors. More than one gene may be involved.

The type of pancreatitis seen in tropical countries in young subjects who are non-alcoholic and without any other well-known etiological factors has been called "tropical pancreatitis". This variety of the disease is very common in Tamilnadu, Andhra Pradesh and Karnataka, south Indian states, and is highest in Kerala. It has been also seen in Orissa in large numbers. When secondary diabetes mellitus due to islet damage is part of the disease spectrum, the condition is often termed "fibrocalculous pancreatic diabetes (FCPD)".

The cardinal symptoms of chronic pancreatitis is pain in the upper abdomen, often severe and continuous. The pain usually radiates to the back and is relieved by doubling forward with pressure over the abdomen. There may be some patients in whom pain may not be a prominent symptom. A history of recurrent episodes of mild abdominal pain in childhood or adolescence is often obtained starting a few years before clinical presentation. In the majority of patients, more than 80%, diabetes mellitus follows years of pain. However, there is a subgroup of patients in whom diabetes may predate the pain. Many patients may be malnourished. It is not clear whether the poor nutritional status plays any role in the etiology of the disease or is simply a consequence of the diabetes and malabsorption.

Fat malabsorption causing steatorrhea and weight loss are common consequences of chronic pancreatitis. This history may not be forthcoming in patients who generally take a diet poor in fat.

Physical examination might show evidence of nutritional deficiencies. Apart from an occasional mild hepatomegaly due to fatty liver, in the vast majority, the physical examination is unremarkable. There may be epigastric tenderness during acute exacerbations of the pancreatitis. Complications of common bile duct obstruction or a pseudocyst may produce physical findings of jaundice, or a palpable swelling in the epigastrium. Ascites may rarely follow a leak from a ruptured pancreatic duct.

INVESTIGATIONS

The hallmark of diagnosis is demonstration of pancreatic calculi by X-ray or still better, ultrasonography. The calculi may be solitary or multiple, and are of varying sizes, usually more in the region of the head, but may be distributed over the body and tail also.

Ultrasound may demonstrate a dilated, irregular main pancreatic duct and an atrophic parenchyma. It also helps to pick up a pseudocyst. Sometimes, the pancreas may be obscured by intestinal gas, when a CT scan will have to be done. A CT is more sensitive in visualizing changes in the pancreas than an ultrasound. Pancreatic function tests such as the classical secretin CCK test, previously thought to be the gold standard in diagnosis, is now rarely employed in routine practice as imaging modalities are quite reliable, easier to perform and less expensive. The oral tests such as bentiromide test or pancreolauryl test serve only as screening tests for pancreatic exocrine deficiency and are positive only with advanced pancreatitis.

A full diabetic work up should be done for all patients with suspected pancreatitis. The vast majority of patients will be diabetic, or they may show impaired glucose tolerance.

Stool fat estimation may show steatorrhea. The Van de Kamer stool fat quantification assay is not necessary in clinical practice. A properly done Sudan III staining of the stool for fat globules will serve in practice to assess steatorrhea.

Liver function tests will help to rule out cholestasis due to CBD obstruction. Se calcium and triglyceride levels should be estimated as elevation of either could cause pancreatitis.

An ERP (endoscopic retrograde pancreatogram) is not routinely done, unless we are planning for surgery, when it might serve as a road map.

MRCP (magnetic resonance cholangiopancreatography) is helpful in certain situations.

EUS (endoscopic ultrasound) is gaining popularity as a test to pick up early changes of chronic pancreatitis. This requires expertise and is now available in specialised centres.

Testing for genetic mutations in pancreatitis is currently outside the purview of clinical protocols.

DIAGNOSIS

A detailed history of alcoholism and smoking (risk for cancer pancreas), dietary habits, and family history of pancreatitis should be elicited.

Physical examination is not of much help in the diagnosis.

The demonstration of pancreatic calculi on imaging is the sina qua non of chronic pancreatitis.

Diagnosis is difficult in early cases of pancreatitis where the patient may have typical pain, but without evidence of pancreatitis on routine imaging. In such cases, an ERP or an EUS, or exocrine function tests, if available, may be helpful.

Complications of Chronic Pancreatitis

1. Pseudocyst.
2. CBD obstruction.
3. Carcinoma pancreas.
4. Splenic vein thrombosis and portal hypertension.

Pseudocysts are less common in tropical pancreatitis than in alcoholic pancreatitis. Asymptomatic pseudocysts are left alone and followed up. If they become symptomatic, they should be tackled by endoscopic means (cystogastrostomy, cystojejunostomy, transpapillary drainage), or surgical excision.

CBD obstruction may be due to edema and fibrosis or may be the presentation of malignancy of the pancreas. If benign, it may necessitate CBD stenting. If due to malignancy, and is operable, some form of pancreaticoduodenectomy is done. Inoperable cases may be palliated by stents.

Carcinoma is one of the dreaded complications of chronic, especially tropical pancreatitis. It occurs in approximately 10% of patients. Generally, it carries a very poor prognosis. Malignancy should be suspected if there is recent aggravation of pain, weight loss, or jaundice or other features of CBD obstruction, or if there is a pancreatic head mass. Often it is difficult to differentiate between a benign and a malignant head mass. CA19-9 estimation or FNAC (fine needle aspiration cytology) may not differentiate between the two in about 50% of instances. When there is a strong suspicion of malignancy, a pancreatico-duodenectomy is the procedure of choice.

Treatment

Treatment of chronic pancreatitis involves:
1. Relief of pain.
2. Management of diabetes.
3. Reversing steatorrhea.
4. Treatment of complications.
5. Correction of nutritional deficiencies.

Relief of Pain

Analgesics and, for severe pain, even narcotics will have to be administrated in adequate doses. Severe continuous pain may necessitate round the clock administration of morphine.

Pancreatic enzyme preparations, particularly those with a high protease content, in tablet form, may, by a negative feedback mechanism, suppress intrinsic enzyme production and thus help to relieve pain.

When pain does not respond to use of analgesics, a celiac plexus block might alleviate pain, even though pain will recur after about six months.

Pancreatic Enzyme Supplements

Pancreatic enzyme supplements serve two purposes in chronic pancreatitis. Firstly, enzyme preparations with high protease content are given to alleviate pain. Secondly, enzyme preparation with a high lipase content help in improving steatorrhea.

Pancreatic enzymes have to be given in large doses of at least 30,000 units of lipase activity, along with each meal. The enzyme activity tends to be degraded by the gastric acid; hence proton pump inhibitors are given in the usual doses.

Newer preparations of pancreatic enzymes, e.g. creon have enzyme particles packed in microspheres of size less than 2mm, enclosed in a capsule, so that the emptying of the enzymes from the stomach into the intestine synchronizes with that of food.

Diabetes Mellitus

A few newly detected diabetics in chronic pancreatitis can be controlled with diet and regular exercise. Another large number is controlled with oral hypoglycemic agents for varying periods . Yet another large group will require insulin for proper control of diabetes, right from the beginning.

Complications of diabetes are common, particularly microvascular complications. Macrovascular complications do occur, though uncommon. Diabetic ketoacidosis is relatively uncommon, one of the reasons being reduced glucagon production.

Endotherapy

Patients with chronic pancreatitis, who have severe pain not controlled with large doses of analgesics, may be considered for endotherapy as a temporary alternative for surgery. Patients with a few small stones in the head region with a dilated proximal duct are the ideal candidates. Sphincterotomy, with pancreatic duct stenting, sometimes undertaken after ESWL (extracorporeal shock wave lithotripsy) to crush the stones, is the usual procedure. Pain-free periods of months to a couple of years have been observed with the procedure. However, this is not yet a widely accepted method.

Surgery

Surgery is indicated in patients with severe, recurrent or continuous intractable pain not responding to full dose of medications.It is also done for complications such as pseudocysts, CBD obstruction and with a head mass with suspicion of malignancy. In patients with a dilated main pancreatic duct (MPD), various types of drainage procedures such as longitudinal pancreaticojejunostomy (PJ), with head coring (particularly with a head mass), or head resection are procedures employed. Surgery is followed by short-term pain relief in 80 to 85% of patients. Long-term pain relief is to the tune of 60 to 75%. In a majority, pain might recur after 5 to 10 years. In patients with a non dilated MPD, some type of resection has to be considered. Subtotal or total pancreatectomy is a very major procedure with often unacceptable sequelae. If there is suspicion of a malignancy in the head, a pancreaticoduodenectomy (classical or modified Whipple's) procedure should be undertaken.

NATURAL HISTORY

A change in the natural history of tropical pancreatitis has been observed during the last few years. The disease is now seen in older subjects, who are usually better nourished, the diabetes is often milder and controllable with oral antidiabetic drugs, and the disease seems to take a more slow protracted course. Many patients can be maintained for longer periods on medical treatment, fewer patients going in for surgery. Longevity seems to have increased by a decade or two. However, the incidence of malignancy has increased, partly due to greater longevity, but may also be due to the ifluence of additional environmental carcinogens. It is also not known whether the same injurious agents that perpetuate the damage to the pancreas might be contributing to the process of malignant transformation too. Another interesting trend is the increasing number of reports, though anecdotal, of so-called "tropical pancreatitis" (? idiopathic pancreatitis) from other parts of India, including northern India.

SUGGESTED READING

1. Mitchell RMS, Byrne MF, Baillie J. Pancreatitis – Seminar. The Lancet; 361: 1447-55.
2. Balakrishnan V. Fibrocalculous pancreatopathy. Int. J. diab. Dis. Countries. 2002; 22: 81-90.
3. Balakrishnan V. (Ed). Chronic Pancreatitis in India 1987. Indian Society. Pancreatology. St. Joseph's Press, Trivandrum.
4. Mohan V, Premalatha G, Pitchumoni CS. Tropical Chronic Pancreatitis. J Clin Gastroenterol 2003: 36(4): 337-46.
5. Whitcomb DC, Gorry MC, Preston RA, Furey W, Jossenheimer MJ, Ulrich CM, Martin SP, Gates JR, Amman ST, Toskers PP, Liddle R, McGrath K, Vomo G, PoRT JC, Ehrlieh GD. Hereditary pancreatitis is caused by a mutation in the cationic trypsinogen gene. Nature genetics 1996; 14: 141-45.
6. Balakrishnan V, Harish Kumar, Sudhindhran S, Unni Krishnan AG. (Eds). Chronic Pancreatitis and Pancreatic diabetis in India 2006. Indian Pancreatitis study group. LG Creations, Bangalore.
7. Balakrishnan V, Nair prem, Radhakrishnan Lakshmi, Narayanan VA. Tropical pancreatitis–a distinct entity, or merely a type of chronic pancreatitis? Indian J gastroenterology 2006;25:74–81.

34

Padmanabhan TK
Pavithran K

Common
Gastrointestinal
Malignancies

CARCINOMA ESOPHAGUS

More than 90% of malignant esophageal neoplasms are squamous cell carcinoma. Primary adenocarcinoma may arise from the submucosal glandular elements within the esophagus or more frequently from columnar epithelium lining distal esophagus. Adenocarcinoma of lower end of esophagus may be due to direct extension of adenocarcinoma stomach. Among the nonepithelial malignant tumors, leiomyosarcoma is the most common tumor.

Epidemiology

In India it is the second most common cancer in males in Bangalore, Mumbai and Chennai, and among the top 5 cancers in males and females.

Etiology

Important causative factors are nitrosamine, polycyclic aromatic hydrocarbon, tobacco, excessive alcohol intake, nutritional deficiency and achalasia cardia. Fifteen percent of cancers occur in upper 1/3rd, 50% in the middle 1/3rd and 35% in the lower1/3rd. Increasing incidence of adenocarcinoma of the lower esophagus has been linked to Barrett's esophagus with intestinal metaplasia of the mucosa.

Clinical Presentation

Initial symptom is dysphagia for solids and eventually for liquids. Pain may be present in 50% of patients. In advanced cases, aspiration pneumonia, hemoptysis, hematemesis, chest pain and back pain may develop.

Diagnosis

Barium swallow may be diagnostic when disease is locally advanced. Esophagoscopy with biopsy is necessary to visualize early lesion and also to get tissue diagnosis. CT scan will be necessary to assess periesophageal extension, lymph node involvement and involvement of liver.

Treatment

Despite advances in surgery, radiotherapy and chemotherapy, cure rate is very poor and the five-year survival is only 5 to 10%.

Surgery

In operable patients surgery in the form of oesophagectomy should be attempted because it gives the best palliation. Esophagectomy includes a cuff of stomach and anastamosis done in the neck.

Radiotherapy

Major advantage of radiotherapy is that it is not associated with acute mortality. Radiotherapy often provides relief of obstruction; but in more than 50% of patients, it is only short term. For patients with localized cancer, who are medically unfit for surgery, curative radiotherapy should be offered. Cure rate is similar to that of surgery. With modern mega voltage X-ray machines like linear accelerator and highly sophisticated CT scan based computer treatment planning, high dose of curative radiotherapy can be delivered without much morbidity. Radiotherapy combined with chemotherapy offers best results but with increased toxicity. External radiotherapy may be boosted by intraluminal brachytherapy. Post-operative radiotherapy is indicated when there is para-esophageal extension, peri-esophageal node involvement or when cut margin is positive.

Chemotherapy

Since more than 75% may harbour occult metastasis, chemotherapy plays a very important role. Cisplatin is one of the most active agents with response rate of 20%. Other drugs are 5 FU, mitomycin, bleomycin and taxol. Most commonly used combination is cisplatin and 5 FU infusion.

Neo-adjuvant Chemotherapy

Chemotherapy can be given before surgery as a neoadjuvant therapy. If there is favourable response, it is continued postoperatively for 2 to 3 cycles.

Concurrent Chemo Radiation

Definitive chemo radiation for localized carcinoma is an alternative to curative surgery and is the standard of care for patients refusing surgery or who are medically unfit.

Endoscopic Palliation

In advanced cases, endoscopic palliation is attempted by de-bulking the tumor by alcohol injection or using laser. Luminal patency can be maintained by endoscopic placement of endoprosthesis. Self-expending metal stents are available.

CARCINOMA STOMACH

Adenocarcinoma is the most common malignant tumor of stomach comprising 97%. Other tumors are carcinoid, lymphoma and leiomyosarcoma.

Epidemiology

Incidence of adenocarcinoma of stomach is highest in Japan, Chile and Iceland. In USA and Europe incidence has decreased over the last few decades. In India it is one of the leading cancers and has highest incidence in males in Banglore and Chennai registries.

Etiology

Common in low socio-economic groups and in those with high starch intake and low fresh fruit and vegetable intake. Asbestos workers and patients with pernicious anemia or atrophic gastritis have a higher incidence. Chronic *H. pylori* gastritis can lead to cancer of the stomach.

Symptoms

Presenting symptoms are vague and consist of anorexia, epigastric discomfort, fatiguability and weight loss. Post prandial abdominal pain, early satiety and vomiting or hematemesis are other features. In advanced stages, there may be palpable mass and ascites.

Diagnosis

1. Barium meal studies can generally identify the malignant ulcer or growth.
2. Gastroscopy and biopsy are essential.
3. CT scan abdomen–secondary nodes and metastasis in liver may be identified. Also helpful to assess extragastric extension.

Treatment

Surgery

Surgery is the treatment of choice. Radical subtotal gastrectomy is the usual surgical procedure. Otherwise total gastrectomy is done. In advanced cases, feeding gastrostomy may be required. Even in the presence of metastasis attempt should be made to resect the primary because this gives the best palliation.

Radiotherapy

Postoperative radiotherapy is recommended after surgery if there is known residual disease or when lymph nodes are involved. Radioopaque clips placed during surgery in areas of known residual disease helps in radiotherapy planning. Radiotherapy with concurrent chemotherapy plays a major role in locally advanced or recurrent stomach cancer. Intraoperative radiotherapy is commonly practiced in Japan, where electron beam therapy is given after gastrectomy before closure of abdomen.

Chemotherapy

Adjuvant chemotherapy: After complete resection, post-operative adjuvant chemotherapy offers slight benefit. Useful agents are 5FU, mitomycin, cisplatin, methotrexate and adriamycin. More recently concurrent chemo radiation is recommended because of better results.

Palliative chemotherapy: In advanced stomach cancer, chemotherapy offers good palliation in 30 to 40% of patients with 6 to 8 months median survival. Various combinations are used with drugs such as 5FU, adriamycin, mitomycin, cisplatin, methotrexate and etoposide. Lymphoma of stomach is usually treated by gastrectomy followed by adjuvant chemotherapy. Post-operative radiotherapy is indicated when residual disease is left behind.

CANCER OF THE PANCREAS

Carcinoma pancreas is one of the most aggressive visceral malignancies. In USA it is the fourth most common cause of cancer death. It is less common in India.

Etiology

There is higher incidence in developed countries. Incidence is high in smokers. Relationship with alcohol and coffee is still not established. Cancer pancreas may arise de-novo, or it may complicate all types of chronic pancreatitis, particularly, tropical pancreatitis.

Diagnosis

Most patients present with asthenia and weight loss. Severe upper abdominal pain is common. There may be jaundice or back pain. Pain is often aggravated by food and causes loss of sleep. Diabetes mellitus may be a complication. Jaundice is usually due to common bile duct obstruction.

Investigations

Blood tests should include CBC, blood sugar, liver function tests, serum amylase and CA19-9 (marker for pancreatic malignancy).

Imaging

1. Ultrasound abdomen is the best initial investigation. It may pick up pancreatic mass and also reveals changes of chronic pancreatitis.
2. Contrast enhanced CT scan (CECT)–Small lesion can be detected and it is useful to assess operability (lymph nodes, invasion of vessels, metastasis). CT guided fine needle aspiration may be helpful.
3. Endoscopic retrograde cholangio-pancreatogram (ERCP).
4. Endoscopic ultrasound (EUS) – Helps to decide on operability.

Pathology

Ninety-five percent of the tumors are adenocarcinomas arising from exocrine pancreas. Most of these tumors arise from the head of the pancreas.

Treatment

Surgery

Surgical resection of localized pancreatic cancer offers the only chance of cure. Most patients will benefit with relief of symptoms with occasional long-term survival. Pancreaticoduodenectomy or Whipple's procedure, or one of its modifications, is the standard operation. It involves en bloc resection of the head of pancreas, neck and uncinate process, duodenum, distal bile duct and gastric antrum. Other techniques are less common. Only 10 to 15% of operable patients will undergo complete resection. The 5-year survival after curative resection is only 10%. Patients who have unresectable cancer may need cholecystojejunostomy or other bypass procedures to relieve bile duct obstruction.

Radiotherapy

Radiotherapy has a major role in the treatment of carcinoma pancreas since majority are locally advanced. 3D conformal radiotherapy and intensity-modulated radiotherapy (IMRT) help to deliver adequate dose to the tumor with relative sparing of adjacent structure. Radiotherapy is recommended in the following situations:

1. After curative resection with positive margins or nodal involvement.
2. Curative radiotherapy in locally advanced diseases.
3. Palliative radiotherapy for local pain and intestinal obstruction.

Adjuvant Therapy

Even after complete resection there is high incidence of local recurrence. Hence concurrent chemoradiotherapy has become widely accepted treatment. Most commonly used drug is 5FU.

Locally Advanced and Metastatic Disease

These patients can be started on chemotherapy with gemcitabine and cisplatin. More often if there is no metastatic disease, concurrent chemo radiation is tried for better local response. 'Clinical benefit response' is more important than objective response, because more emphasis is given to the quality of life.

CANCER OF THE HEPATOBILIARY SYSTEM

Epidemiology

Incidence is high among orientals and African Bantu. In India it is among the highest 15 cancers in males, but is quite low in women.

Etiology

In a large number of patients with primary hepatocellular carcinoma (HCC), cirrhosis is present. Hepatitis B infection is responsible for 80% of liver cancers. In younger patients, who have acquired the infection in infancy, the cancer occurs in a normal liver. Chronic hepatitis C infection is also a cause of liver cancer. Cholangiocarcinoma may complicate sclerosing cholangitis, either primary, or secondary to inflammatory bowel disease. In the far East, liver fluke infection is a cause of cholangiocarcinoma. Aflatoxin from certain fungi in food is also implicated in HCC.

Pathology

- Hepatocellular carcinoma (HCC)
- Cholangio carcinoma
- Hepatoblastoma (mostly in children).
- Liver metastases (from colon, stomach, pancreas, etc.).

Diagnosis

Initial symptoms are non-specific with complaints of weakness, anorexia, abdominal fullness and dull upper abdominal pain. Later, liver may be palpably enlarged and tender. Ascites, portal hypertension and jaundice may appear in due course.

Investigations

1. Liver function tests-elevation of alkaline phosphatase out of proportion to SGOT, SGPT and bilirubin is characteristic.
2. Ultrasound of liver may show solitary irregular hyperechoic lesion in HCC. Sometimes, the lesion may be multifocal involving one or both lobes. Metastases are usually multiple.
3. Elevated AFP (alpha fetoprotein) is useful in diagnosis (values > 500 µg/dl). However, false-negative and positive results are common.
4. CT scan will clearly reveal the anatomical situation and extent of disease, and vascular invasion.
5. MRI may be necessary to assess resectability.
6. Surgeons discourage a pre-operative liver biopsy/fine needle aspiration for fear of needle track spread.

Treatment

Surgery

Only curative treatment is surgical resection. Recommended surgery is total hepatic lobectomy. Total hepatectomy and liver transplantation is possible in occasional cases. Five year survival can be about 30% after hepatic resection.

Radiotherapy

Since the radiation tolerance of liver is much below cancericidal dose, radiotherapy has no curative role. But pain may be relieved by palliative radiotherapy in inoperable case.

Chemotherapy

Systemic chemotherapy may be the only option for vast majority of these patients. These tumors are not chemosensitive and hence response rate is only 10 to 20%. 5FU and doxorubicin are commonly used. New drugs are gemcitabine, irinotecan and combination containing interferon. Local chemo embolisation of tumor or intra-arterial chemotherapy may produce marginal response.

Other modalities of palliation are alcohol injection into the tumor nodule, and radiofrequency ablation.

BILE DUCT CANCERS (CHOLANGIOCARCINOMA)

This may involve the proximal common bile duct (CBD) or hepatic ducts (Klatskin tumor), or the distal CBD.

Most common presentation is obstructive jaundice.

Diagnosis

Evaluation of obstructive jaundice leads to diagnosis.

Investigations

1. Liver function tests show features of obstructive jaundice with high conjugated bilirubin levels and alkaline phosphatase.
2. Ultrasound – Ultrasound shows dilated gall bladder and hepatic ducts. It may suggest a mass.
3. CT scan may reveal a hilar cholangiocarcinoma, mass lesions of liver or pancreas.
4. Transhepatic cholangiogram and ERCP–This will define the area of obstruction and transhepatic drainage is possible and ERCP may define lower extent of completely obstructing lesions.
5. MRC (magnetic resonance cholangiography).

Treatment

Surgical treatment is the only therapy that offers a chance of cure. For proximal tumor, decompression of biliary tree is done by direct anastamosis to gastrointestinal tract, since curative resection is rare. For periampullary carcinoma, surgery in the form of pancreaticoduodenectomy (Whipple's), or pylorus preserving dudenectomy is recommended.

Palliation may be obtained by placing stents in the obstructed ducts to facilitate drainage and to relieve jaundice.

GALLBLADDER CARCINOMA

Cholelithiasis predisposes patients to gall bladder carcinoma. In south-India incidence is less than that of liver cancer. But in north-India, incidence is much higher.

Signs and Symptoms

Pain in right hypochondrium, nausea, vomiting and weight-loss and later on jaundice may develop. Physical examination may show hepatomegaly and a mass in the gallbladder region in many patients.

Investigations

1. Ultrasound may show enlarged gallbladder, thickening of gallbladder walls, or sometimes a mass may be visualised.
2. CT scan often shows a mass in the GB region. Associated gallstones are commonly seen.

Treatment

Surgery

In operable cases, cholecystectomy along with node dissection in porta hepatis and common bile duct is the treatment of choice. In most of the cases only palliative anastomosis is possible.

Radiotherapy

Since curative resection is rare, radiotherapy plays a very important role. Radiotherapy is indicated after curative surgery since it improves survival. It can offer excellent palliation in inoperable tumor. With modern high dose rate brachy therapy system transcatheter irradiation through transhepatic external biliary drainage tube is possible and gives high local dose. This can be supplemented with external radiotherapy in suitable patients.

Chemotherapy

Chemotherapy is same as for cancer liver and offers only palliation. Sometimes concurrent chemo radiotherapy offers better results.

CANCER OF THE DUODENUM AND SMALL INTESTINE

Incidence is low and uniform world-wide. Possible protective factors are alkalinity of small bowel contents, rapid transit of food, liquid consistency of food, high immunoglobulin and lack of bacteria in the small bowel.

Pathology

Sixty-percent of malignant tumors are adenocarcinomas. Other malignant tumors are carcinoid, leiomyosarcoma and lymphoma.

Diagnosis

Colicky pain is the most common symptom. Other symptoms are weight loss, cachexia, intestinal obstruction and palpable mass. Some patients present with melena due to bleeding from the mass. Duodenal tumor may produce obstructive jaundice, lymphadenopathy in lymphoma and carcinoid syndrome in carcinoid tumor.

Investigations

Contrast GI Studies

Contrast x-ray studies of GI tract with small bowel follow through may show the tumor. Barium enema studies may be useful in distal ileal lesion. Enteroclysis (small bowel enema) helps delineate a mass lesion better than a barium meal.

Endoscopy

Upper GI endoscopy should be done and will reveal mass in the duodenum. Distal ileum may be visualized by colonoscopy. Biopsy is always done if the lesion is visualized.

CT Scan

CT scan will show tumor extension beyond bowel wall, lymph node metastasis and liver involvement.

Enteroscopy will help to visualize a mass beyond the reach of the upper GI endoscope.

Capsule endoscopy is a newer modality to visualize ulcerations, masses or bleeding in the small bowel, but biopsy is not possible.Bowel obstruction is a relative contraindication.

Treatment

Surgery

Surgery is the main treatment for all tumors of small intestine. For non-resectable tumors surgical bypass is necessary if obstruction is present.

Radiotherapy

Radiotherapy has little role to play except in palliation of pain or obstruction. Radiotherapy may be needed for lymphoma after bowel resection and chemotherapy. Carcinoids are treated by surgical resection.

Chemotherapy

Role of chemotherapy is not well established as an adjuvant treatment. Agents which are used for GI tumors have been used in a palliative setting. Drugs like 5FU and nitrosoureas have been used.

COLORECTAL CANCER

Epidemiology

Incidence of colorectal cancers is very high in USA and other western countries; however, it is low in Japan and Africa. In India the incidence is 1-3/1,00,000.

Etiology

Predisposing Factors

- Low fibre diet has a high correlation probably due to the long transit time
- Diet that is high in fat content
- Bile acids produce their carcinogenic effect as a promoter
- Familial adenomatous polyposis (FAP) and hereditary non-polyposis carcinoma of colon (HNPCC)
- Chronic ulcerative colitis, and to a lesser extent, Crohn's disease
- Adenomatous polyp, especially larger than 1 cm diameter
- Obesity and sedentary life style increases the risk
- Genetic mutations e.g. APC gene.

Pathology

Majority are adenocarcinomas. Less common tumors are lymphoma, carcinoids, leiomyoma, etc.

Symptoms

Bleeding per rectum, change in bowel habits, weight loss, cachexia, and obstruction. Generally, left sided lesion present with bleeding and obstructive symptoms. Right sided, especially cecal lesions, may present with non-specific symptoms including weight loss, anemia or melena.

Investigations

1. Barium enema double contrast studies should be done if colonoscopy is not available. This will reveal mass lesion or obstruction.
2. Colonoscopy with biopsy is the most important investigation.
3. Ultrasound of liver – for thickening or narrowing of bowel wall, mass lesson in bowel and, metastasis in liver.
4. Serum markers like CEA and CA19-9 are not diagnostic. However, CEA is very useful for follow-up after surgery.
5. CT scan helps in detecting gross tumor extension outside bowel wall and to detect liver metastasis and regional lymphnodes.
6. Stool examination for occult blood is useful (in screening of susceptible population).

Treatment

The disease is classified according to modified Duke's classification based on extent of tissue invasion into A, B_1, B_2, C_1, C_2 and D.

Surgery

Resection of primary tumor with safe margin and end-to-end anastamosis is the standard treatment. Associated mesocolon with lymph nodes is also removed. Depending upon the site of tumor, surgery may be right or left hemicolectomy, total or sub-total colectomy, sigmoid colectomy, anterior resection or abdominoperineal resection. Review colonoscopy should be done for recurrence six months after surgery and then yearly. Rise in CEA levels post operatively usually suggests recurrence.

Radiotherapy

Radiotherapy has no role when complete curative resection has been done in mobile colon. But it is useful when tumor is in immobile part of colon, when margin of resection is minimal, when there is pericolic extension, when tumor invades adjoining tissues, when cut ends are positive or close to the tumor or when there is perforation or fistula. Radiation is also given when regional nodes are involved. Patients with fixed tumor or locally advanced tumor may benefit from pre-operative radiotherapy, which may make tumor resectable.

Chemotherapy

Chemotherapy of metastatic disease is with combinations of 5FU, leucovorin, and irenotecan. Metastasis in liver are to be looked for, and small lesions < 5 cm, if solitary, or < 3 cm if 2 to 3, are amenable for surgical resection.

CANCER OF THE RECTUM

Epidemiology

Cancer of the rectum is also a disease of the industrialized western countries; Czech Republic has the highest incidence, 24/1,00,000, followed by UK and USA. In India the incidence is 1.5-3.3/1,00,000. The incidence is higher than that of carcinoma colon.

Diagnosis

Common symptoms are rectal bleeding and change in bowel habit. There may be palpable mass on digital examination. Commonly patients consult the doctor complaining of piles. These patients should have a proper digital rectal examination and proctosigmoidoscopy with biopsy to rule out rectal carcinoma.

Investigations

1. Endoscopy and biopsy. Rigid proctoscopy is better than flexible endoscopy for visualization and biopsy.
2. CT scan of the pelvis and abdomen is useful to assess nodal disease, perirectal extension and to rule out liver metastasis.

Pathology

Adenocarcinoma is the most common malignant tumor. Rarely malignant melanoma can occur.

Treatment

Surgery

Upper 1/3rd carcinoma is treated with anterior resection thus maintaining natural passage. For mid1/3rd cancer anterior resection is done when sufficient length of distal rectum is available for anastamosis. Lower 1/3rd cancers will require abdominoperineal resection with colostomy. Total mesorectal excision of lower 1/3rd tumor reduces the risk of loco-regional recurrence.

Radiotherapy

Pre-operative radiotherapy, either short course of five days, or long course of 25 days, is recommended for locally advanced operable tumor. In inoperable tumors radiotherapy may downstage the tumor and surgery may be possible. Post-operative radiotherapy is indicated when surgical clearance is incomplete or if the stage is more advanced than anticipated. Even in early cancer, postoperative addition of radiotherapy and chemotherapy reduces the incidence of local relapse, when compared to adjuvant chemotherapy alone. Inoperable tumors are always treated with combined chemoradiotherapy.

Chemotherapy

Patients with stages II and III disease require adjuvant chemotherapy after surgery, usually along with radiotherapy. Standard chemotherapy regime is 5 FU with leucovorin. High-risk patients benefit from oxaliplatin and 5FU based chemotherapy every two weeks for 12 cycles. In metastatic disease combination chemotherapy with oxaliplatin, or irinotecan with 5FU and leucovorin are the drugs of choice. Recent trials using antiangiogenesis agent bevacizumab and epidermal growth factor inhibitor (cetuximab), in combination with irinotecan and 5 FU containing regimen, have shown good response.

SUGGESTED READING

1. Stein HJ, Brucher BL, Sendler A, Slewert JR. Esophageal cancer: Patient evaluation and pretreatment staging. Surg Oncol 2001; 10: 03-111
2. Fuchs CS, Mayer RJ. Gastric carcinoma. N Engl J Med 1995; 333(1): 32-41
3. Gores GJ. Cholangiocarcinoma: current concepts and insights. Hepatology 2003; 37(5): 961-9
4. S D Ryder. Guideline for the diagnosis and treatment of Hepatocellular carcinoma (HCC) in adults. Gut, 2003; 52: 1-8.
5. Levy MJ, Wiersema MJ. Pancreatic neoplasms. Gastrointest Endosc Cli N Am 2005; 15(1): 117-42
6. Chareton B, Coiffic J, Landen S, et al: Diagnosis and therapy of ampullary tumors. World J Surg 1996; 20: 707-12

35

Ramesh H

Acute Abdomen: A Challenge to the Surgeon and Physician

INTRODUCTION

By definition, acute abdomen denotes an abdominal pathologic condition, which if left undiscovered and untreated, would have a deleterious effect on the patient's health status. An acute abdominal condition may present in the most dramatic or the most insidious manner; in each case the underlying condition may be life-threatening. Prompt diagnosis and decisive management may be the difference between life and death. If surgery carried no risk and did not adversely affect the course of some diseases, it would be safe to say "if in doubt, operate." Unfortunately, laparotomy itself carries risks and the course of some disorders such as acute pancreatitis and paralytic ileus is adversely influenced by anesthesia and surgery.

The diagnosis of acute conditions, therefore, frequently resolves itself into arriving at a fairly immediate judgment derived from an accurate and detailed history, a careful physical examination and a few selected lab tests and x-ray studies. While gathering the evidence, changes should be evaluated in terms of pathophysiologic alterations rather than specific diagnoses, and attention must be given to the need for supportive measures while investigation is underway.

A narrative of the various causes of acute abdomen and their management is beyond the scope of this chapter. Rather, the aim of this chapter is to highlight ten issues, which confront the clinician who treats patients with an acute abdomen.

WHO SHOULD TREAT AN ACUTE ABDOMEN?

Traditionally, an acute abdomen has been the domain of the surgeon. Most causes of acute abdomen are surgical. However, a number of non-surgical conditions present with acute abdominal pain and they must be considered in every case (Table 35.1).

Table 35.1: Nonsurgical causes of acute abdomen

- Heart: Myocardial infarction, acute pericarditis, dissecting aneurysm
- Lung: Pneumonia, pleuritis
- Digestive system: Acute pancreatitis, acute gastroenteritis, acute hepatitis
- Endocrine system: Acute adrenal insufficiency, diabetic ketoacidosis
- Metabolic: Acute porphyria, hyperlipidemia
- Skeletal: Rectus muscle hematoma
- Nervous system: Tabes dorsalis, nerve root compression
- Genitourinary: Acute pyelonephritis, acute salpingitis
- Hematologic: Sickle cell crises.

HOW EMERGENT IS THE CONDITION?

A triage system has been recommended for the management of acute abdomen.

Priority I: This is the catastrophic presentation, which may be caused by perforation of a hollow viscus, massive hemorrhage or by acute sudden arterial occlusion with extensive tissue necrosis, all of which are characterized by sudden onset of severe prostrating continuous pain, moderate to extreme abdominal tenderness and muscle spasm; and rapid development of shock. There is marked tissue damage and fluid loss from traumatic, chemical or vascular insult. Hypotension, oliguria, acidosis, respiratory distress and mental obtundation may occur. Immediate institution of supportive and resuscitative measures (i.e. intravenous correction of fluid and electrolyte imbalance, blood replacement, gastric suction, vasopressor agents, oxygen, narcotics) are imperative. Emergency operation as soon as the patient's condition permits, must be done to repair a perforated viscus, to restore blood supply by relief of strangulation-obstruction, or to control hemorrhage in a ruptured ectopic pregnancy, ruptured spleen and (hopefully when conditions permit) a dissecting aneurysm.

Acute pancreatitis, which may have a sudden catastrophic onset, is treated nonoperatively with supportive and resuscitative measures, as outlined above, with nasogastric suction to control or prevent paralytic ileus, and with antibiotics to control or prevent infection.

It may be difficult to differentiate acute pancreatitis from other catastrophic conditions. The clinical picture and markedly elevated serum amylase will be helpful. Imaging such as ultrasonography (USG) or CT scn usually gives the diagnosis. Diagnostic laparoscopy may be of benefit in this situation, and may help avoid an unnecessary laparotomy. Laparotomy in the first week of acute pancreatitis increases the risk of subsequent infected pancreatic necrosis by over 25%.

In this catastrophic group, emergency treatment is imperative. Without treatment, rapid and progressive deterioration of the patient occurs, and the prognosis is very guarded.

Priority II: It includes conditions associated with vigorous smooth muscle contractions in an attempt to propel luminal contents past an obstruction. This is the so-called colic group, which is characterized by severe intermittent recurrent cramping pain and serious disturbance in gastrointestinal function when the obstruction is in the small bowel.

Marked systemic reactions are not generally encountered in the early stages of gut obstruction, but become severe as the process advances. In bowel obstruction the need for surgical treatment is urgent to prevent ischemic necrosis of the gut, but not as critical as in the catastrophe category. There is more time for studies and preparation of the patient. Diagnosis can usually be established by careful clinical evaluation of the patient, characteristic hyperactive bowel sounds and demonstration by x-ray of distended loops of gut above the level of obstruction. Fluid and electrolyte imbalance must be corrected and distention relieved by nasogastric suction before operation. The prognosis is good in cases seen early but much more serious when ischemic necrosis of gut occurs and resection of gangrenous bowel is required.

Biliary and renal colic are treated conservatively with use of drugs for relief of pain and relaxation of smooth muscle spasm to facilitate passage of the calculus. Both renal and biliary colic are treated medically with diet, fluids and narcotics, and surgery is usually not required, at least for the acute episode of colic.

At times a marked gastroenteritis or a fecal impaction may cause severe colicky pain, but history, physical examination, and the benign course will obviate any serious consideration of ill-advised surgery.

Priority III: The lowest category of urgency, includes inflammatory conditions associated with abdominal pain and a possible acute abdomen. The progression of inflammatory changes occurs over a period of several hours to a few days. Initially the systemic and abdominal manifestations are not severe and there is considerably more time to observe and evaluate the patient. With progression of inflammation and infection, pain and tenderness increase, become more localized, and fever and leukocytosis increase. Without treatment, there is further tissue damage, and perforation and peritonitis may ensue. Clinical diagnosis is usually possible on the basis of clinical feature and tests.

WHAT ABOUT THE USE OF NARCOTIC ANALGESICS IN THE INITIAL STAGES OF MANAGEMENT OF AN ACUTE ABDOMEN?

The age-old maxim was that "until a diagnosis or a decision to operate is made, narcotic analgesics should not be used lest they mask the pain which is such an important diagnostic feature of the disease". However, there has been considerable debate on the subject. There is no doubt that Nissman et al's suggestion that good communication between emergency physicians and surgeons is crucial to quality patient care; however, there is general disagreement with their contention that the administration of analgesia for acute abdominal pain "cannot be undertaken with any certainty of safety." Tintinalli's, *Emergency Medicine: A Comprehensive Study Guide* advocates the "judicious use of opioid analgesia in the emergency department management of acute abdominal pain." There is no doubt however, that accurate documentation of findings by the emergency physician prior to administration of the narcotic is necessary, as also good communication between the emergency physician (EP) and the surgeon.

IS THERE A GREATER DEPENDENCE ON IMAGING DATA TODAY AS COMPARED TO YESTER YEARS?

Over the past decade, significant advances in technology, new applications, changed protocols and considerable accumulated experience have prompted an increased use of imaging techniques in patients with acute abdomen. Multidetector (multislice) CT, sonography, and MR imaging—that were previously not available or were not commonly used in the evaluation of patients with acute abdominal complaints—have changed the approach of the EP. This increase in imaging from plain x-rays to more complex tests have permitted more accurate diagnosis of conditions before surgery and has enabled many medical conditions to be identified and treated without operation. In reality, however, the selection process is strongly influenced by past experience and skills, the quality and availability of equipment, and the cost of examination, and is therefore often institutionally dependent. It must be emphasized however, that imaging may delay the process of treatment. Too often patients with intra-abdominal bleed and hemodynamic instability languish in a CT suite while needing emergency surgery. Resuscitation, achievement and maintenance of hemodynamic stability, correction of fluid, electrolyte and acid-base imbalances must proceed hand-in-hand.

WHAT IS THE BEST CLINICAL APPROACH?

There are really only four pathologic processes that occur in the GI tract: hemorrhage, ischemia, obstruction and infection. Most abdominal pathology involves one or a combination of these processes. Despite this apparent simplicity, the diagnosis of abdominal complaints is often so imprecise. Co-existing non-gastrointestinal pathology is often responsible, as is the tendency on the part of the clinician to narrow the field of diagnostic possibilities too soon. Further, diverse disease processes often present with overlapping, nonspecific symptoms such as nausea, vomiting, fever, diarrhea and anorexia. Assessment of these symptoms might be helpful, but most abdominal conditions that require surgery produce abdominal pain, and it is the evaluation of abdominal pain that is most often the key to the diagnosis.

The clinical approach to patients who have abdominal pain is the same as that of any emergency. An initial overview is accomplished rapidly to determine that the airway is patent and protected, that air exchange is adequate, and that the patient has adequate systemic perfusion. In some cases, the need for resuscitation precludes the more conventional approach of obtaining a patient history and physical examination before proceeding.

The tools for evaluating abdominal complaints are patient history, physical examination, imaging studies and laboratory tests. By far the most important of these is the patient history. The most common pitfall in evaluating abdominal pain is probably the failure to obtain a sufficiently detailed and accurate history. As in the management of abdominal trauma, the evaluation of nontraumatic abdominal pain is severely hampered when the patient is unable to provide adequate history. Consequently, confused elderly patients, preverbal children, patients who have a language barrier, and intoxicated or spine-injured patients constitute a significant "red-flag" and need to have particular attention paid to abdominal evaluation, even when the initial presentation seems only marginally related to the abdomen.

HOW SHOULD THE HISTORY BE TAKEN?

The essential elements of the history are to determine (1) the nature, onset, location and radiation of abdominal pain; (2) the presence and sequence of onset of associated symptoms such as fever, nausea, vomiting, urinary symptoms and pelvic symptoms (in women); and (3) pertinent details in the review of systems including bowel movements, appetite, weight changes, and menstrual history. It is also important to inquire about previous similar episodes, prior medical and surgical history and current medication use. Although every medical student learns this basic approach, it is surprising how often basic elements of the history are omitted in "puzzling cases," and when the diagnosis proves to be elusive, obtaining further history is usually the key to clarifying the situation.

WHAT ARE THE KEY POINTS IN CLINICAL EXAMINATION?

Physical examination of the abdomen is used to confirm the initial diagnostic impression and to detect signs of peritoneal irritation. It is useful to proceed in a standard fashion beginning with inspection, auscultation, percussion, and palpation, in that sequence. "Inspection" can reveal important information including the presence of distension, masses, surgical scars, discoloration by ecchymosis (Cullen's and Gray-Turner's signs) and skin abnormalities such as spider angiomata, petechiae, jaundice and rashes. "Auscultation" for bowel sounds and bruits should precede palpation because the latter can induce peristalsis artificially. Bowel sounds are probably the least helpful element of the abdominal examination because reflex ileus can occur with virtually any painful abdominal condition and might persist for a time, even with intra-abdominal catastrophes. High-pitched, tinkling bowel sounds are suggestive of small bowel obstruction but are not a reliable indicator of such. The presence of bruits is important in older patients because it might indicate the presence of vascular insufficiency or abdominal aortic aneurysm. "Percussion" can help to distinguish gaseous from solid or fluid causes and rebound tenderness can also be elicited. Percussion of the flanks might demonstrate tenderness consistent with pyelonephritis.

"Palpation" is saved for last and should be performed gently, beginning with the quadrant most remote from the patient's pain, moving toward the painful area. Deep palpation and the classically described test for rebound tenderness have limited utility and might be misleading. Many patients will report pain with deep palpation of the abdomen and most will react to the sudden release of deep pressure with pain or surprise. Experienced clinicians use gentler methods of eliciting peritoneal signs such as the cough test, rocking the patient's bed from side to side (Bed-shaking test of Bapat), or gentle percussion to diagnose peritoneal irritation. Performing deep palpation and sudden release in patients who have clear signs of peritonitis or a "board-like" abdomen can only be considered to be sadistic and provides no additional information.

Other aspects of the physical assessment include rectal and pelvic examinations. Rectal examination is useful for detecting gross or occult blood and rectal masses or lesions, but it is of questionable utility in differentiating between the various causes of abdominal pain . Repeated rectal examinations by multiple physicians are not indicated. Pelvic examination is mandatory in any circumstance in which the cause of the pain might be pelvic pathology, which includes most cases of abdominal pain in women.

LABORATORY TESTS AND OTHER INVESTIGATIONS

While simple laboratory tests are useful and may reveal anemia, co-existing diabetes or reveal the patient to be pregnant, a shotgun approach is not recommended. Depending upon the symptom complex and the clinical likelihood, emergency departments dealing with acute abdomen should create investigation "panels" which may serve to guide the junior physician and also prevents the clinician from overlooking essential tests. In pain per se and gastrointestinal bleeding, abdominal x-rays have shown to be very ineffective. US scan for biliary and liver disease and CT scan have revolutionized the approach to acute abdomen—both traumatic and non traumatic. Perforations of the bowel, bowel ischemia due to vascular obstructions, pancreatitis and other conditions can easily be made out by scanning after oral and IV contrast administration. While radiographic tests should be focused and obtained to confirm a diagnostic suspicion rather than used as a broad search for unexpected pathology, there is no doubt that an empirical CT scan often throws up an unexpected diagnosis which has major implications on patient recovery.

DECISION MAKING

Despite advances in the understanding of pathologic processes and the availability of imaging tests, it may not be possible for patients to be rushed into a diagnosis and further onto a therapeutic algorithm. There is a genuine need to retain patients in the emergency department and in some of these cases, periodic re-examination alone is helpful in clinching the diagnosis. Care must also be taken during this period to identify co-morbid illnesses and extra-abdominal conditions which may have a bearing on diagnosis or therapy.

THE TEAM CONCEPT

Many diseases like perforated duodenal ulcer, which present as an acute abdomen are purely surgical–they need emergency surgery. There are others, which are managed medically for the most part such as acute pancreatitis. Intensive care is a critical part of the process of recovery and the role played by an internist, anesthesiologist, pulmonologist, physiotherapist and nephrologist in the management of these patients can not be overemphasized. Further, diseases such as ulcerative colitis have a spectrum of presentation, which requires both medical and surgical management with appropriately timed interventions from both specialists (Figure 35.1). Diagnosis and treatment of acute abdomen is now a multidisciplinary task, which brings out the best of skills of many medical and surgical specialties.

THE FUTURE

Increasing use of medical simulators, trauma life support courses, robotics and virtual reality will pave the way for an increasingly aware and capable medical

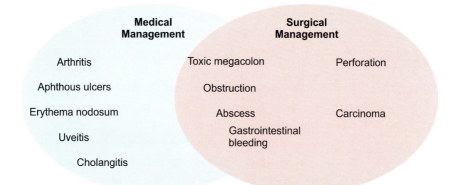

Fig. 35.1: Spectrum of disease

professional in dealing with acute abdominal conditions. It is no longer possible for every emergency physician to have experienced each and every cause of acute abdomen and thus develop the necessary skills required to manage these difficult problems. Telemedicine is also likely to bridge the distances between the specialist in the tertiary care center and the emergency physician in a somewhat remote smaller hospital. Thus, technology may help improve diagnosis and management. Computerized scoring systems have come and gone, but there is no doubt that good clinical history taking, a thorough clinical examination, repeated re-examination over a short period of time, and judicious investigations will alone enable physicians and surgeons to diagnose acute life-threatening abdominal conditions and manage them in an expeditious manner.

SUGGESTED READING

1. Stamos MJ. Acute abdomen: Current controversies and unresolved issues. In Current Critical Care: Diagnosis and Treatment, Eds. Bongard FS, Sue DY. Tata New Delhi. McGraw-Hill Publishing Company Limited, 748-55.
2. Diethelm AG, Stanley RJ, Robbin ML.The acute abdomen. In Sabiston DC (eds): The Textbook of Surgery – Biological Basis of Modern Surgical Practice, 15th ed, Bangalore, WB Saunders Company and Prism Books Ltd, 1997, pp 825-46.
3. Saini S. Acute abdomen: Diagnostic imaging in the clinical context. N Engl J Med 1996; 335:1775.
4. Gore RM, Miller FH, Pereles FS, et al. Helical CT in the evaluation of the acute abdomen. AJR Am J Roentgenol (United States), 2000; 174(4):901-13.

36

Deepak Suvarna

Getting Rid of
Intestinal Parasites

INTRODUCTION

Intestinal parasitic infections are ubiquitous and infect millions of people. These infections are spread most commonly through the ingestion of food or water contaminated with human or animal feces as a result of poor sanitation

PROTOZOAN PARASITES

Protozoan parasites commonly cause asymptomatic infections among indigenous residents of developing and tropical countries, particularly among children.

Protozoan pathogens commonly encountered include *Giardia lamblia*, *Entamoeba histolytica*, *Cryptosporidium parvum*, and *Cyclospora cayetanensis*. *Giardia*, *Cryptosporidium* and *Cyclospora*, may cause an acute self-limited illness with profuse watery diarrhea in immunocompetent hosts; chronic diarrhea and malabsorption lasting for weeks to months in untreated, inadequately treated or immunocompromised hosts.

Entamoeba histolytica is a potentially tissue-invasive organism and can cause hemorrhagic colitis, fever, or basic absces; However, amebic infections may also be present in asymptomatic hosts and in persons with watery diarrhea as the chief complaint.

The role of *Blastocystis hominis* in human disease remains controversial, because this microorganism has been found in stools of healthy asymptomatic human hosts and in those with symptoms.

A summary of common intestinal protozoa associated with travellers' diarrhea, risk groups, transmission, and manifestations is presented below:

Giardia Lamblia

Risk groups: Residents of endemic areas, international travellers, children, and caretakers.

Transmission: Fecally contaminated water and food.

Manifestation: Acute diarrhea, chronic diarrhea, malabsorption, weight loss, fatigue.

Entamoeba Histolytica

Risk groups: Residents of endemic areas, international travellers.

Transmission: Fecally contaminated water and food.

Manifestation: Acute diarrhea, dysentery, chronic diarrhea, abdominal pain, amebic abscess.

Cyclospora Cayetanensis

Risk groups: Residents of endemic areas, international travellers, immuno-compromised persons.

Transmission: Fecally contaminated water, food, internationally shipped fish products.

Manifestation: Watery diarrhea, cramping, abdominal pain; self-limited in immunocompetent persons; chronic diarrhea in immunocompromised.

Diagnosis

Stool specimens should be collected within one hour of submission to the laboratory. Stool should be immediately suspended in polyvinyl alcohol or other preservatives for microscopic diagnosis of characteristic morphologic (cysts and trophozoites) forms by wet-mount and trichrome stain.

Antigen-detection tests such as ELISA, immunofluorescent antibody tests, and special stains (e.g. acid-fast stain for detection of oocysts of *Cryptosporidium* and *Cyclospora*) may be performed. Intracellular microsporidia species are detected by immunofluorescent antibody tests of stool specimens and histochemical stains (Giemsa, fluorochrome stains) of tissue preparations.

Treatment

Treatment regimens for protozoan parasites are outlined in Table 36.1.

Table 36.1: Treatment regimens for protozoan parasites			
Infection	Drug	Adult dose (non-pregnant)	Pediatric dose
Giardia	Metronidazole	500 mg tid or 5–10 days	5–7 mg/kg tid ×5–10 days
E. histolytica—asymptomatic cyst passers	Diloxanide furoate	500 mg tid ×10 days	20 mg/kg/d in 3 doses ×10 days
E. histolytica—intestinal or invasive disease	Metronidazole Tinidazole	750 mg tid ×10 days 800 mg tid ×5 days	35–50 mg/kg/d in 3 doses ×10 days 60 mg/kg (maximum, 2 g)/d ×5 days
Cyclospora	Cotrimoxazole (trimethoprim plus sulfamethoxazole)	Trimethoprim 160 mg plus sulfamethoxazole (800 mg) twice daily ×7–10 days	Trimethoprim 5 mg/kg plus sulfamethoxazole 25 mg/kg twice daily ×7–10 days

Prevention

The cyst forms of *Giardia* and *Cryptosporidium* are relatively resistant to chemical disinfection by chlorine. Filters with a pore size of one mm remove cyst forms. Heating water and food to 100°C is the most reliable way to destroy protozoan parasites.

Intestinal Helminth Infections

Symptomatic disease caused by intestinal worms and flukes is associated with heavy parasite burdens, tissue migration of larval stages, ectopic eggs or extra-intestinal adult parasites. Abdominal pain, diarrhea, allergic symptoms (particularly associated with tissue migration of larval stages through the lungs), inflammation due to ectopic eggs or adult parasites in extra-intestinal tissues, anemia due to microscopic intestinal bleeding and acute intestinal obstruction are all possible complications of a heavy infection.

Intestinal Roundworms (nematodes)

Commonly encountered members of this phylum causing disease in human beings include *Ascaris lumbricoides* (common roundworm), *Ancylostoma duodenale* or *Necator americanus* (hookworm species), *Trichuris trichiura* (whipworm), *Enterobius vermicularis* (pinworm) and *Strongyloides stercoralis*.

Transmission

The intestinal roundworms are common soil-transmitted helminths. *Ascaris* and *Enterobius* usually are acquired through ingestion of soil containing mature parasite eggs. Hookworm species and *Trichuris* are acquired through contact of bare human skin with damp soil containing infective larvae. Human infections with *Trichinella spiralis* usually occur in settings where human beings ingest undercooked or raw pork butchered from pigs fed on raw garbage.

The transmission factors and common symptoms associated with infection with intestinal roundworms are summarized below:

Common Roundworm: *Ascaris lumbricoides*

Mode of infection: Raw fruits and vegetables.

Clinical features: Pneumonitis, colicky epigastric pain, nausea and vomiting, passage of a mature pencil-sized worm.

Hookworm (Old world): *Ancylostoma duodenale,* (New world): *Necator americanus*

Mode of infection: Percutaneous or perioral infections from contaminated soil or vegetation.

Clinical features: "Ground itch" (rash), pneumonitis, abdominal pain, diarrhea, anemia.

Strongyloides: *Strongyloides stercoralis*

Mode of infection: Skin contact with wet, infected soil.

Clinical features: Rash on buttocks or thighs, abdominal pain, nausea and vomiting, weight loss, eosinophilia, recurrent bacterial systemic infections with gastrointestinal flora in immunocompromised patients, malabsorption.

Whipworm: *Trichuris trichiura*

Mode of infection: Raw fruits and vegetables, soil contact, flies on food.

Clinical features: Mild anemia, bloody diarrhea, rectal prolapse in heavy infections.

Pinworm: *Enterobius vermicularis*

Mode of infection: Anus-finger-mouth cycle or from clothing, bedding, dust.

Clinical features: Perianal itching, irritation, restlessness, sleeplessness.

Trichinosis: *Trichinella*

Mode of infection: Undercooked or raw domestic pig, wild boar.

Clinical features: Non-typical symptoms in the enteral phase followed by fever, muscular ache, headache, edema, disorder of vision and rash.

Diagnosis

Morphologic identification of adult worms, larvae and eggs in stool samples or other specimens are the standard for diagnosis of *Ascaris*, hookworm, and whipworm. For *strongyloides* infection, a combination of stool examination, duodenal biopsy, duodenal aspirate and strongyloides antibody tests may be needed. Trichinosis is diagnosed acutely by the history of eating raw or undercooked meat, later by histologic examination of tissue biopsy specimens of affected organs and by serum antibody tests.

Treatment

Table 36.2 shows the drugs commonly used in the treatment of human helminthic infections.

Parasite	Pyrantel pamoate	Mebendazole	Albendazole	Thiabendazole	Ivermectin	Niclosamide	Praziquantel
Table 36.2: The drugs commonly used in the treatment of human helminthic infections							
Common roundworm	X	X	X				
Hookworm	X	X	X				
Whipworm		X	X				
Pinworm	X	X	X				
Strongyloidiasis				X	X		
Trichinosis		X	X				
Tapeworm						X	X
Schistosomiasis							X
Liver flukes							X

Prevention

Hygienic measures, such as thorough cleansing of the hands and under the fingernails (especially before food preparation), wearing shoes, building and using latrines, avoiding skin contact with damp sandy soil in endemic areas, instituting drug treatment of infected individuals, and eating well-cooked meat and fish can interrupt the cycle of transmission of these infections in endemic areas.

Cestodes (tapeworms)

Taenia saginata (beef tapeworm), *T. solium* (pork tapeworm), *Diphyllobothrium latum* (fish tapeworm) and *Hymenolepis nana* and *H diminuta* (dwarf tapeworms) are common tapeworms causing human intestinal infections.

Transmission

Beef and pork tapeworms usually are acquired from eating raw or undercooked meat and meat products; and fish tapeworms are acquired from raw or undercooked fish. *Hymenolepis nana* and *H diminuta* are common parasites of rats and mice. The dwarf tapeworms commonly affect children living in warm climates who have the opportunity to swallow dirt or fleas.

Symptoms

Most commonly, persons with tapeworm infections are asymptomatic and become aware of their infection when a ribbon or tape of proglottid segments is passed by way of the rectum. In other cases, a stool ova-and-parasite examination ordered for work-up of anemia or eosinophilia reveals the presence of a tapeworm infection. Chronic infection with *D. latum* is associated with macrocytic anemia secondary to vitamin B_{12} deficiency. Heavy infection by *H nana* and *H diminuta* may cause diarrhea, abdominal distress and poor appetite.

Diagnosis

Diagnosis can be made by finding characteristic eggs in a stool specimen or by morphologic characteristics of the proglottids.

Treatment

Tables 36.2 and 36.3 show the drugs used in the treatment of intestinal helminthic infections.

Prevention

Prevention of *T saginata* or *T. solium* infection depends on eating well-cooked beef and pork respectively. *D. latum* can be prevented by eating only well-cooked marine fish. Environmental sanitation, flea control, and treatment of infected persons contribute to prevention of *H. nana* and *H. diminuta* infections.

Trematodes (flukes)

Fluke infections present usually in the chronic stage because signs and symptoms of acute infections may not be noted, and disease results from chronic inflammation and fibrosis around the flukes and eggs retained in the tissues.

Transmission

Intestinal flukes, liver flukes and lung flukes usually are acquired by eating raw or lightly cooked, pickled, salted or smoked seafood and aquatic plants in endemic areas. *Schistosoma mansoni*, *S haematobium*, *S japonicum* and *S mekongi*

Table 36.3: Dosing regimens

Drug	Dosage
Pyrantel pamoate	Ascaris: 11 mg/kg (maximum 1 g) once Hookworm: 11 mg/kg (maximum 1 g) ×3 days Pinworm: 11 mg/kg (maximum 1 g) once, repeat dose in 2 weeks
Mebendazole	Ascaris, hookworm, whipworm: 100 mg twice daily ×3 days
Albendazole	Ascaris, hookworm: 400 mg once (adults and children) Whipworm: 400 mg daily ×3 days (adults and children)
Thiabendazole	*Strongyloides:* 50 mg/kg divided in two doses (maximum, 3 g/d) ×2 days (adults and children)
Ivermectin	*Strongyloides:* 200/kg/d 1–2 days (adults and children)
Niclosamide	Adults: a single dose of 2 g (four tablets) chewed thoroughly Children: 50 mg/kg once
Praziquantel	*Taenia saginata, T. solium, Diphyllobothrium latum, Dipylidium caninum, Hymenolepis diminuta:* a single dose of 5–10 mg/kg *H. nana:* a single dose of 25 mg/kg *Schistosomiasis:* 20 mg/kg twice daily ×1–3 days Intestinal flukes: 25 mg/kg thrice daily ×1 day *Paragonimus sp:* 25 mg/kg thrice daily ×2 days
Oxamniquine	*S. mansoni:* 15 mg/kg once (adults); 20 mg/kg/d divided in two doses ×1 day (children)
Triclabendazole	*Paragonimus* sp: 5 mg/kg once daily ×3 days *Fasciola hepatica* : 10 mg/kg once

infection occur when intact human skin is splashed or immersed in freshwater contaminated with infected snails shedding the infective larval stage of schistosomiasis (cercariae).

Symptoms

A pruritic macular-papular rash (*swimmer's itch*) follows after schistosomal cercariae penetrate the skin. Subsequently *S haematobium* localizes to mesenteric venules of the urinary bladder; *S. mansoni, S. japonicum* and *S. mekongi* to the mesenteric venules of the colon.

A clinical syndrome consisting of fever, abdominal pain, and bloody diarrhea (Katayama fever) may present in hepatosplenic (*S. mansoni, S. japonicum, S. mekongi*) schistosomiasis. Late-stage infections can manifest with ascites and variceal bleeding due to liver fibrosis and portal hypertension.

Liver fluke infections with *Clonorchis sinensis* and *Opisthorchis viverrini* may cause chronic intermittent abdominal pain. Infection with intestinal flukes is associated with acute diarrhea and abdominal discomfort, with chronic diarrhea being reported in chronic untreated infections.

Diagnosis

Diagnosis of fluke infections usually is made by identification of species specific eggs in stool specimens. Characteristic eggs also can be identified in tissue samples from rectal snips, biopsy of the bladder or colon in cases of schistosomiasis. Species specific serum tests for schistosomiasis are also available.

Treatment: See Table 36.2 and 36.3.

Prevention

Cooking fish, seafood, and aquatic vegetables thoroughly before eating is the most direct way to prevent infection with lung and liver flukes. Freshwater snail control is important to control the spread of schistosomiasis, as is avoiding of skin contact with snail-infested waters in endemic areas.

SUGGESTED READING

1. Hotez P J, Brooker S, Bethony J M, Bottazzi M E, Loukas A, Xiao S. Current Concepts: Hookworm Infection. N Engl J Med 2004; 351:799-807,
2. Liu L X, Weller P F Drug Therapy: Antiparasitic Drugs. N Engl J Med 1996; 334:1178-84.
3. Haque R, Huston C D, Hughes M, Houpt E, Petri W A Jr. Current Concepts: Amebiasis. N Engl J Med 2003; 348:1565-1573.
4. G R, Li Y, Williams G M, McManus D P. Current Concepts: Schistosomiasis Ross A GP, Bartley P B, Sleigh A C, Olds N Engl J Med 2002; 346:1212-20.
5. R Knight, MG Schultz, DW Hoskins, and PD Marsden. Intestinal parasites. Gut, 1973; 14:145-68.
6. Jong E. Prim Care. Intestinal parasites. 2002; 29(4):857-77.

37

Prakash Zacharias

Nutrition in Gastrointestinal Diseases

INTRODUCTION

A balanced diet is essential for maintaining good health. Malnutrition can adversely influence the outcome in a variety of diseases and dietary modifications are required in some of them. Obesity is also emerging as an important issue.

ANATOMY AND PHYSIOLOGY OF DIGESTION AND ABSORPTION

In order to unravel the mysteries of malnutrition, the anatomy and physiology of digestion and absorption need to be understood. The ingested food is chemically complex and is broken down by digestion and then absorbed and assimilated into the body.

The carbohydrates are broken down into simple sugars by various enzymes such as salivary amylase, pancreatic amylase and later by disaccharidases located at the intestinal epithelial surface. The sugars are absorbed anywhere along the intestinal surface. Thus diseases of pancreas and intestinal mucosa can adversely affect carbohydrate digestion and absorption.

The complex process of protein digestion is carried out by gastric pepsin and pancreatic trypsin and culminates at the intestinal epithelial layer. Proteins are thus broken down into peptides and amino acids. Peptides are preferentially absorbed by the intestine. Passive diffusion, facilitated diffusion and active transport are various mechanisms by which these peptides are absorbed. Understandably pancreatic diseases and intestinal pathology can cause protein maldigestion and malabsorption respectively.

The intricate process of fat digestion is carried out by lingual, gastric and pancreatic lipases along with colipases. The triglycerides are broken down into monoglycerides and fatty acids. These water insoluble products are made water soluble with the aid of bile salts by the formation of "micelles" and then absorbed by the intestine. Following absorption, the triglycerides are reconstituted and transported to the liver. The liver cannot produce such enormous amounts of bile salts, and this problem is solved by reabsorption in the terminal ileum. Diseases or surgery involving terminal ileum may adversely affect fat absorption.

All water-soluble vitamins except Vitamin B_{12} are absorbed unchanged throughout the intestines. An intact fat digestive mechanism is required for fat-soluble vitamins. Vitamin B_{12} has a different absorptive mechanism. The food bound Vitamin B_{12} is initially cleaved in the stomach. B_{12} then binds to R proteins in the stomach forming an R protein—B_{12} complex, which is cleaved later in the upper small intestine by the pancreatic enzymes. The B_{12} then binds to intrinsic factor produced by gastric parietal cells. The intrinsic factor-B_{12} complex binds to specific receptors in the terminal ileum. After absorption, it is transported to the liver attached to a transport protein, transcobalamin II. Hence problems anywhere along this path can result in B_{12} deficiency.

Micronutrients and divalent cations (iron, calcium, magnesium, zinc, copper, manganese) are absorbed in the proximal small intestine. These micronutrients are required for critical enzymatic reactions in the body.

ASSESSMENT OF NUTRITIONAL STATUS

Unfortunately, no single test provides an accurate assessment of a patient's nutritional status. Various methods used are mentioned in Table 37.1.

Table 37.1: Tests for nutritional assessment

Tests	Comments
Anthropometry	
Triceps and subscapular skinfold thickness	Inaccurate, lacks specificity
Creatine-height index	False positive results with diuretics, renal and liver disease
Immunocompetence	
Delayed cutaneous hypersensitivity	Affected by severe malnutrition, infection, immune deficiency and medications
Serum Proteins	
S Albumin	Lacks specificity
Prealbumin	Affected by renal disease and infection
Serum transferrin and S. cholesterol	Lacks specificity
Combination of multiple parameters	
Prognostic nutritional index (PNI)	Replaced by SGA
Subjective global assessment (SGA)	Patients categorized as well, moderate and severe malnutrition

A good history including recent weight loss, dietary history, physical examination and biochemical tests would give a clue to the nutritional status of the patient. "Subjective Global Assessment" (SGA) is a particularly useful guide, which incorporates history, physical findings, the muscular strength and stamina, and also the metabolic demands. In hospitalized patients, poor outcome predictors include history of more than 10% weight loss in the recent past, low serum albumin and abnormal SGA.

Nutritional Requirements

To administer nutritional therapy, the nutritional requirements need assessment. The energy needs can be assessed by determining patient's BMR (basal metabolic rate) using Harris-Benedict equation.

Men: BMR (kcal/day) = 66.4+ [13.75 x weight (kg)] + [5 x height (cm)]-[6.8 x age]

Women: BMR (kcal/day) = 65.5+ [9.7 x weight (kg)] + (1.8 x height (cm)]-[4.7 x age]

Another useful method would be to provide 25 to 30 kcal/kg/d for men and 20 to 25 kcal/kg/d for women. Adjustments in BMR are made based on stress factors and hypermetabolism. Critically ill medical patients require energy requirements of 1.0 to 1.15 times the BMR. Protein requirements are met by giving 0.8g/kg/d for healthy individuals, 1.2 to 1.5g/kg/d for hospitalized patients and 1.5to 2.0g/kg/d for critically ill patients. As mentioned earlier, the need for micronutrients should not be ignored.

Balanced Diet

Balanced diet is one which contains various foods such as energy yielding foods (carbohydrates, pure fats), body building foods (proteins) and protective foods (vitamins, micronutrients) in such proportions that an individual is assured of his minimum nutritional requirements. This is influenced by the age, sex, physical activity and physiological state viz. pregnancy, lactation etc. The (ICMR) Nutrition Expert Group (1968) has recommended guidelines for balanced diets depending on the age, economic status etc in India. One such diet is given in Table 37.2.

Nutritional Diseases

Nutritional diseases can be broadly classified into:
1. Dietary deficiency
   -Protein energy malnutrition
   -Avitaminosis
   -Deficiency of minerals and micronutrients.
2. Hyperalimentation and obesity

Nutritional deficiencies in gastrointestinal and hepatic disease can be due to:
1. Inadequate oral intake secondary to dysphagia, anorexia, nausea, vomiting, restrictive diets, etc.

Table 37.2: Balanced diets for various groups (Low Cost) (I.C.M.R Nutrition Expert Group)

Food Item	Adult man			Adult woman			Children			Boys	Girls
	Sedentary work	Moderate work	Heavy work	Sedentary work	Moderate work	Heavy work	1-3 yrs	4-6 yrs	10-12 yrs	10-12 yrs	10-12 yrs
Cereals	400	475	650	410	440	575	175	270	420	380
Pulses	70	80	80	40	45	50	35	35	45	45
Leafy veg	100	125	125	100	100	50	40	50	50	50
Other veg	75	75	100	40	40	100	20	30	50	50
Roots and tubers	50	60	80	50	75	100	10	0	30	30
Milk	200	200	200	200	200	200	300	250	250	250
Oil and fat	35	40	50	30	35	40	15	25	40	35
Sugar or jaggery	30	40	55	30	30	40	30	40	45	45

2. Maldigestion and malabsorption; e.g. mucosal disease like tropical/celiac sprue, pancreatic insufficiency etc.
3. Gastrointestinal losses from diarrhea, bleeding, fistulas, or protein-losing enteropathy.
4. Hypercatabolic states like inflammatory bowel disease, severe pancreatitis, etc.

Obesity has reached epidemic proportions in the western population and this trend is catching on in developing countries as well. Obesity is defined as a body mass index (BMI) >30 kg/m^2. A BMI >30 kg/m^2 is associated with significant morbidity and mortality. These include gastroesophageal reflux, gallstones, pancreatitis, colon cancer fatty infiltration of the liver, hepatic fibrosis and cirrhosis. The treatment of obesity is often difficult and unsatisfactory. About two-thirds of persons who lose weight will regain it within one year, and almost all of them will regain it in five years time. Epidemiological studies reveal that even a modest weight loss of 5 to 10% has considerable health benefits and reduces morbidity significantly. For a successful outcome, a multipronged approach incorporating behavior modification, nutrition education, physical activity, pharmacotherapy and surgery (when BMI >35-40) may be required.

Food-borne Illness

Illness caused by contaminated food (e.g. typhoid, food poisoning, acute hepatitis etc.) can contribute towards ill health or even death. Pyrrolizidine alkaloids have been implicated in epidemics of hepatic veno occlusive disease reported from India. Aflatoxin induced liver cancer is another example. Provision of good sanitation, clean food and drinking water, avoidance of contamination of the food chain and health education or can help in eradicating these diseases.

Nutrition in Gastrointestinal and Liver Diseases

As alluded to earlier, various gastrointestinal diseases have nutritional consequences and some modifications in the diet or even nutritional therapy may be needed. These include chronic liver disease, pancreatitis, inflammatory bowel disease (IBD), post-gastrectomy syndromes celiac disease etc.

Chronic Liver Disease

Malnutrition and micronutrient deficiencies are common in patients with liver disease. In alcoholic cirrhosis, protein energy malnutrition is seen in 34 to 82%

of patients. Regardless of the etiology, poor nutritional status is associated with a bad prognosis. Factors contributing to malnutrition include anorexia, vomiting, early satiety due to ascites, restrictive diets, fat malabsorption in cholestatic liver disease, glucose intolerance and hypercatabolic state. Nutritional supplementation therapy can produce short and long-term benefits, which is reflected in improved nitrogen balance and liver function, decreased incidence and severity of encephalopathy, and may even prolong survival. Protein restriction is not required in cirrhosis unless the patient has encephalopathy. Normal protein intake should be resumed as soon as the encephalopathy is controlled. Sodium and water restriction is required only if ascites or edema are present. Frequent small meals, bedtime snack, multivitamins, calcium, zinc and magnesium supplements are also beneficial. Contrary to popular belief, branched chain aminoacid formulae offer no advantage over standard aminoacids in the treatment of hepatic encephalopathy.

Pancreatitis

Most attacks of acute pancreatitis are mild and self-limiting which resolve with supportive treatment. Nutritional support is unnecessary in these patients as they can resume a diet within 5 to 7 days .The medical treatment is generally supportive and consists of decreasing pancreatic stimulation, providing intravenous hydration and analgesia. Approximately 5 to 15% of patients may develop necrotizing pancreatitis, which has a mortality rate of 5 to 20%. Severe acute pancreatitis induces a catabolic state characterized by increased energy needs, proteolysis and glucose production. Nutritional support in patients with severe pancreatitis would prevent nutrient deficiencies and preserve lean body mass and functional capacity (Table 37.3).

Table 37.3: Nutrition in acute pancreatitis		
	Enteral	*Parenteral*
Indication	Moderate to severe pancreatitis (≥3 Ranson Criteria) Normal gut integrity	Moderate to severe pancreatitis Complications of pancreatitis
Preferred route	Nasojejunal	Central venous catheter
Type of diet	Elemental or semielemental Low fat content	Total nutrient mixture ≤30% lipid (Triglycerides <400mg/dl)

Recent evidence suggests that the less expensive enteral nutrition delivered beyond the ligament of Treitz is as effective as parenteral nutrition with fewer infectious complications. It also preserves gut integrity, gut barrier and immune function. Enteral feeding also facilitates transitional feeding. Enteral feeding may be abandoned if it increases pain, ascites or fistulous output.

Malnutrition seen in chronic pancreatitis is multifactorial. Chronic abdominal pain, anorexia, diabetes and ongoing alcohol intake may all contribute. Pancreatic enzyme therapy is the mainstay of treatment. In addition to alcohol abstinence, replacement of fat-soluble vitamins and zinc would help in restoring the nutritional status.

Inflammatory Bowel Disease (IBD)

Inflammatory bowel disease has an impact on the nutrition of patients. This is more pronounced in Crohn's disease of the small bowel and is less frequent when the involvement is limited to colon, and in ulcerative colitis.

Table 37.4. Nutritional deficiencies in IBD

	Crohn's disease (%)	Ulcerative colitis (%)
Weight loss	65-78	18-62
Growth retardation	40	-
Hypoalbuminemia	25-80	26-50
Anemia	60-80	-
Calcium deficiency	13	-

The anemia in these patients can be due to iron, vitamin B_{12} or folate (therapy related) deficiency. Zinc deficiency is the most common mineral deficiency in these patients. Malabsorption of vitamin D, calcium and corticosteroid therapy predisposes these patients to osteoporosis.

Nutritional therapy in IBD patients is useful in reversing growth failure, correcting nutritional deficiencies and improving nutritional status in peri-operative period. It is also useful in maintaining nutrition in those with the short bowel syndrome (See 37.4). Parenteral and enteral nutrition as a primary modality has been attempted in the treatment of IBD patients but evidence in this regard has not been convincing.

Post Gastrectomy State

Deficiencies of divalent cations, vitamin B_{12} and fat malabsorption can occur in the post-gastrectomy state and may need supplementation.

Celiac Disease

This chronic disorder of proximal small intestine due to permanent gluten intolerance may present with diarrhea and malabsorption or systemic manifestations without gastrointestinal symptoms. These patients can present with iron deficiency anemia, psychological disturbance or infertility. Gluten-free diet (avoiding wheat, barley, and rye) is the cornerstone of treatment.

Parenteral and Enteral Nutrition

These should be considered in those who requires supplementation or who cannot or will not eat. Enteral nutrition is preferred if the gut is accessible and functional. Parenteral nutrition eliminates the enteral stimulation and the "first pass" through the liver. It is recommended if enteral intake is inadequate or if the gut is unavailable for feeding. This can be administered through a central vein or a peripheral vein. The principle is to provide adequate calories and nutrients in the form of a mixture of aminoacids, lipids and dextrose. Nowadays commercial preparations are available. Parenteral nutrition can be associated with mechanical, vascular, metabolic, infectious and gastrointestinal complications.

Table 37.5: Methods of enteral feeding delivery

Nasogastric	
Nasojejunal	Endoscopic or fluoroscopic
Gastrostomy	Percutaneous endoscopic gastrostomy (PEG), surgical or radiologic
Jejunostomy	Surgical or endoscopic (PEJ)

Nasogastric or nasoenteric tubes are appropriate for short-term (<30 days) feeding and for long term (>30days) feeding gastrostomy tubes are recommended (Table 37.5). Mechanical obstruction is the only absolute contraindication for enteral feeding. Tubes placed beyond the ligament of Treitz codecrease the risk of aspiration. PEG is preferable as it can be performed with local analgesia and with fewer complications than operative gastrostomy. Apart from a few complications like wound infection, aspiration, diarrhea, and alterations in drug absorption, tube feeds are very safe. The potential causes of diarrhea include medications such as antibiotics or sorbitol-containing products, altered bacterial flora, formula composition (including osmolality), infusion rate, hypoalbuminemia and bacterial contamination of the enteral fluid.

Elemental Diets and Immunonutrition

Elemental diets are chemically defined diets, which may be useful in patients with poor small bowel nutrient absorption.

Immunonutrients are dietary components which influence immunologic response mechanisms. These include glutamine, omega-3 fatty acids, arginine and ribonucleic acid. The claims that these agents lower septic complications have not been substantiated.

CONCLUSION

Over the last three decades considerable knowledge has been gained on the impact of nutrition on various diseases. This has influenced the management of many gastrointestinal diseases such as cirrhosis, pancreatitis and inflammatory bowel disease with consequent reduction in morbidity and mortality. Because of many advantages, enteral nutrition is preferred over the parenteral route. Immunonutrition may open up new avenues for therapeutic intervention.

Acknowledgement: I wish to thank my colleagues Dr. Ajith Mathew, Dr. Anish Kumar and Dr. Vidyadhara Prasad Gupta who helped me in the preparation of this manuscript.

SUGGESTED READING

1. ICMR Nutrition Advisory Committee (1981). Recommended daily allowances of nutrients and balanced diets. Indian Council of Medical Research, New Delhi.
2. Swaminathan. M (2003). Advanced Textbook Food and Nutrition Bappco, Bangalore
3. FP Antia and Philip Abraham (2001). Clinical Dietetics and Nutrition-Fourth Edition.Oxford University Press
4. Ronald L Koretz, Timothy O Lipman, Samuel Klein. AGA Technical review on parenteral nutrition. Gastroenterology 2001;121:970-1001
5. American Gastroenterological Association Medical Position Statement: Guidelines for the use of enteral nutrition. Gastroenterology 1995;108:1280.

38

Elango EM

Genetics in Gastroenterology and Hepatology

INTRODUCTION

In clinical practice, the prime significance of genetics is in elucidating the role of genetic variation and mutation in the etiology of a large number of disorders. For any disease the cause is genetic predisposition or acquired mutation in combination with environment. The genetic factors are classified into three categories.

1. Single gene disorders
2. Chromosome disorders
3. Multifactorial disorders.

In the post era of Human Genome Project, it is possible to obtain the DNA sequence of any gene to study the basic genetic defects for a patient with specific disease. Proteomics is the present field wherein the functional aspect of the gene product is analyzed in correlation with environmental factors. This chapter is an overview of genetics in general with a specific focus on hereditary diseases in gastroenterology and hepatology (Table 38.1).

CHOLESTATIC LIVER DISEASES

Progressive Familial Intrahepatic Cholestasis (PFIC 1)

It is an autosomal recessive form of severe cholestatic liver disease. This disease is caused by mutation in the gene designated ATP8B1 which is mapped to chromosome 18. Mutations in ATP8B1 lead to defective bile acid transport. Genetic heterogeneity was observed in this disorder, which revealed that mutations in other genes are also involved in the pathology. A second form of progressive familial intrahepatic cholestasis (PFIC2) is caused by mutation in a liver-specific ATP-binding cassette (C) transporter (ABCB11). PFIC3 is caused by mutation in the class III multidrug resistance P-glycoprotein (MDR3). PFIC4 is caused by mutation in 3-beta-hydroxy-delta-5-C27-steroid oxidoreductase (HSD3B7).

A gene for Benign Recurrent Intrahepatic Cholestasis (BRIC, Summerskill Syndrome) is also mapped to chromosome 18. This suggested that both PFIC1 and BRIC are allelic because of a defect in the same enzyme. Later it was found that they are caused by mutations in the same ATP8B1 gene on chromosome 18q21-q22. An autosomal dominant form of BRIC which is unlinked to the ATP8B1 gene has also been found.

Dubin-Johnson Syndrome

Dubin-Johnson syndrome (Hyperbilirubinemia II) is caused by mutations in the canalicular multispecific organic anion transporter (CMOAT) and the gene is mapped to 10q24. This disease is inherited as autosomal recessive with reduced penetrance. Minor abnormalities may occur in heterozygotes. Urinary coproporphyrin I is a good indicator of the genotype of the individual in the Dubin-Johnson syndrome since the excretion is based on the homozygotic or heterozygotic condition of the individual.

Wilson's Disease

Wilson's disease is a hereditary, autosomal recessive disorder caused by mutation in the ATP7B gene. The worldwide prevalence of Wilson disease is estimated to be of the order of 30 per 1 million, with a gene frequency of 0.56% and a carrier frequency of 1 in 90, and a higher prevalence seems to exist in Sardinia, where approximately 10-12 new cases per year are identified. There was evidence of severe mitochondrial dysfunction in the livers of patients with Wilson disease. Animal models have been developed to study mutational analysis and gene therapy for this disease.

Hemochromatosis

Classic hemochromatosis (HFE), an autosomal recessive disorder, is caused by mutation in a gene designated HFE on chromosome 6p21.3. Juvenile hemochromatosis or hemochromatosis type 2 (HFE2) is also autosomal recessive. One form, designated HFE2A, is caused by mutation in the gene encoding hemojuvelin, which maps to 1q21. A second form, designated HFE2B, is caused by mutation in the gene encoding hepcidin antimicrobial peptide (HAMP), which maps to 19q13. Hemochromatosis type 3 (HFE3), an autosomal recessive disorder, is caused by mutation in the gene encoding transferrin receptor-2 (TFR2), which maps to 7q22. Hemochromatosis type 4 (HFE4), an autosomal dominant disorder, is caused by mutation in the SLC11A3 gene, which encodes ferroportin and maps to 2q32.

Colorectal Cancer

In colorectal cancer more than one gene locus is involved alone or in combination. Hereditary colorectal cancer (HCC) is a multistep carcinogenesis process, progressing from normal epithelium to metastatic carcinoma through hyperplastic epithelium—early adenoma—intermediate adenoma—late adenoma—and carcinoma. The genes in which mutations occur at steps in this process include APC on chromosome 5, K-ras on chromosome 12, TP53 on 17p, and DCC on chromosome 18. Inheritance of a single altered gene predisposes to colorectal cancer in 2 distinct syndromes, familial adenomatous polyposis (FAP) and hereditary nonpolyposis colorectal cancer (HNPCC). The genetic defect in FAP involves the rate of tumor initiation, by targeting the gatekeeper function of the APC gene. In contrast, the defect in HNPCC largely affects tumor aggression by targeting the genome guardian function of DNA repair.

Familial Polyposis of the Colon (FPC)

Familial adenomatous polyposis (FAP) is an autosomal dominant disorder, and the APC gene maps to 5q21. Gardner syndrome—colonic polyposis with extrabowel tumors, especially osteomas, and a rather characteristic retinal lesion—is now known to be a phenotypic variant of FAP, caused by mutation in the APC gene. Mutations in the APC gene are an initiating event and most of these mutations accumulate in the central region of the APC gene, which is called the mutation cluster region (MCR), resulting in expression of COOH-terminally truncated proteins. APC mutations in the first or last third of the gene are associated with an attenuated polyposis with a late onset and a small number of polyps. Mutations in the central region of the gene correlate with a severe phenotype of thousands of polyps at a young age and with additional extracolonic manifestations. Nonneoplastic cells of FAP patients are expected to retain normal APC function due to the presence of 1 wild type allele, irrespective of the mutation's position in the affected allele. Consistent with the Knudson 2-hit model, the wild type APC allele is lost in a great majority of colorectal tumors of both sporadic and FAP patients.

Peutz-Jeghers Syndrome

Peutz-Jeghers syndrome (PJS) is an autosomal dominant disorder due to mutations in the serine/threonine kinase (STK11) gene at locus 19p13.3. STK11 is a tumor suppressor gene that acts as an early gatekeeper regulating the development of hamartomas in PJS suggesting that hamartomas may be pathogenetic precursors of adenocarcinoma. Additional somatic mutation events underlie the progression of hamartomas to adenocarcinomas. Some of these mutations are common in the later stages of tumor progression seen in the majority of colorectal carcinomas.

Inflammatory Bowel Disease (IBD)

IBD is subdivided into Crohn's disease and ulcerative colitis phenotypes. The prevalence of inflammatory bowel disease is increased in individuals with other autoimmune diseases. Crohn's disease and ulcerative colitis are considered complex genetic traits, as inheritance does not follow any simple Mendelian models. IBD has been linked to chromosomes 16p12-q13 (IBD1), 12p13 (IBD2), 6p (IBD3), 14q11-q12 (IBD4), 5q31 (IBD5), 19p13 (IBD6), 1p36 (IBD7), and 16p (IBD8) not linked to CARD15.

Crohn's Disease

Mutations in the caspase recruitment domain-containing protein 15 (CARD15) gene also known as NOD2 mapping to chromosome 16 are associated with susceptibility to Crohn's disease. An allele of the ABCB1 gene is also associated with susceptibility to Crohn's disease. Polymorphism in the DLG5 gene, which maps to 10q23, is associated with the risk of developing IBD; genetic interaction studies suggested interactions between the 113A variant of DLG5 gene and risk-associated CARD15 alleles. Nonperforating Crohn's disease, the more benign form, was associated with increased interleukin-1-beta (IL1B) and interleukin-1 receptor alpha (IL1RA) mRNA expression. Possibility of a Mycobacterium (*M. paratuberculosis*), as a cause of Crohn's disease was evidenced by RT-PCR and DNA sequencing from mucosal specimens in humans with Crohn's disease. The source of *M. paratuberculosis* was potable water supply, which may be a reservoir of infection. Mouse models of colitis offer an avenue for identifying IBD genes or pathways that may lead to identification of the human orthologs.

PANCREATITIS

Hereditary Pancreatitis

Association of germline mutations in cationic trypsinogen gene (PRSS1), mapped to chromosome 7, with pancreatitis was first reported in hereditary pancreatitis (HP). The autosomal dominant mutations with high penetrance have been reported, of which, R122H mutation eliminates autocatalytic cleavage site in trypsin. This protects trypsin from autolysis thus generating supertrypsin. Autosomal recessive mutations have also been reported. In contrast HP families with no trypsinogen mutations have been found which revealed heterogeneity in this disease.

Chronic Pancreatitis

Most patients with idiopathic (ICP) or tropical (TCP) chronic pancreatitis, however, do not have mutations in PRSS1, and have rather presented with mutations in pancreatic secretory trypsin inhibitor gene (PSTI / SPINK). SPINK1 provides first line of defense against prematurely activated trypsinogen within the pancreatic acinar cells up to 20%. SPINK1 mutations act as disease modifier and the mechanism is more complex than a simple autosomal recessive one.

Mutations in cystic fibrosis transmembrane conductance regulator (CFTR) causing cystic fibrosis (CF) have also been reported in association with pancreatitis. Of the 900 mutations so far identified, a single mutation, i.e. deletion of phenylalanine (Δ F508) is known to occur in 66% of the CF patients in both the alleles. Several mild mutations CFTR – R117H and 5T/7T/9T alleles in the intron 8, are associated with ICP. Compound heterozygotes are more strongly linked with ICP than CF.

CONCLUSIONS

New insights into the genetic basis of disease are being generated, thanks to technological advances, such as the PCR, real time PCR and automated DNA sequencing. Although its promise is great, the integration of genetics into the everyday practice of medicine remains challenging. This chapter discussed in brief the role of genetics in hereditary diseases in gastroenterology and hepatology. The application of molecular genetics in everyday clinical practice is hampered by the difficulties like prediction of disease penetrance, the presence of multiple mutations of a particular gene with varying functional consequences and the exogenous factors modulating disease expression. To date, the most significant impact of genetics has been to increase our understanding of disease etiology and pathogenesis and to reliably identify siblings of affected patients who carry the risk to develop symptomatic disease.

Foundation for heterogeneity is at the primary genetic level, and expression of genetic susceptibility requires environmental triggers.

SUGGESTED READING

1. Giardiello FM, Brensinger JD, Paterson GM. AGA Technical Review on Hereditary colorectal cancer and Genetic Testing. Gastroenterology 2001: 121: 198-213.
2. Solomon C, Pho L, Neklason D, Burt R. Genetic counselling for gastrointestinal patients. In Textbook of Gastroenterology, Yamada T, (Ed.): Lippincot Raven; Philadelphia 2003.
3. Bacon BR. Hemochromatosis: Diagnosis and management. Gastroenterology 2001; 120: 718-725.
4. Giardiello FM, Brensinger JD, Paterson GM. American Gastroenterology Association Medical Position Statement: Hereditary Colorectal Cancer and Genetic Testing. Gastroenterology 2001; 121: 195-197.

39

Thankappan KR

Newer Drugs in Gastroenterology and Hepatology

NEWER ANTIVIRAL AGENTS

Adefovir Dipivoxil

Adefovir dipivoxil (AD) is an oral diester of adefovir, which is a cyclic nucleotide analogue with activity against hepatitis B virus. Adefovir diphosphate causes termination of viral DNA chain by competitively inhibiting natural substrate, deoxyadenosine triphosphate of DNA polymerase. AD significantly improves histological, biochemical, and virological outcomes in patients chronically infected with hepatitis B virus (HBV) and is effective in both HBe Ag positive and negative patients. The available data suggests that HBV mutations conferring resistance to AD emerge infrequently and slowly, unlike that with lamivudine. It is an attractive option for patients infected with lamivudine resistant HBV and failing to respond to lamivudine therapy. AD is also found to be useful when added to lamivudine or other existing therapy in various patient groups infected with lamivudine resistant HBV. This includes patients with decompensated liver disease, patients co-infected with HIV and patients awaiting or recovering from liver transplantation. It is indicated in chronic HBV infection with elevated ALT/AST or histologically active disease. The recommended daily dose is 10 mg and the duration of treatment is not defined at present.

Other Newer Antiviral Agents

There are more than half a dozen other potent HBV anti virals under trial. The prominent ones under these are: (1) famcyclovir (2) emtricitabine (3) lobucavir (4) entecavir (5) gancyclovir.

Combination therapy

Exploring the efficacy and safety of combining various agents such as interferon alfa + lamivudine, lamivudine + famcyclovir and adefovir/lobucavir + lamivudine is comparatively a newer approach for better results which seems encouraging.

Pegylated Interferon

The modification of interferon (IFN) with polyethylene glycol (PEG), which are amphophilic polymers, results in a decreased clearance and increased serum half life with sustained levels of IFN over the course of one week. It thus prevents the oscillations of serum HCV RNA seen with standard IFN alfa. This is the rationale for its weekly injection. The two PEG IFN that have been studied include the long branched 40 kd alfa 2a and short linear 12kd alfa 2b with no significant difference in efficacy. In genotype 2 and 3 of HCV (India falls in this group) the sustained viral response rate (SVR) is 76-82% when used in combination with ribavirin (with both PEG IFN alfa 2a and alfa 2b). But the response rate of genotype 1 is only 42-46 %. It also appears that 24 wks (as against the 48 wks of usual course) of treatment and lower dose of ribavirin is adequate for genotype 2 and 3. The merits of PEG IFN over the standard IFN are the once weekly dosing and high sustained virological response, but its high cost is a disadvantage. PEG IFN monotherapy alone is two-fold more efficacious than standard interferon monotherapy in a dose dependant fashion. Dose of PEG IFN alfa 2b is 1.5 µg/kg weekly plus ribavirin 800 mg per day.

Terlipressin in Hepatorenal Syndrome

This synthetic analogue of vasopressin has intrinsic vasoconstrictor activity. It has the advantage over vasopressin of a longer biological half-life, allowing administration as a 4 hourly bolus.

In various studies on hepatorenal syndrome (HRS), terlipressin in average dose of 1 mg 12 hourly showed initial improvement, but relapsed when treatment was discontinued. When it is used along with human serum albumin infusion, better results are reported but there are no recommendations for its use so far. Other agents tried or under study for HRS are: (1) octapressin (2) ornipressin (3) octreotide (4) dopamine (5) misoprostol (6) endothelin antagonist (7) N-acetyl cysteine.

All these trials are better justified when used as a pre-liver transplant plan.

Urso-deoxy Cholic Acid (UDCA)

UDCA, a dihyroxy bile acid, is a major constituent of the bile of the Chinese black bear. In humans it constitutes 3% of total bile acid pool. The spectrum of its clinical applications in various cholestatic liver diseases is increasing. This drug shows varying results, some of which are promising, in the following conditions:

1. Primary biliary cirrhosis (drug of choice)
2. Primary sclerosing cholangitis
3. Intrahepatic cholestasis of pregnancy
4. Liver disease in cystic fibrosis
5. Graft versus host disease

6. Chronic hepatitis C
7. Acute rejection after liver transplantation
8. Alcoholic liver disease
9. Non-alcoholic steatohepatitis
10. Benign recurrent intrahepatic cholestasis
11. Caroli's disease
12. Auto immune hepatitis and
13. Gallstone dissolution (for smaller cholesterol stones without calcification).

Mechanisms of Action of UDCA

UDCA is a hydrophilic non-hepatotoxic compound that acts by attenuating the effects of endogenous hydrophobic bile acids, some of which are believed to be hepatotoxic. Alterations in bile acid pool may occur by competition for ileal uptake sites or by direct action at the hepatocyte level. In addition UDCA may reduce class I and class II HLA antigens expression on hepatocyte and biliary epithelial cells. Dosage for various conditions is 15-20 mg/kg/day.

Silymarin in Liver Diseases

Silymarin, an extract of the plant silybum marianum is a mixture of silybin, silydianin, silychristin, and isosilybin of which silybin is the most active agent. Its postulated mechanisms of actions are (1) antioxidant (2) stabilization of mast cells (3) increasing hepatocyte protein synthesis (4) inhibiting lipid peroxidation.

Dose: 140 mg three times daily for treatment and 70 mg tree times daily for maintenance in alcoholic hepatitis, acute hepatitis and toxic hepatitis.

Even though many clinical trials are favouring its beneficial effects for the treatment of various liver diseases, its exact role in clinical medicine is yet to be decided.

BIOLOGICAL THERAPY OF INFLAMMATORY DISEASE

Anti-tumor Necrosis Factor Antibody

Infliximab is an FDA approved anti-TNF antibody for the treatment of Crohn's disease. It is used in moderate to severely active Crohn's disease when other treatment modalities fail and is also indicated in fistulizing Crohn's disease. The results are encouraging when used in the dose of 5 mg/kg at 0, 2, 6 wks intervals to induce remission. For maintenance of remission the dose is 5 mg / kg at 8 weeks intervals.

Other newer drugs in this group are Etanercept, CDP 571, Adalizumab, interleukins etc. Contraindications for the use of infliximab are:
1. Patients with clostridium difficile infection
2. Known strictures
3. History of autoimmune disease
4. Malignancy particularly lympho-proliferative disorders.

Balsalazide

Balsalazide is an oral prodrug of 5-aminosalicylic acid, which is azo-bonded by an inert substance, aminobezoyl beta alanine (ABA). In the colon the azo bonding will be split by the colonic bacterial azo-reductase into 5-ASA and ABA. Because of this targetted delivery of the drug effective action is expected. Many studies favour this better efficacy of balsalazide which is more seen with left sided colitis in the dose of 6.75 gram/d in three divided doses for 8-12 wks.

Itopride

The prokinetic drug itopride has a dual mode of action-by dopamine D2 antagonism and by the inhibition of the enzyme acetyl choline esterase . It is useful for the management of gastric motility disorders, gastroparesis, non-ulcer dyspepsia and chronic gastritis. It can be a useful adjunct in the management of gastroesophageal reflux disease. Itopride is metabolized by N-oxidation and so unlikely to alter the pharmacokinetics of concomitantly administered drugs. There are no clinically significant cardiovascular side effects unlike that of cisapride. In the dose of 50 mg three times daily itopride is a promising prokinetic agent for the management of gastric and esophageal motility disorders.

Mosapride also is another comparatively newer prokinetic agent with actions closer to that of itopride, again without significant cardiac side effects.

Probiotics in Clinical Medicine

Probiotics are microbial food supplements, which beneficially influence the health of humans. Probiotics such as lactobacilli, bifidobacilli, streptococcus thermophilus, and saccharomyces boullardi are found to be useful in some studies as an adjunct for the management of antibiotic associated diarrhea, rotavirus diarrhea in children, irritable bowel syndrome and in various other gastrointestinal disorders including inflammatory bowel disease. The mechanism of action is thought to be by: (1) maintaining the microbial mileu to host's advantage (2) decreasing the load of pathogenic bacteria (3) competing for nutrients (4) producing acidification (5) the production of inhibitory substances (bacteriocins) (6) immunomodulation. Probiotics can be taken as curd, yoghurt, fermented milk or freeze dried cultures.

It should be remembered that the effect of all the probiotics are not identical and may also vary with different socioeconomic groups and various geographical areas.

Racecadotril

This enkephalinase inhibitor is an antisecretory anti-diarrheal agent useful for all age groups starting from two months of age for acute diarrhea. It is less likely to alter gastrointestinal motility.

Adult Dose: 100 mg three times daily

Pediatric dose: 1.5 mg/kg body weight

Tegaserod

Tegaserod is a partial agonist of serotonin 5HT4 receptors. In constipation predominant irritable bowel syndrome (IBS) it may stimulate peristalsis, increase intestinal secretion and may alter associated pain by acting on three major physiological abnormalities of IBS namely altered gut motility, visceral hypersensitivity and altered intestinal secretion. In various studies the efficacy of the drug range from 5-20% over placebo in the dose of 6 mg twice daily.

SUGGESTED READING

1. Akobeng AK; et al. Cochrane database syst rev 2004;(1): CD3574
2. Fiocchi C; NEJM 2004;350 (9): 934-6
3. Rutgeerts et al, Gastroenterology 2004 Feb 126-(2): 402-13
4. Marteu P, et. al Endoscopy 2004;36 (2):130-6 Review
5. Li L H et, al. Bio Pharm Bull 2004;27 (7):1031-6
6. Kang J S, et al. Biochem Phamacol 2004;1;67 (1):175-81
7. Agreus, et al. Gut 2002;50: 2-9.
8. Galsky J. l Clin Gastreterol 1999; 28: 249-53.
9. Conn. Current Therapy. WB Saunders 2001.

40

Sudheer K

Conventional Imaging in Gastroenterology

INTRODUCTION

An overview of conventional radiological techniques, its usefulness, limitations and scope is briefly covered in this chapter.

The primary aim in imaging is to image the organs in their normal and abnormal states. Imaging can be real time or static. Real time imaging includes X-ray fluoroscopy and ultrasound scanning. Rest of the imaging techniques are static in nature. An example of this is screening examination of chest, which shows cardiac activity and diaphragmatic movements, while chest radiograph gives a static picture at a particular given time. A plain X-ray of the pregnant uterus shows the foetus as a static image while ultrasound shows foetal activities like limb movements, heartbeats, swallowing, etc.

The imaging investigation should be appropriate for the clinical situation. In order to choose the right investigation, a thorough knowledge of the clinical problem is mandatory for the radiologist and the clinician. It must be very clear in their mind as to the diagnostic yield from a particular investigation for a given clinical problem. The radiologist and the clinician are equally responsible for the time, money and energy expended in every investigation.

Conventional radiology uses mainly plain X-rays and contrast studies. The radiographs are obtained by the qualified technologist under the supervision of the radiologist. The radiologist may have to do fluoroscopy and compression techniques as and when required. It is customary to do a preliminary radiograph before contrast is given. The plain X-rays usually give a clue as to the nature of the lesion namely impacted foreign body, abnormal gas pattern, bowel obstruction (small/large/complete/incomplete, etc.), impending perforation and free gas under the diaphragm as in perforation. The role of plain X-rays as far as the solid organs are concerned is limited. However, gross organomegaly, stones in urinary tract, pancreas and gall bladder may be diagnosed.

The contrast media usually employed are negative contrast (air, carbon dioxide and other gases), which have low atomic number than the soft tissues and hence appear dark and black. The positive contrast media (barium sulfate and iodinated compounds) have high atomic number than the soft tissues of the body and appear bright and white. The positive contrast media can either be water-soluble (solutions of organic iodine compounds) or water insoluble (aqueous suspension of insoluble barium sulfate) (Fig. 40.1).

Ionic contrast media dissociate in water into electrically charged particles named ions. Non-ionic contrast media are electrically neutral like water molecules.

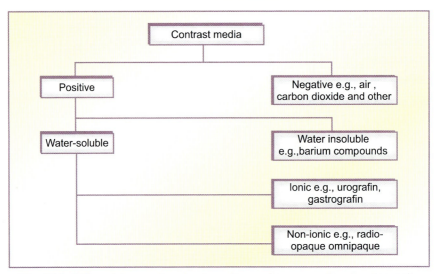

Fig. 40.1: Different types of contrast media used in conventional radiography

Routinely, in the investigation of GIT, a compartmentalization is applied. (Table 40.1).

Investigation	Parts visualized	Patient preparation
Barium swallow Thick paste (consistency of tooth paste)	Cervical, thoracic and sub-diaphragamatic parts of the esophagus, fundus of the stomach	No preparation is needed
Barium meal 200 ml of undiluted barium sulfate suspension	Esophago-gastric junction, stomach, duodenum and duodeno-jejunal flexure	Overnight fasting
Barium meal follow through 300 ml of barium sulfate suspension diluted	Duodeno-jejunal flexure, jejunum, ileum and ileocecal junction	Overnight fasting
Barium enema 1 litre of barium solution	Entire length of the colon, cecum and terminal ileum	Thorough cleansing of bowel by laxatives or wash out

Table 40.1: Showing different forms of barium studies, parts visualised and patient preparation

The jejunum and ileum can be alternatively imaged by small bowel enema by introducing a tube beyond the DJ flexure and injecting diluted contrast continuously till the ileocecum is obtained.

Esophagus, stomach, duodenum and the colon can be outlined with barium and air (double contrast) with or without smooth muscle relaxants like buscopan or glucagon. With single contrast investigation the lumen alone is studied; however, with double contrast, the surface mucosa can be evaluated and mural lesions can be identified. Ulcerations and infiltrations can also be identified.

In clinical situations, where perforation of hollow viscus or post-operative leak from anastomotic sites are evaluated, iodinated water soluble contrast media like gastrografin is used. If barium sulfate is used there is chance of production of granulomas.

In subacute small bowel obstruction, since we use non-flocculating barium suspensions, the chances of it progressing to acute bowel obstruction are very rare.

For diagnostic detail it is always preferable to use barium sulfate suspension over water-soluble iodinated contrast agent because of its radiographic detail. Water-soluble contrast usually gets diluted and dissipated and hence the radiographic detail is very poor.

Adverse Effects

Oral barium sulfate may outline bronchial tree by aspiration or through tracheo-esophageal fistula, and enter into the mediastinum or peritoneal cavity via perforation. Barium in the bronchial tree is less harmful than aspiration of food and seldom causes any problem. In the mediastinum and peritoneal cavity, barium sulfate may produce adhesion and/or granulomas. The passage of barium sulfate with food, intestinal and pancreatic enzyme and fecal matter is considered more damaging than the passage of barium sulfate alone.

Constipation may follow oral barium sulfate and can be treated with fluid and laxatives. If perforation of GIT is suspected, water-soluble iodinated contrast medium is used as it will be reabsorbed into the blood stream and excreted through the kidneys. There is no risk of granuloma formation.

Pediatric Imaging

In pediatric practice, special emphasis is given to radiation doses. Indication for examination should be well founded. Radiation protection is critical, lead shielding of gonads is used whenever possible. Examination of GIT upto the age of three months requires no preparation. In older children, the same preparation as that of adults is used. In newborn, the contrast agent should be prepared in isotonic solutions due to the risk of water intoxication.

Hepatobiliary System

Investigations such as oral cholecystogram/intravenous cholangiogram are outdated. Sonological evaluation has virtually replaced cholecystography in gall bladder and related problems. CT and MRI give a global anatomy of the biliary tree so that treatment planning can be very accurate.

SUGGESTED READING

1. Ronald L Eioenberg, Gastrointestinal Radiology, Lippincott-Ravew, New York. 3rd Edn. 1996
2. Alexander R, Margulis, H Joachim Burhenne, Alimentary Tract Radiology 4th Edn. (1st Indian Edn. 1990).

41

Srikanth Moorthy
Sreekumar KP

Imaging in
Gastroenterology:
Newer Modalities

ULTRASONOGRAPHY

Ultrasonography (USG) is the best primary imaging technique for evaluating a wide range of gastrointestinal disorders. Its advantages are that it is free of potentially harmful ionizing radiation, relatively inexpensive, widely available and sufficiently sensitive to detect many solid organ pathologies. A number of bowel diseases, which result in mural thickening or mass can also be detected with USG.

ULTRASONOGRAPHY OF LIVER AND BILIARY SYSTEM

Ultrasound is the usual first imaging examination done in patients with suspected liver mass, obstructive jaundice or liver enzyme abnormality. USG clearly distinguishes a simple hepatic cyst or hydatid cyst from a solid mass or abscess. An abscess, typically, will be well defined and hypoechoic with mobile internal echoes (Fig. 41.1). Combined with typical clinical features, the diagnosis can be made with a fair degree of certainty. Multiplicity of lesions, hypoechoic or hyperechoic, in a background of normal liver raises the suspicion of metastasis. Definite diagnosis rests on a guided fine needle aspiration cytology. A large hypo and hyperechoic mass with portal vein thrombosis is typical of hepatocellular carcinoma. In advanced cirrhosis, the liver has a coarse echotexture, which can mask underlying hepatocellular carcinoma. In these patients, clinical suspicion and/or raised alpha fetoprotein levels should prompt a spiral CT or MRI.

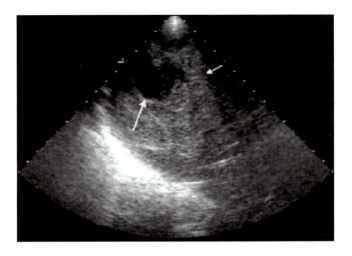

Fig. 41.1: Ultrasound abdomen showing liver abscess in the right lobe of liver.

USG has a high sensitivity and specificity for detecting biliary ductal dilatation. The site and cause of obstruction can also be assessed with a slightly lesser degree of accuracy. USG is the most sensitive imaging technique for detecting gallbladder (GB) calculi. Both calcified and non-calcified calculi can be seen. Presence of GB wall thickening and peri-cholecystic fluid indicates cholecystitis. USG is less sensitive for calculi within the bile duct.

COLOR DOPPLER

Doppler refers to blood flow imaging using the shift in frequency of ultrasound created by moving blood (Doppler effect). Stationary tissue does not produce the Doppler shift. In everyday clinical parlance, Doppler refers to the waveforms generated by the moving blood (Doppler spectrum). In a colour Doppler image, the complex Doppler information is simply represented in colour (blue for flow in one direction and red representing flow in the opposite direction) and superimposed on the usual black and white images. Doppler and color doppler are becoming an integral part of the ultrasound scan of liver. The color Doppler demonstration of flow within a mass can differentiate it from an abscess. Hepatocellular carcinomas tend to show marked internal vascularity characterized by low resistance arterial flow. The portal vein and its branches can be easily mapped using color Doppler. In portal hypertension USG shows increased portal vein size (> 11mm) with loss of the normal phasic variation of portal blood flow in the Doppler wave form. Flow reversal in the portal vein and extrahepatic portosystemic collateral can also be detected using a combination of USG and Doppler. In a suspected Budd-Chiari syndrome USG and Doppler are used to assess the patency of the IVC and hepatic veins.

COMPUTED TOMOGRAPHY (CT)

Over the last decade CT technology has been revolutionized by spiral or helical CT. As opposed to the 'slice by slice' approach of the conventional CT, in spiral CT, the patient moves through the gantry while the CT X-ray tube rotates continuously around the patient. This enables faster scanning, which in turn allows organs to be captured in various phases of vascular enhancement. The scan can be done in a single breathhold minimizing patient motion artifacts. Moreover, since no data is lost in between two slices, the scan has more precise anatomical detail. Reconstructions, if required, are more 'life-like'. (Figs 41.2 and 43.3)

SPIRAL CT OF LIVER

The ability to obtain scans rapidly allows the liver to be imaged in the arterial, portal venous and hepatic venous phases separately with a single injection of

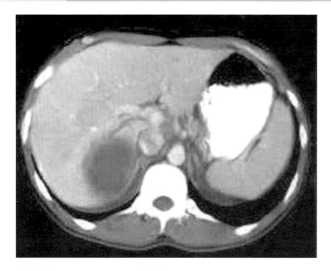

Fig. 41.2: Contrast enhanced CT scan showing large liver abscess
in the right lobe of the liver

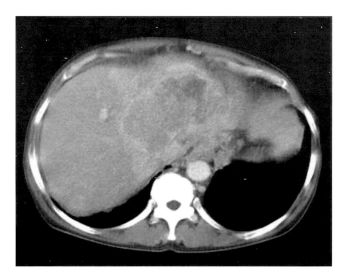

Fig. 41.3: Contrast enchanced spiral CT-scan showing hypervascular lesion
in the left lobe of the liver with left portal vein obstruction
suggesting hepatocellular carcinoma

contrast. The arterial phase (scan starts 30 seconds after start of injection) can
detect hypervascular lesions like hepatocellular carcinomas, vascular
metastases and hemangiomas. The portal venous phase (about 50 seconds
delay) scans produce maximum enhancement of the liver parenchyma and
clearly depicts relatively hypovascular mass lesions like most metastatic

deposits, cysts and cholangiocarcinomas. Moreover, the relationship of the mass lesions to the hepatic vasculature can be clearly shown allowing precise segmental localization and accurate surgical planning.

CT ARTERIOPORTOGRAPHY (CTAP)

CTAP is an invasive procedure done to detect small nodules of HCC in a patient with cirrhosis. It is reported to have a higher sensitivity than contrast enhanced MRI. Two catheters are placed in the common hepatic artery and superior mesenteric arteries respectively. CT of Liver is performed while injecting contrast into the hepatic artery first (arterial phase). Then contrast is injected into the SMA and the liver is scanned again in the portal venous phase. The procedure helps to plan and select patients for surgery, chemoembolisation and radiofrequency ablation.

ULTRASONOGRAPHY AND CT OF PANCREAS

Ultrasonography: It is the best initial screening imaging tool in suspected pancreatic disease. Adequate visualization of the entire gland may be hampered by presence of overlying bowel gas, body habitus of patient and presence of large calculi in the gland. Scanning through water filled stomach is generally required to delineate the distal body and tail. Pancreatic mass lesions, pancreatic duct dilatation and intraductal calculi can be readily seen on USG. Small lesions, which do not alter the contour of the gland, like insulinomas can be missed. Subtle peripancreatic fat infiltration by inflammation or tumor can also be missed and is best evaluated with CT.

Computed tomography: Spiral CT allows complete, consistent evaluation of the entire gland and adjacent vessels (portal vein, splenic vein, superior mesenteric artery and vein) and the retroperitoneum in all patients. In pancreatic mass lesions, CT is indicated for surgical planning. Involvement of adjacent vascular structures, regional lymphadenopathy and liver metastases can be clearly visualized. Arterial phase spiral CT is the imaging technique of choice for small functioning endocrine tumors of pancreas like insulinomas. CT is more sensitive than USG in detecting early changes of pancreatitis i.e., focal non-enhancing areas, peripancreatic fat stranding, fluid collections and necrosis. The severity of the disease can be graded using CT findings and this has been shown to correlate with the prognosis. CT is exquisitely sensitive to the presence of calcifications and, hence, is indicated in the initial work up of suspected chronic pancreatitis.

SPIRAL CT FOR BOWEL PATHOLOGY

The capability of faster scanning has expanded the traditional indications of CT in the abdomen to include imaging of bowel pathology. Spiral CT allows the entire small and large bowel to be seen in continuity. Segments of thickened or collapsed bowel can be localized accurately making CT an essential tool in the investigation of suspected inflammatory, infiltrative and ischemic bowel disease. Spiral CT has virtually replaced oral contrast examinations in the imaging of intestinal obstruction.

ABDOMEN SCAN–CT OR ULTRASOUND

Ultrasound does not have ionizing radiation, is inexpensive and widely available. It is the best imaging modality to detect GB pathology. It is highly sensitive in detecting intrahepatic biliary radicular dilatation and focal lesions in the liver. Sensitivity for detecting mass lesions may be less in the background of cirrhosis. The evaluation of structures outside the liver like the distal CBD, pancreatic body and retroperitoneum can be suboptimal due to overlying bowel gas. CT, on the other hand, allows consistent visualization of the pancreas and other retroperitoneal structures unhindered by bowel gas. CT is thus, essential for pre-op staging of tumors and is better than ultrasound in evaluating a suspected focal lesion in cirrhotic liver. Spiral CT done with arterial and venous phase scans has a higher sensitivity than ultrasound for detecting liver metastases. However, metastatic deposits, which enhance to the same extent as the liver parenchyma can be missed on CT while these lesion may be apparent on USG. It must be borne in mind that the CT examination carries a significant radiation risk and hence should be used judiciously in patients, especially children. It is advisable to use ultrasound for follow up studies and for screening when there is only a low index of suspicion for disease.

MAGNETIC RESONANCE CHOLANGIOPANCREATOGRAPHY (MRCP)

MRCP is a non-invasive MRI technique, which provides projection images of the biliary and pancreatic ductal system comparable to an endoscopic view or a percutaneous cholangiogram. MRCP is performed in breathhold using special fast heavily-T2 weighted sequences which renders fluid (bile, urine, ascites, cyst) very bright and suppresses signal from other tissues. A typical MRCP examination consists of 1) Conventional T1 and T2 axial scans through area of interest 2) Breathhold 'thick slab' projection images obtained in AP, lateral and oblique planes 3) Breath hold thin section T2 weighted scans (HASTE scan) in coronal and axial planes to delineate finer anatomic details of the ductal system. (Fig. 41.4)

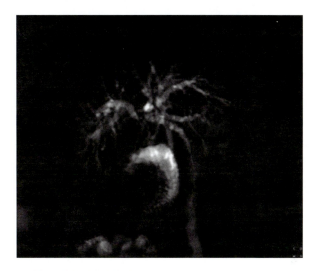

Fig. 41.4: MRCP film showing normal biliary tree

COMMON INDICATIONS FOR MRCP

1. Hilar cholangiocarcinoma: The involvement of the common hepatic duct, confluence of the left and right hepatic ducts and extension of tumor along segmental ducts can be seen. This helps plan surgery and percutaneous drainage.
2. High CBD injury post cholecystectomy
3. Evaluation of hepaticojejunostomy stricture, where there is no endoscopic access
4. Follow up of patients with chronic pancreatitis. To assess duct size before pancreaticojejunostomy surgery
5. Congenital anomalies of CBD (Choledochal cyst) and pancreatic duct (pancreas division.).

MRCP VERSUS ERCP

Unlike ERCP, MRCP is non-invasive and free of ionizing radiations. MRCP would be ideal for follow-up imaging and when there is only a low index of clinical suspicion. ERCP involves X-ray exposure and carries a small, but significant risk of procedure related complications. ERCP, however, allows biliary drainage, biopsy or other appropriate interventions to be performed, in one step. MRCP is generally not required in lower CBD obstructions.

MRI OF LIVER

The advantages of MR imaging in the investigation of liver diseases are well documented. The lack of ionizing radiation and safety of gadolinium chelates are important considerations. The recent developments in MR including fast imaging breath hold sequences and new MR contrast media have revolutionized the capabilities of MR.

Studies comparing MRI with dynamic contrast enhanced CT and spiral CT have shown that MR is more accurate.

Liver imaging protocols include axial T1 and T2 sequences. Breath-hold sequences are available in the newer generation MR scanners. Contrast enhanced sequences are invariably used. Depending on the clinical question, acquisitions in the coronal or sagittal planes are added.

Intravenous contrast agents can potentially increase the sensitivity and specificity of MR imaging for detection and characterization of liver lesions. The most commonly used contrast agent is the extra cellular gadolinium chelate. RES (reticulo endothelial system) specific and hepatocyte selective agents have recently been developed and used.

Gadolinium is administered as a rapid intravenous bolus (10 ml) and imaging is performed with a T1 weighted breath hold acquisition that is repeated dynamically. The gadolinium after intravenous administration is rapidly distributed to the extra cellular space from the vascular compartment prior to renal excretion. Gadolinium has paramagnetic property that reduces T1 relaxation to a much greater extent than T2 relaxation resulting in increased signal intensities on T1 images.

The main application of MR is in evaluation and characterization of focal liver lesions in cirrhosis. A combination of T1 weighted, T2 weighted and dynamic gadolinium enhanced scans can accurately define most of the lesions in cirrhotic liver as regenerating nodules, dysplastic nodules or hepatocellular carcinoma (HCC).

Regenerating nodules are hypo intense to hyper intense in T1 images and iso-intense to hypo-intense in T2 images. On post contrast images they appear hypo intense as the hepatic parenchyma enhances more than the nodule. Iron accumulation can be seen in up to 25% regenerating nodules facilitating their identification as low signal intensity lesions in T2 images.

Dysplastic nodules appear hyper intense in T1 and hypo intense in T2. Mild enhancement can be present in the early arterial phase.

As hepatocellular carcinoma develops in a dysplastic nodule, hyper intensity appears in T2 images. Nodule within a nodule sign has been described for a hypo intense dysplastic nodule harbouring a small hyper intense HCC in T2 images. Post contrast images show intense enhancement in the early arterial phase with contrast washout in the late phase. MR imaging features that suggest presence of HCC are

1. Lesion size greater than 3 cm
2. Hyper intensity in T2
3. Intense enhancement in the arterial phase
4. Contrast washout in the late phase.
5. Presence of a capsule

Another application of MR is in differentiating metastasis from other benign focal lesions like cysts and hemangioma. All of these lesions appear hypointense in T1 and hyper intense in T2. But maximum hyper intensity is for hemangioma (light bulb sign). Long TE images (TE 120 to 180 milli seconds) will show that hemangiomas have a signal similar to CSF whereas most malignant lesions will not be as bright as CSF. Differentiation of cyst from hemangioma is unimportant as both are benign lesions. Post contrast dynamic studies can confirm a hemangioma. Peripheral nodular enhancement of the same intensity as the major vessels is a characteristic finding.

PERCUTANEOUS TRANSHEPATIC CHOLANGIOGRAPHY (PTC)

The combination of MRCP and ERCP has almost completely replaced the need for diagnostic PTC. PTC today is done only as a prelude to percutaneous biliary drainage. PTC is done under conscious sedation and local anesthesia. A special 15 cm long flexible needle (Chiba needle) is introduced into the liver percutaneously through the right flank. Dilated bile ducts are opacified with contrast.

PERCUTANEOUS TRANSHEPATIC BILIARY DRAINAGE (PTBD)

PTBD is of three types. (1) External drainage: A simple pigtail drainage catheter drains the bile out into a bag. (2) Internal-external drainage: A special catheter is placed across the obstruction with its endholes in the duodenum jejunum and proximal holes in the dilated system above the obstruction. The proximal end of the catheter lies outside at the puncture site. If this end is closed, bile drains internally and if it is kept open, external drainage occurs. (3) Stent: Once an obstructing lesion is crossed, an internal stent (usually metallic self-expandable) can be placed eliminating the catheter and external bag.

MOST COMMON INDICATIONS FOR PTBD

1. Biliary obstruction with cholangitis-temporary external drainage
2. Hilar and upper CBD obstructions where ERCP is technically more difficult-Internal-external drainage and subsequenty stent.
3. Post-operative hepaticojejunostomy stricture where there is no endoscopic access-internal-external drainage and balloon dilatation for benign strictures and stent for malignant stricturer.

ANGIOGRAPHY

Diagnostic gastrointestinal angiography involves selective catheterization of the celiac axis, superior mesenteric and inferior mesenteric arteries. Following a pressure injection of iodine containing contrast, images have to be acquired into the venous phase. Indications for angiography in the modern era are restricted to (1) investigation of GI bleed occult to upper and lower GI endoscopy (2) as a prelude to endovascular therapeutic embolization of liver tumors, (3) for the diagnosis and therapy of pseudoaneurysms in the GI tract which may be post-traumatic, post-operative or spontaneous in a background of pancreatitis. (Fig. 41.5)

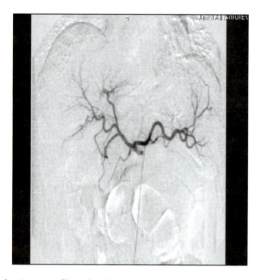

Fig. 41.5: Aortogram film showing normal celiac trunk with its branches

ANGIOGRAPHY OF OCCULT GI BLEED

Lower GI bleed occurring in the small bowel or in the right colon is frequently difficult to localize with endoscopy. If the rate of bleed is at least 1ml/mt, angiography will show an extravasation at the bleeding point. These patients require definite surgery. Emobolization can stop torrential bleeding and help stabilize a sick patient. The common etiologies are small or large bowel angiodysplasias, non-specific ulcers, diverticula and gastrointestinal stromal tumors. Spiral CT with oral contrast is a useful investigation in a patient with occult GI bleed who is not actively bleeding.

EMOBOLIZATION OF LIVER TUMOR

Metastatic deposits from carcinoids and functioning endocrine tumors of pancreas tend to produce distressing symptoms due to production of vasoactive substances. These symptoms can be effectively palliated by embolizing (blocking) the feeding hepatic arterial branches. Inoperable hepatocellular carcinomas can be palliated by selectively injecting cancer chemotherapeutic agent into the arterial branch feeding the tumor-which in then embolised with gelfoam. This procedure is called chemoembolization. A very high concentration of the chemotherapeutic agent can be achieved at the target site while significantly reducing the systemic side effects. It has been shown that in properly selected patients chemoembolization offers both survival benefit and improvement of quality of life.

SUGGESTED READING

1. Balthazar EJ, Robinson DL, Megibow AJ, et al. Acute pancreatitis: Value of CT in establishing prognosis. Radiology 1990;174:331-336.
2. Withers CE, Wilson SR: The liver. In Rumack CM, Wilson SR, Charboneau JW eds. Diagnostic ultrasound, 2nd ed. New York: Mosby, 1998;87-154.
3. Koehler RE, Memel DS, Stanley RJ. Gastrointestinal tract. In Lee JAT, Sagel SS, Stanley RJ, Heiken JP eds. Computed body tomography with MRI correlation, 3rd ed.Philadelphia:Lippincott and Raven 1998;637-700.
4. Heiken JP. Liver. In Lee JAT, Sagel SS, Stanley RJ, Heiken JP eds. Computed body tomography with MRI correlation, 3rd ed.Philadelphia:Lippincott and Raven 1998;701-777.

42

Nandakumar R

Gastrointestinal Endoscopy: The Basics

INTRODUCTION

Flexible endoscopes consist of a control head and a flexible shaft with a manoeverable tip. The head is connected to a light source via an umbilical cord, through which pass other tubes transmitting air, water, suction, etc. The suction channel is used for the passage of various accessories.

There are two types of endoscopes – fibreoptic scopes and videoscopes. In fibreoptic scopes, the image is transmitted by optical fibre bundles whereas in videoscopes this is by charged couple device (CCD). The image quality of present videoscopes equals that of fibreoptic scopes in both colour and resolution. The advantage of videoscopes lies in the fact that many persons can view the image simultaneously and there is less eye strain for the endoscopist.

The control head has the knobs for up/down and right/left movements. An operating channel of 2-4 mm diameter allows the passage of fine flexible accessories like biopsy forceps, cytology brushes, and sclerotherapy needles. In side-viewing scopes the tip of the channel incorporates an elevator, which permits directional control of the accessories. The channel size varies with the instrument's function. Therapeutic endoscopes with large channels allow better suction and larger accessories.

PREPARATION AND SAFETY

The physician should ensure that the examination is indicated, that there are no major contraindications, and that the patient understands and consents to it. Complex endoscopies (e.g., therapeutic ERCP) carry more risks than simple ones (e.g., diagnostic OGD). There are patient factors also. The American Society for Anesthesiology (ASA) score can be used to give a crude measure of overall fitness or illness.

1. Healthy
2. Minor problems, no systemic effects or continuous medications
3. Significant illness, currently controlled by medication
4. Major systemic illness, poorly controlled or uncontrolled
5. Moribund.

Informed consent should be obtained in writing before all endoscopic procedures. All patients should sign a form stating that they understand the nature and purpose of the procedure, possible risks and the alternatives.

SEDATION

Pharyngeal anesthesia is useful as a routine. Lignocaine spray or gargle is applied to the posterior pharyngeal wall to suppress the gag reflex. The usual intravenous agents used are diazepam, midazolam, pethidine and fentanyl. For conscious sedation the usual starting dose is about 2 mg midazolam with gradual titration. The patient should be carefully monitored once sedatives are administered. Resuscitation equipments should be readily available in the endoscopy suite. General anesthesia may be required in special situations such as in young children.

CLEANING AND DISINFECTION OF ENDOSCOPES AND ACCESSORIES

Thorough mechanical cleaning of the endoscopes should be done immediately after the procedure to remove all blood, mucus, body secretions and organic debris. After this, formal cleaning and disinfection procedures should take place. A variety of endoscope reprocessors – manual, semiautomatic and automatic are available. The most widely used disinfectant is 2% gluteraldehyde.

UPPER ENDOSCOPY

The entire esophagus, stomach and proximal duodenum can be examined (Figs 42.1 and 42.2)

COMMON INDICATIONS

Evaluation of
- Dysphagia
- Heartburn

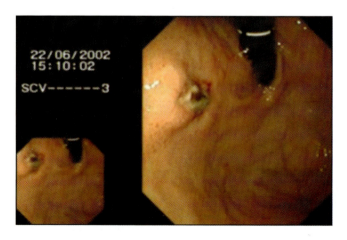

Fig. 42.1: Endoscopic picture showing gastric ulcer

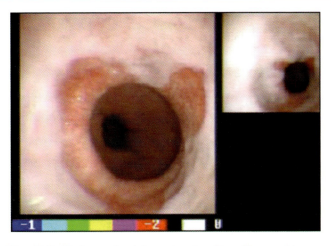

Fig. 42.2: Endoscopic picture showing Barrett's esophagus

- Upper GI bleed
- Upper abdominal pain—in suspected ulcer disease
- Anorexia and early satiety
- Recurrent vomiting

The common lesions that can be diagnosed includes esophagitis, esophageal carcinoma, esophageal varices, gastric and duodenal ulcers and gastric carcinoma.

No specific preparation other than fasting for 6-8hours is required for the procedure. Dentures, if used, should be removed.

The therapeutic upper endoscopic procedures include esophageal variceal ligation (EVL), esophageal sclerotherapy (EST), esophageal stricture dilatations, achalasia dilatation, esophageal stent placements, removal of esophageal and gastric foreign bodies, and percutaneous endoscopic gastrostomy tube placements.

ENDOTHERAPY OF ESOPHAGEAL VARICES

In EVL the preloaded bands mounted to endoscopic tip is applied over the varices after suctioning them into the cap over which the bands rest. In EST sclerosing agents like sodium tetradecyl sulfate, ethanolamine oleate and sodium morhhuate are injected into the varices.

STRICTURE DILATATION

There are two types of dilators-balloon dilators which can be passed through the scope (TTS balloons) and PVC coated plastic dilators (e.g; Savary Guilliard dilator), which are passed over a guidewire.

Achalasia dilatation is done with a specially designed non-compliant balloon-rigiflex balloon dilator.

NON-VARICEAL BLEED

These include bleeding gastric and duodenal ulcers, angiodysplasias, Mallory-Weiss tear and Dieulofoy's lesion, etc. A variety of endoscopic modalities are available to treat non-variceal bleeding.

Thermal
> Monopolar coagulation
> Bipolar coagulation
> Argon plasma coagulation
> Heater probe
> Laser

Non thermal
> Injection-adrenaline, normal saline
> Hemoclips

COLONOSCOPY

In a routine examination anal canal to cecum is examined. It is possible to examine the terminal ileum for a few centimeters with the regular colonoscope.

COMMON INDICATIONS

- Diagnosis, to assess extent of disease and treatment response in Inflammatory bowel disease – Crohn's disease, ulcerative colitis
- Diagnosis of intestinal tuberculosis
- Colonic polyps – diagnosis and surveillance
- Evaluation of lower gastrointestinal bleed
- Diagnosis and post operative surveillance in colon cancers (Figs 42.3 and 42.4)

PREPARATION

A well-planned preparation is absolutely essential as fecal material obscures the mucosal details. The patient is advised to take a semi-solid or liquid diet on the day prior to the procedure. One of the bowel-cleaning agents used contains polyethylene glycol marketed as PEGLEC. The whole content of the pack is dissolved in about 1.5 liters of water and consumed in two hours' time starting at 5am on the day of procedure. Another agent is EXELYTE, which is a sodium phosphate preparation, which can be consumed with a much smaller quantity i.e., about 300 ml of lemon juice.

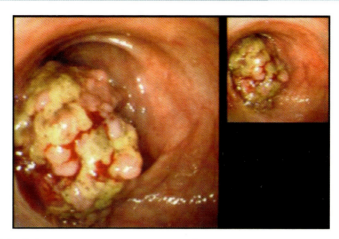

Fig. 42.3: Colonoscopy showing large proliferative mass in the sigmoid colon suggesting sigmoid colon malignancy

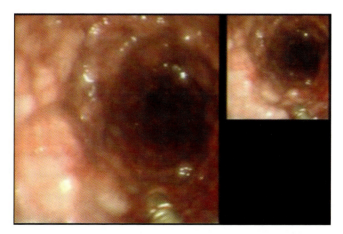

Fig. 42.4: Colonoscopy showing diffuse small polypoidal lesions in entire colon suggestive of familial adenomatous polyposis coli

The therapeutic procedures performed include polypectomy, balloon dilatation, stent placement, etc.

COLONOSCOPIC POLYPECTOMY

The polyps are snared near the base of the stalk using a colonoscopy snare of appropriate size. After this, polypectomy is achieved with electrocautery combining coagulation and cutting. It is prudent to inject the stalk with 1:10000 adrenaline to decrease the risk of bleed (Fig. 42.5)

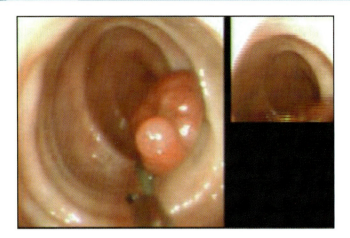

Fig. 42.5: Colonoscopy showing colonic polyp

Complications

Even though rare, complications can occur, especially with therapeutic procedures. It is extremely important to recognize this and take necessary action. The important complications are bleeding and perforation. Bleeding is encountered in polypectomy, especially when snaring is attempted without sufficient coagulation. Perforation can result from attempted passage across tight strictures.

ERCP

The sideviewing scope is specially designated for examining the papilla and performing various biliary and pancreatic therapeutic procedures.

Preparation

Patient should be fasting 6-8 hours prior to the procedure. Coagulation parameters, if abnormal, should be corrected by vitamin K injections or fresh frozen plasma infusions prior to the procedure. Patient should receive prophylactic antibiotics (e.g., cefotaxime IV) one hour prior to the procedure.

The biliary therapeutic procedures include removal of common bile duct stones, biliary stricture dilatation, nasobiliary drainage and biliary stenting. The pancreatic procedures performed are nasopancreatic drainage, stone extraction, stricture dilatation and pancreatic stenting.

THERAPEUTIC BILIARY PROCEDURES

Sphincterotomy

The biliary sphincter has to be divided to ensure adequate access into the biliary tree for therapeutic procedures. The sphincterotome has a cutting wire, which is connected to the diathermy plate. Over a zebra guidewire the sphincterotome is placed with the wire in 11-12 0' clock position for biliary sphincterotomy and current is applied. The length to be cut depends on the indication.

CBD Stone Removal

After the sphincterotomy stone removal is effected by using baskets of various designs and biliary balloons of varying sizes, which can be inflated in the CBD.

Stricture Dilatation

Biliary strictures may be benign-bile duct injury during surgery, or due to malignant disease. Biliary balloon dilators and push dilators of graded sizes are available for the purpose.

Endoscopic Placement of Prosthesis

Stenting is one of the therapeutic options in palliation of cholestatic symptoms in inoperable malignancy involving biliary system, e.g., cholangiocarcinoma. It is also indicated in benign conditions in certain instances-incomplete stone clearance in a case of choledocholithiasis. Both plastic and metallic stents of various designs are available.

Therapeutic Pancreatic Procedures

The pancreatic sphincterotomy is performed in a similar method as mentioned earlier but in a 1 O'clock direction. There are baskets and balloon dilators designed for the pancreatic duct. Endoscopic stent placement through major or minor papilla to relieve obstruction is similar to biliary stent placement.

Complications

The most common complication of sphincterotomy is acute pancreatitis. This is related to the number of attempts at cannulation and number, volume and pressure of injection of the pancreatic duct. The most serious complication is perforation, which is usually retroduodenal. The anatomical factors predisposing to perforation includes small papilla, juxtapapillary diverticula, intradiverticular papilla, narrow duct and past Billroth II operation. Most perforations respond to conservative management. Post sphincterotomy bleed is another complication, which, if severe, requires adrenaline injection or hemoclip application to achieve hemostasis.

SUGGESTED READING

1. Infectious disease complications of GI endoscopy: part II, exogenous infections. Nelson DB Gastrointest Endosc 2003 May; 57(6): 695-711.
2. American society for Gastrointestinal endoscopy – Society of Gastroenterology Nurses and Associates Endoscope Reprocessing Guideliness. Walter VA; Di Marino AJ; Gastrointest Endosc Clin N Am 2000 Apr;10(2):265-73
3. Patient controlled analgesia and sedation in gastrointestinal endoscopy. Kulling D; Bauerfeind P; Fried M; Biro P Gastrointest Endosc Clin N Am 2004 Apr;14(2):353-68

43

Ramesh GN

Advances in Gastrointestinal Endoscopy

INTRODUCTION

Progress in the practice of clinical gastroenterology has been made possible, in many respects, by rapid advances in gastrointestinal endoscopy. However, clinically important endoscopic advances are not routinely met with rapid acceptance and utilization by the general endoscopic community. Reasons for this delay include the cost of acquiring new technology, the difficulty in obtaining additional training once one's clinical practice has become established, and the (at times appropriate) skepticism regarding any new technology.

This review focuses on new developments that are likely to change the day-to-day practice of gastroenterology.

ADVANCES IN ESOPHAGOGASTRODUODENOSCOPY

Sedation-less Endoscopy

A substantial proportion of procedure-related complications are related to sedation and analgesia. One method to improve the safety and reduce the cost of endoscopy is to perform procedures without sedation. With the development of **ultrathin endoscopes with** smaller calibre (outer diameter 5.3 mm for fibreoptic endoscopes or 5.9 mm for videoendoscopes) compared to the larger caliber of standard endoscopes (outer diameter 9 mm) sedation-less endoscopy is possible, reducing the direct and indirect costs of the procedure.

Endoscopic Control of Non-variceal Bleeding

Two significant technological advances have impact in the treatment of non-variceal bleeding over the past few years: the availability of metallic clipping devices and the expanded use of band ligation for non-variceal gastrointestinal bleeding. Metallic clips have important theoretical advantages over previously available hemostatic methods providing definitive occlusion of the vascular lumen with minimal, if any, risk of perforation and immediate visual documentation of therapeutic efficacy. A related device, the detachable snare, has therapeutic potential in the management of post polypectomy bleeding.

Band ligation has recently been used in the treatment of hemorrhage caused by arteriovenous malformations, Mallory-Weiss tears, Dieulafoy lesions, postpolypectomy bleeding and bleeding colonic diverticula.

Endoscopic Control of Variceal Bleeding

Endoscopic band ligation (EBL) is now considered superior to traditional variceal sclerotherapy for the management of active esophageal variceal hemorrhage.

EVL is associated with less rebleeding, fewer local complications, and improved short-term survival. Recent data suggest that ligation may be superior to β-blockers for the primary prophylaxis of esophageal variceal hemorrhage.

For the treatment of gastric varices cyanoacrylate injection has yielded excellent results.

Botulinum Toxin Injection for the Treatment of Achalasia

The injection of botulinum toxin (Botox) directly into the lower esophageal sphincter was shown to result in significant symptomatic improvement in many patients with achalasia. The toxin results in paralysis of smooth muscle, thereby relaxing the hypertensive sphincter and allowing improved esophageal emptying. However the benefit is short term and the procedure is best reserved for patients with high operative risk.

Endoscopic Mucosal Resection

Endoscopic mucosal resection (EMR) is a technique that allows the minimally invasive removal of larger portions of non-pedunculated gastrointestinal mucosa than previously possible. The basic steps include performing a submucosal injection of saline beneath the area of lesion of interest, suctioning the lesion into a cap or other device attached to the distal portion of the endoscope and resecting the mucosa/lesion using a standard or modified snare. EMR has been used to resect superficial mucosal neoplasms (particularly early gastric carcinoma), remove small submucosal tumors, and obtain larger, deeper histological specimens when forceps biopsies are non-diagnostic.

Improved Imaging of Mucosa

Newer technologies with the potential to enhance the diagnostic yield of gastrointestinal endoscopy even further include vital dye staining, fluorescence spectroscopy and optical coherence tomography.

Vital dye staining: Tissue staining involves either the selective cellular uptake of a dye by different tissue types (absorptive staining) or a change in color in response to specific cellular products (reactive staining), as in the case of pH indicators. Chromoscopy or contact staining, uses a stain to highlight topographic aspects of the mucosal surface. The use of tissue staining techniques has yet not gained wide acceptance.

Tissue staining shows promise as an adjunctive method to enhance the detection of pathology during gastrointestinal endoscopy. It is relatively inexpensive and simple to perform. The dyes commonly used are methylene blue, lugol's solution and toluidine blue.

Spectroscopic images: Tissue spectroscopy is based on the evaluation of characteristic patterns of light emission or reflection from superficial tissue. Laser-induced fluorescence (LIF) spectroscopy uses laser energy to stimulate endogenous tissue fluorophores to emit light (fluoresce). Analysis of the wavelength and intensity of fluorescence provides information regarding subtle differences in the chemical substrates and morphology of tissue. In patients with Barrett's esophagus, LIF spectroscopy has been applied to the detection of dysplasia and carcinoma. LIF spectroscopy was able to detect esophageal cancer (both squamous cell and adenocarcinoma) with a sensitivity of 100% and specificity of 98%.

Light-scattering (reflectance spectroscopy) uses an analysis of the intensity and wavelength of light reflected from the surface of a given tissue to estimate the size and degree of crowding of surface epithelial nuclei. This technique generally uses white (non-laser) light. In patients with Barrett's esophagus, enlargement and crowding of cell nuclei are morphological changes that signal the progression from benign metaplasia through dysplasia to cancer.

Optical coherence tomography (OCT): Optical coherence tomography (OCT) is a method that provides two-dimensional cross-sectional images of the gastrointestinal tract. OCT provides true anatomic images corresponding to the layers of the gastrointestinal tract (mucosa, submucosa, muscularis propria, and serosa/adventitia). However, by using light instead of ultrasound waves, the resolution of OCT is nearly 10-fold greater than that of high frequency EUS and approaches that of light microscopy.

The potential applications for OCT include endoscopic surveillance of high-grade dysplasia in patients with Barrett's esophagus or ulcerative colitis, and diagnosis of microscopic inflammatory conditions such as collagenous or lymphocytic colitis. OCT could also be used to distinguish hyperplastic from adenomatous polyps. However at present OCT is not sufficient to replace histological diagnosis.

ADVANCES IN TISSUE ABLATION

Selective tissue ablation has clinical use in endoscopic hemostasis, palliation of malignant obstruction, and curative eradication of superficial malignant or pre-malignant lesions. Several methods for accomplishing this goal have been developed in recent years.

Argon Plasma Coagulation

Argon plasma coagulation (APC) is a novel technique that allows noncontact, tangential tissue ablation. Using APC, the space between the target tissue and probe is infused with ionized argon gas. The gas provides a medium through which electrical energy is transferred. APC has considerable potential for achieving hemostasis of lesions not associated with bowel wall thickening (e.g., superficial vascular ectasias) and ablation of superficial neoplastic and preneoplastic tissue.

Photodynamic Therapy

The theoretical success of photodynamic therapy (PDT) as a non-thermal, laser-assisted ablative technique is based on the ability of photosensitizers to produce cytotoxicity in the presence of oxygen after stimulation by light of an appropriate wavelength.The most commonly used photosensitizer is hematoporphyrin derivative, or dihematoporphyrin ether.

Visible red light of 630 nm is typically used because it both activates the photosensitizer and penetrates the tissue to a depth that produces the clinically desired effect.

PDT is an attractive alternative to standard endoscopic (thermal) laser therapy in Barrett's epithelium. The retention of the photosensitizer by malignant or dysplastic cells promotes selective destruction of the target tissue.

PDT provides equivalent palliation to Nd:YAG laser for malignant esophageal obstruction and may be easier to perform. In addition, it may be possible to use PDT with curative intent for superficial esophageal malignancies or dysplasia.

Barrett's Esophagus (BE)

The screening, prevention, and early detection of esophageal adenocarcinoma has become the focus of intense clinical and endoscopic research. Significant advances have been achieved in the screening and management of this problem.

Screening Recommendations

Endoscopy is advised for patients with a long-standing history of symptomatic gastroesophageal reflux, particularly for those patients over the age of 50 years. Approximately 8-20% of patients with these symptoms will be found to have Barrett's esophagus, and the annual incidence of adenocarcinoma in these patients is approximately 0.5-1%. Tissue staining techniques, as discussed above, may soon contribute to earlier detection of dysplasia and early cancer in patients with Barrett's esophagus.

Although the prevalence of dysplasia or cancer is greatest in patients with long-segment Barrett's esophagus (31%), the prevalence of cancer in patients with short-segment Barrett's esophagus (10%) and esophagogastric junction – specialized intestinal metaplasia (6.4%), is not negligible. In the light of these findings, serial screening in patients with lesser extent of Barrett's metaplasia may be cost effective.

Selective Ablation of Barrett's Esophagus

Once a high-risk lesion has been identified, the treatment required (e.g., esophagectomy) is highly invasive and associated with potentially significant post-operative morbidity. Another strategy currently undergoing critical assessment is the endoscopic elimination of regions of Barrett's mucosa. Preliminary studies have documented regeneration of squamous epithelium after ablation.

Despite encouraging endoscopic results most published reports have documented that foci of residual intestinal metaplasia persist beneath the regenerated squamous epithelial layer in about one third of cases.

Endoscopic Treatment of Gastroesophageal Reflux Disease (GERD)

This is one area where tremendous progress has been achieved. Over the past decade, there has been refinement of surgical techniques, and endo therapeutic options for GERD. The endoscopic sewing machines have undergone modifications that have made them user-friendly. The availability of polymers (Enterix) that solidify on injection into the muscular layer, thus increasing the sphincter tone has added one more dimension. The long term results with these techniques are comparable to those achieved by surgery, but are more expensive. Laparoscopic fundoplication will, however, remain the procedure of choice.

Palliation of Malignant Obstruction

Although criteria for surgical resection of gastrointestinal malignancies continue to evolve, a large percentage of such neoplasms are considered unresectable at the time of diagnosis. Luminal obstruction occurs commonly with esophageal carcinoma, distal gastric carcinoma, pancreatic carcinoma, and colorectal carcinoma. Effective endoscopic palliation can provide symptomatic relief without the need for a more invasive surgical approach. Approaches to achieving longer lasting relief have focused on either the removal of tissue (debulking) or the placement of expandable endoprostheses.

Tissue destruction can be performed by various methods including bipolar electrocautery, injection of absolute alcohol, laser photoablation, argon plasma coagulation (APC), and PDT. Endoscopically insertable endoprostheses were previously made of rigid materials of a fixed diameter that were forcibly advanced through the stenosis. The self-expanding metallic stents (SEMS) have changed the concept of palliation. These stents can be compressed to a narrow diameter, advanced through the stenosis, and then rapidly expanded to achieve luminal patency.

Expandable stents with longer delivery devices that allow deployment distal to the esophagus have been developed recently. Encouraging results show effective palliation of malignant pyloric, duodenal and colonic obstruction.

Endoscopy of the Small Intestine

The small intestine can be evaluated by endoscopy in three ways: push enteroscopy, operative endoscopy, or sonde (passive) enteroscopy. In push enteroscopy, the tip of a long endoscope (colonoscope, pediatric colonoscope, or specially designed enteroscope) is passed beyond the ligament of Treitz. An overtube may be used to facilitate passage into the small intestine by preventing looping of the enteroscope in the stomach. The push enteroscopic technique does not permit visualization of the distal portions of the small intestine.

In hospitals without the availability of push enteroscopy, the next best method for evaluating bleeding from the small intestine is Laparoscopic Assisted Pan Enteroscopy (LAPE), during which a surgeon advances the endoscope manually through the surgically exposed intestine. Unlike push or sonde enteroscopy (see below), intraoperative endoscopy permits visualization of the entire length of small bowel mucosa in the majority of cases. Intraoperative endoscopy may be performed using a standard gastroscope, colonoscope (pediatric, if available), or enteroscope.

Another method of small bowel endoscopy is sonde enteroscopy, during which the tip of a small caliber enteroscope is allowed to move along the small intestine passively. Unlike push enteroscopy, the sonde method allows visualization of the distal portions of the small intestine but offers little or no therapeutic capabilities. Indications for sonde enteroscopy are limited. Newer methods are being tried. Self propelled enteroscopes and double-balloon enteroscopes hold great promise.

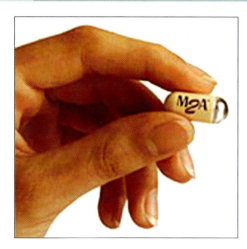

Fig. 43.1: Picture showing capsule endoscope

The wireless capsule endoscopy is an 11 x 26 mm capsule that encases a digital camera, light emitting diode, batteries and a transmitter. Images are taken twice per second and transmitted to a recording device worn on a belt by the patient. Thousands of images are transmitted to the recording device and then evaluated after the study is completed. This new technology has its greatest utility in the evaluation of obscure GI bleeding and disorders of small intestine like Crohn's disease and tumors (Fig. 43.1)

Colonoscopy and Sigmoidoscopy

Most of the advances in this area have been related to the understanding of the significance of small polyps in relation to the presence of colonic malignancies. Surveillance programs have also been fine tuned.

Screening Colonoscopy—Time to take a Deeper look

Because sigmoidoscopy fails to detect some significant neoplastic lesions (even in average-risk patients), what is a reasonable alternative? Recently published guidelines have suggested that screening colonoscopy may be an acceptable option. However, this approach has not yet been universally accepted; the reasons suggested include the perceived risk of complications with colonoscopy and the greater expense when compared with sigmoidoscopy.

As with endoscopy, radiologic technology continues to improve. The recent development of "virtual colonoscopy" (or more accurately computerized tomographic colography) is a case in point. Virtual colonoscopy involves the computerized reconstruction of images obtained via high-resolution computerized tomographic imaging. The resulting images are displayed on a video monitor as though viewed through an imaginary (virtual) colonoscope.

Pancreaticobiliary Endoscopy

The most significant advances in pancreaticobiliary endoscopy made in the past few years have been related to improved outcomes rather than advances in technology. Although new methods have been applied to the management of biliary obstruction and unique biodegradable expandable stents are on the horizon, the most clinically important advances involve the recognition of at least some of the causes of endoscopic retrograde cholangiopancreatography (ERCP)-related complications (Figs 43.2 and 43.3)

Predictors of ERCP-related Complications

ERCP is an extremely useful modality, but it is clearly not without risk. Expected complications vary depending on the diagnostic indication and intervention performed. The most common complications include pancreatitis, bleeding and infection. Fatal complications are rare but can occur. A recent large-scale multicenter prospective cohort study evaluated numerous proposed risk factors for complications of endoscopic sphincterotomy and identified the following as independently significant-suspected sphincter of Oddi dysfunction, cirrhosis, difficult bile duct cannulation, use of precut (access) sphincterotomy and use of combined percutaneous and endoscopic technique.

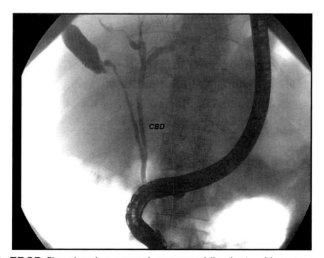

Fig. 43.2: ERCP film showing normal common bile duct, with common hepatic duct and long cystic duct

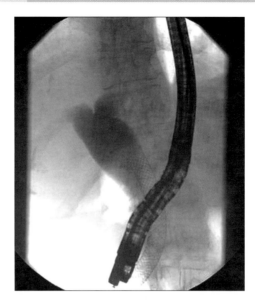

Fig. 43.3: ERCP film showing biliary metal prosthesis in situ

Endoscopic Necrosectomy

The role of endoscopic cystogastrostomy in the management of pancreatic pseudocysts is well established. The ability to make use of the cystogastric stoma to enter the pseudocyst and excise/extract the necrotic material from the pseudocyst (endoscopic necrosectomy) promises to be an exciting therapeutic option in the management of pancreatic pseudocysts.

Endoscopic Ampullectomy

Patients with an adenoma in the periampullary region, or a small periampullary growth in a patient who is at high risk for surgery, can now be offered endoscopic resection of the ampulla. The role of the procedure is, however, quite limited, and should be done only by endoscopists with great expertise.

Advances in Endoscopic Ultrasonography (EUS)

EUS has become an important adjunct to standard endoscopy and other traditional imaging techniques. Published reports have continued to validate the clinical use of EUS in the evaluation of known or suspected pancreatic adenocarcinoma and the diagnosis of gastrointestinal subepithelial tumors. New applications of EUS include the evaluation of suspected choledocholithiasis, staging of non-small cell lung cancer, and diagnosis of chronic pancreatitis. Additionally, EUS-guided tissue sampling has greatly expanded the diagnostic use of this technology. Endosonography can provide useful clinical information not available by other imaging modalities. Perhaps the most exciting development in EUS has been its evolution from a simply diagnostic modality to a useful therapeutic tool.

The Evolving role of EUS in Esophageal Cancer

Esophageal cancer staging is determined according to the TNM classification system by evaluating the depth of penetration of neoplastic cells through the Esophageal wall (T), the presence or absence of metastatic lymph nodes (N), or the presence or absence of distant metastases (M). Staging has been shown to be one of the most accurate predictors of clinical outcome and has been essential in determining optimal treatment of some cancers. EUS is the only currently available imaging technology that allows visualization of the distinct histological tissue layers of the esophageal wall.

Evaluation of Suspected Choledocholithiasis

Neither transabdominal ultrasonography nor computerized tomography scan can reliably exclude the presence of choledocholithiasis. EUS is well-suited to the evaluation of suspected common bile duct stones because EUS can image the common bile duct as it passes posterior to the duodenal bulb and there is little, if any, risk of pancreatitis. Recent data have shown that EUS is equivalent to ERCP with regard to sensitivity and overall accuracy for the detection of common duct stones but that EUS is more cost-effective than ERCP for patients with a low to intermediate likelihood of stones (Fig. 43. 4)

In addition to EUS, magnetic resonance cholangiopancreatography (MRCP) has recently been shown to be useful for the exclusion of choledocholithiasis. EUS and MRCP seem to be approximately equivalent in terms of sensitivity and accuracy, but MRCP has the advantage of being less invasive than EUS.

EUS for the Diagnosis of Suspected Chronic Pancreatitis

EUS provides extremely detailed imaging of the pancreatic parenchyma and thus has some use in the evaluation of patients in whom chronic pancreatitis is clinically suspected. Several studies have recently shown that, using a variety of endosonographic criteria, EUS can reliably identify patients with early changes of chronic pancreatitis.

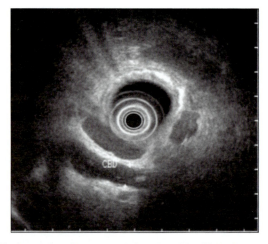

Fig. 43.4: Endoscopic ultrasonography showing dilated common bile duct with calculus in it

EUS-guided Celiac Neurolysis

In the majority of cases, adenocarcinoma of the pancreas will be unresectable at diagnosis. In these patients, the clinical focus changes from potential cure to effective palliation. Although the celiac ganglia are not directly visualized via EUS (or any other imaging modality), they are known to be located adjacent to the lateral surfaces of the celiac axis. This site is readily accessible to needle puncture under endosonographic guidance because the needle path required is quite short (1-2 cm) and generally free of intervening structures. In addition, EUS provides real-time imaging of the needle tip and adjacent vascular structures, making inadvertent vascular trauma unlikely. After needle puncture, a variety of substances may be injected, depending on the clinical situation. In general, performing a celiac plexus block adds less than 5 minutes to the examination time.

Recent data suggest that EUS-guided celiac block is safe and provides effective, long-lasting pain relief for a majority of patients with pain caused by malignancy. EUS-guided celiac block may provide effective pain relief for some patients with chronic pancreatitis, although the frequency of effective relief is lower than that for malignancy and the relief rarely persists more than 6 months.

SUMMARY

Advances in gastrointestinal endoscopy have altered the practice of clinical gastroenterology and, we anticipate, will continue to do so into the next millennium. At the turn of the century, unprecedented developments in endoscopic technology suggest that even greater achievements in diagnosing and treating gastrointestinal disorders are possible. The future of therapeutic endoscopy is without limits. Possibilities in the not-too-distant future include endoscopic closure of perforations, colonoscopic resection of small colonic growths and transnasal percutaneous endoscopic gastrostomy. The availability of such novel procedures, however, needs to be greeted with a careful understanding of the merits and demerits of each. The success of an endoscopist and of an endoscopic procedure lies not in overt aggression, but in cautious optimism.

SUGGESTED READING

1. Novel endoscopic therapies for gastrointestinal malignancies: endoscopic mucosal resection and endoscopic ablation. Med Clin North Am 2005 Jan; 89(1):159-86, ix.
2. Review article: The advent of capsule endoscopy – a not-so-futuristic approach to obscure gastrointestinal bleeding. Lewis B, Goldfarb N Aliment Pharmacol Ther (England), May 1 2003; 17(9) p1085-96.
3. Optional biopsies, "bioendoscopy", and why the sky is blue: the coming revolution in gastrointestinal imaging. Pasricha PJ, Motamedi M . Gastroenterology (United States), Feb 2002; 122(2) p571-5.
4. Endoscopic fluorescence spectroscopic imaging in the gastrointestinal tract. Gastrointest Endosc Clin N Am 2004 Jul;14(3):487-505, viii-ix.
5. Small-bowel endoscopy. Rossini FP; Pennazio M Endoscopy 2002 Jan;34(1): 13-20.
6. Perspectives of chromo and magnifying endoscopy: how, how much, when, and whom should we stain? Kiesslich R; Jung M; Di Sario JA; Galle PR; Neurath MF J Clin Gastroenterol 2004 Jan; 38(1):7-13.

44

Shanmuga Sundaram P
Padma S Sundaram

Radionuclides in Gastroenterology

INTRODUCTION

Nuclear Medicine diagnostic techniques involve use of gamma emitting radioactive isotopes, which are administered parenterally or orally to the patient. Radioisotopes tagged with organ specific pharmaceuticals, when administered, emit gamma rays, so that the sodium iodide crystal of gamma camera can perceive this, as scintillations. The scintillations (photons) get converted to electrical signals thereby forming an image. Most commonly used radioisotope is technetium (^{99m} Tc), having a physical half-life of six hours.

The basis of nuclear medicine investigations is purely physiological; hence the functional de-arrangements are detected much earlier when compared to anatomical imaging modalities. This is best suited for the study of gastrointestinal disorders, which will be discussed briefly in this chapter.

Nuclear Gastrointestinal Procedures

1. Esophageal transit study
2. Gastroesophageal reflux scintigraphy – Milk scan
3. Gastric motility scintigraphy
4. Gastrointestinal bleed scintigraphy
5. Ectopic gastric mucosa (Meckel's diverticulum) scintigraphy
6. Intestinal motility studies
7. Breath test – H.pylori infection detection
8. Schilling test – Vitamin B12 deficiency.

Nuclear Hepatobiliary and Liver Reticuloendothelial System Imaging

1. Hepatobiliary scintigraphy
2. RBC blood pool liver scintigraphy
3. Reticuloendothelial sulfur colloid scintigraphy of liver.

Esophageal Motility Studies

Esophageal scintigraphy can distinguish organic from nonorganic diseases and it is possible to quantitate esophageal transit. After an overnight fast, around 100 – 200 uCi of technetium labelled sulfur colloid or DTPA in 15 ml of water is ingested in a single swallow and subject continues to "dry swallow" at 15 seconds interval for a period of 10 minutes. Images are recorded in a dynamic fashion and analyzed. This procedure is easy to perform and has a good patient tolerance. Indications are achalasia, scleroderma and diffuse esophageal spasm.

Using esophageal manometry as the gold standard, sensitivities and specificities up to 95% and 96% respectively have been reported. Some investigators found esophageal scintigraphy to be more sensitive than esophageal manometry and contrast radiology.

Gastroesophageal (GE) Reflux Scintigraphy (Milk scan)

This procedure is performed in children having symptoms such as failure to thrive, and recurrent chest infections where gastroesophageal reflux is suspected. It is also indicated in adults having heartburn and regurgitation symptoms. The tracer (i.e. ^{99m}Tc labeled sufhur colloid/DTPA) is instilled into stomach through a nasogastric tube in case of children or through a capsule along with an acidified juice (300 ml) in case of adults. Any reflux of tracer into esophagus is considered as a positive study for GE reflux and in case of adults, abdominal binders are used to increase the intra abdominal pressure during the study. When compared to studies like acid reflux testing and esophageal manometry, this procedure is noninvasive and better tolerated.

Gastric Emptying Studies

Scintigraphy studies are performed to evaluate gastric emptying patterns for solids and liquids separately as they empty at different rates and fashion. While liquids empty in an exponential fashion, solids empty in linear fashion. Scintigraphy with a radiolabeled test meal represents the gold standard for evaluating solid gastric emptying. Preparation of a standardized meal labeled with radioactive tracer mimicking solid food is important to correctly interpret gastric emptying studies. Patients with dyspepsia, postgastrectomy dumping, gastric dysfunction as seen in diabetes, parkinsonism, multiple sclerosis and supranuclear palsy, and myasthenia gravis are some of the ideal candidates for this test.

Many centers prefer to do only a solid phase study. Although many varieties of labeled food are described, for the Indian setup either scrambled, cooked egg labeled with ^{99m}Tc Sulfur colloid or labeled mashed potatoes/bread and jam (for vegetarians) is preferred. For the liquid phase of study 10% dextrose labeled with ^{99m}Tc DTPA can be used. After an overnight fast and administration of labeled meal, dynamic imaging is done and an emptying curve is generated so that t ½ value (i.e. emptying time) in minutes can be obtained.

Meckel's diverticulum Imaging (for Ectopic Gastric Mucosa)

Meckel's scintigraphy is based on identification of ectopic gastric mucosa that is present in Meckel's diverticulum. When ^{99m}Tc–pertechnetate is injected intravenously it accumulates within the mucus producing cells of ectopic gastric mucosa as in normal gastric mucosa. An area of at least 2 cm^2 of mucosa is necessary for successful scintigraphic visualization. Sensitivity over 80-90% in children has been reported. Pharmacological interventions with H$_2$ receptor antagonists, pentagastrin or glucagon have been used to enhance the sensitivity. Any cause of focal hyperemia, renal pelvis activity, or uterine blush can cause false positive scans (Fig. 44.1)

GI Bleed Scintigraphy

Scintigraphy is the preferred non-invasive diagnostic procedure in evaluation of lower GI bleeding, which can be performed even in acutely ill patients and requires no real patient preparation.

It can aid in timing the angiographies, and scans the entire intestinal loops. While ^{99m} Tc labeled RBC scintigraphy is the preferred procedure, sulfur colloid scintigraphy also can be performed. In case of labeled RBC scintigraphy the extravasated technetium tagged RBCs in the lumen of intestinal loops are imaged. This procedure can detect bleeding rates as low as 0.1 to 0.5 cc/min and a sensitivity of 90% and specificity of 95% have been reported. Delayed imaging is recommended to identify the correct site of bleeding. Scintigraphy is about 10 times more sensitive than angiography for the detection of GI bleeding. The main advantage of using ^{99m}Tc labeled RBCs is that the agent remains in the intravascular space for 24 hours, thus it is excellent for imaging intermittent or slow GI bleeds.

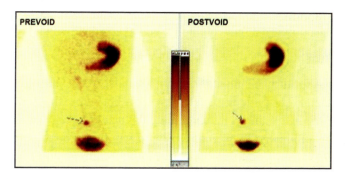

Fig. 44.1: Meckel's scan using ^{99m}Technetium labelled pertechnate showing ectopic gastric mucosa suggestive of Meckel's diverticulum

Small and Large Intestinal Motility Studies

Assessment of colonic transit has traditionally been performed using radiological marker techniques although recently radionuclide techniques have become important. Confirmation of the presence and knowledge of severity of slow colonic transit can help to differentiate simple, normal-transit constipation from more severe idiopathic slow –transit constipation and obstructive defecation.

[111]Indium labeled cation—exchange resin particles are used as oral tracers. Imaging may have to be extended for three days in constipated patients. Small intestinal transit studies use [99m] Tc DTPA or sulfur colloid or I-131 fibre as radiopharmaceuticals. Imaging is performed in different positions ranging from supine to 45 degree to upright posture and may have to be acquired continuously for three hours.

Breath Test for Gastric H.pylori Infection

Presence of active *Helicobacter pylori* infection in gastric mucosa can be diagnosed non-invasively with C-14 urea breath test. It is based on the detection of enzyme urease, produced by *H. pylori*. Since urease is not present in normal human tissues, and since other urease-producing bacteria do not colonize the stomach, presence of urease in stomach can be equated with *H.pylori* infection.In presence of urease, orally administered C-14 urea will be hydrolyzed into ammonia and $^{14}CO_2$. $^{14}CO_2$ is absorbed into circulation and exhaled by the lungs. Presence of a significant amount of $^{14}CO_2$ in the exhaled breath indicates active infection.It consists of oral administration of C-14 urea, followed by sampling of exhaled breath at timed intervals. Breath samples are then analyzed in a liquid scintillation counter.This procedure is now extensively used to detect presence of *H.pylori* in the stomach and also to document its eradication post therapy (after one month) .

Schilling Test

This is used to study GI absorption of vitamin B_{12}, which requires presence of intrinsic factor. The patients usually fast the night before the test, and 0.5 μg of Cobalt 57-labeled vitamin B_{12} containing 0.5 uCi is then given orally. This is immediately followed by intramuscular injection of 1000 mg of non-labelled vitamin B_{12} (given to saturate liver and blood binding sites, thus promoting urinary excretion of labeled vitamin B_{12}). A urine sample collected after 24 hrs is assessed for the presence of labeled B_{12} (normal value is in the range of 10-40%

of administered dose). Values lower than 7% indicate the presence of pernicious anemia and malabsorption. To differentiate these two, a 2-stage schilling test is required (labeled B_{12} and intrinsic factor).

Liver/Spleen Imaging

Although space occupying lesions of liver are now preferentially evaluated by CT imaging, for diffuse liver dysfunction colloid liver scintigraphy is preferred. The physiological principle behind this imaging is phagocytosis of colloid particles by reticuloendothelial system. Radiocolloids like ^{99m} Tc Sufur colloid (or ^{99m} Tc Phytate) are injected intravenously, which is trapped by reticulo-endothelial cells in liver, spleen and marrow. Normally marrow is not imaged, but in the presence of severe liver dysfunction as in cirrhosis of liver with portal hypertension, bone marrow will be visualized. It is possible to quantitate the shift in colloid uptake from liver to spleen and bone marrow (colloid shift). This procedure is very sensitive in detecting and following up early hepatocellular dysfunction due to diabetes, alchoholic liver disease and fatty infiltration.

Another condition in which colloid liver scan is diagnostic is hepatic vein occlusive disease (Budd Chiari syndrome). The scan shows classical findings of a "hot spot" (i.e. increased tracer uptake) in the caudate lobe due to collateral venous return along the obliterated umbilical vein facilitating direct venous drainage of the caudate lobe into the inferior vena cava with relatively decreased colloid distribution throughout the rest of the liver. While space occupying lesions of the liver like primary hepatoma, focal nodular hyperplasia, hepatic adenoma, abscess, cyst, hemangiomar etc. may all show a non specific finding (cold defect) in liver colloid scintigraphy, a ^{99m}Tc labeled RBC blood pool liver imaging is ideal for evaluating liver hemangioma. Classically a focal cold defect in liver colloid scan shows good RBC tracer accumulation in a positive case of hemangioma.

Hepatobiliary Scintigraphy

While colloid liver scintigraphy depicts the distribution of reticuloendothelial system component of liver, a hepatobiliary scintigraphy performed with ^{99m}Tc Imino Diacetic Acid (IDA compounds) traces the biliary tree. IDA compounds are cleared from circulation by hepatic cells and secreted into bile by carrier mechanisms in the same way as bilirubin. Early images demonstrate the hepatic parenchyma and delayed images show the progression of tracer into hepatic outflow tract. Although a number of IDA compounds are available for this imaging, the most preferred one is being Mebrofenin as its uptake is optimum even in presence of high serum bilirubin levels.

Hepatobiliary scintigraphy is indicated in the diagnosis of acute or chronic cholecystitis, gallbladder dyskinesia, postoperative biliary leak, choledochal cyst and in the evaluation of neonatal hyperbilirubinemia. Hepatobiliary scintigraphy is best suited for post-liver transplant evaluation also.

Acute Cholecystitis

If one were to pathologically examine all acutely inflamed gallbladders, over 95% would have obstructed cystic duct. In this group of patients IDA compounds secreted into bile cannot enter the inflamed gallbladder. This provides the theoretical basis for this diagnostic procedure. Visualization of biliary system with non-visualization of gallbladder even at 4 hours is considered diagnostic of acute cholecystitis. Intravenous morphine augmentation can be performed to shorten the duration of the cholescintigraphy examination. Sensitivity and specificity for diagnosing acute cholecystitis by this modality is greater than 95% and 98% respectively. Negative predictive value of a normal exam (visualization of gall bladder within 1 hour) in excluding acute cholecystitis is greater than 99%.

Chronic Cholecystitis

The majority of patients with chronic cholecystitis exhibit visualization of the gallbladder (85-90%) albeit delayed. Delayed visualization of the gallbladder (between 1 to 4 hours of the exam) is considered fairly characteristic for chronic cholecystitis, but delayed visualization can also be seen in a very small number of patients with acute cholecystitis. The longer the delay in visualization, the higher the correlation with chronic cholecystitis.

Gallbladder Dyskinesia

Patients suspected to have gallbladder dyskinesia also can be evaluated by hepatobiliary scintigraphy. Patients with chronically inflamed, partially obstructed, or functionally impaired gallbladders (gallbladder dyskinesia) will demonstrate an abnormal gallbladder ejection response to cholecystokinin (CCK). An abnormal gallbladder ejection fraction is considered when less than 35% is ejected and is not affected by age. To determine gallbladder ejection fraction, IV infusion of sincalide (0.02 µg/kg) slowly over 3-5 min can be done and if it is not available it can be performed with a fatty meal stimulus.

Neonatal Hyperbilirubinemia

Although there are several causes of hyperbilirubinemia in the newborn, it is very important to identify biliary atresia, as early surgery is the only therapeutic option for this condition. Hepatobiliary scintigraphy is a good, non-invasive screening procedure to exclude biliary atresia. A hepatobiliary scan with ^{99m}Tc Mebrofenin showing good progression of tracer from CBD into intestinal loops virtually excludes biliary atresia. If there is non-progression of tracer into intestinal loops even in delayed images both neonatal hepatitis and biliary atresia are to be considered and only a liver biopsy can resolve this issue. It is preferable to pretreat these babies with 0.5 mg/kg body weight phenobarbitone orally at least for 5 to 7 days prior to hepatobiliary imaging.

Sensitivity and specificity of this test is 97-100% and 82-94%, with an accuracy of 91%. In addition to biliary atresia, other anomalies of biliary tract such as choledochal cysts, and Caroli's disease can also be evaluated by hepatobiliary scintigraphy.

Hepatobiliary scintigraphy is also used to assess the biliary enteric patency in postoperative cases. Dilated intrahepatic ducts and delayed bowel visualization can point to partial obstruction at anastomotic site. The same way any biliary leak also can be evaluated. Serial biliary scintigraphy has a role in evaluating postoperative biliary tract complications and in assessing rejection of liver transplants.

Oncological Applications

Positron Emission Tomography (PET Scan) with ^{18}F Fluro-deoxy glucose (FDG) is extensively used in identification of secondary deposits of gastrointestinal primary tumors thereby aiding in management. Monoclonal antibody imaging such as ^{99m}Tc and ^{111}In labeled anti carcino-embryonic antigen (CEA) antibody scintigraphy are used in follow-up of colonic cancers. Neuroendocrine tumors of gastrointestinal tract can be assessed by ^{111}Indium labelled octreotide scintigraphy.

SUGGESTED READING

1. Essentials of Nuclear Medicine Imaging, 4th edition, Mettler, and Guiberteau, (Eds.) WB Saunders Company, Philadelphia 1998.
2. Handbooks in Radiology: Nuclear medicine, 1©st edition, Fredrick L Datz, Year Book Medical Publishers Inc. Chicago 1988.
3. Nuclear Medicine in clinical diagnosis and treatment, 2nd edition, P C Murray P J Ell, Churchill Livingstone, Edinburgh 1998.
4. Diagnostic Nuclear Medicine by Martin P Sandler, 3rd edition, Lippincott Williams and Wilkins 1996.
5. Diagnostic Nuclear Medicine, 2nd Edition (Eds.) A Gottschalk, PB Hoffer, EJ Potchen, Williams and Wilkins 1998.
6. Clinical Nuclear Medicine, 2nd Edition, MN Maisey, KE Britton DL Gilday (Eds.): Lippincott; Philadelphia, PA 1991.

45

Vinod Kumar V

The Gastroenterologist and the Internet

INTRODUCTION

Internet is the most economical, vast and convenient resource for current medical information offering physicians, medical students and patients up-to-date medical information at the click of a mouse. Internet offers an ideal tool for medical literature search, physician education, patient education and telemedicine.

The number of medical sites on the internet is growing everyday. The purpose of this article is to highlight what is there on the net specifically for the person interested in gastroenterology. The intention is not to review each and every site in detail but to present an overview of sites useful to a gastroenterologist.

Problems with Medical Information on the Internet

One of the biggest problems with the internet is that anybody with access to a computer and the net can put up any information on the net claiming authenticity irrespective of qualifications and credibility. So the challenge today is to assess how credible a piece of medical information found on the internet is. There have been several attempts to standardize the requirements for a credible medical web site and assign a credibility rating both internally and externally. One of the easier ways to ensure this is by checking whether the site fulfills the following criteria:

1. Information is current and frequently updated
2. Reference sited
3. Purpose and intentions of the site are clearly stated
4. Disclosures of the sponsors
5. Interests are declared and there is no conflict of interest
6. Contents are balanced with both advantages and disadvantages
7. Level of evidence is clearly stated
8. Site is backed by renowned faculty.

Internet Sites for the Gastroenterologist

There are an enormous number of medical sites, both general and specialty related, for the gastroenterologist. In general, these can be subdivided into the following categories:

1. Medical resources sites
2. Societies and organizations
3. e-journals and e-books

4. Imaging
5. Medical search engines
6. Medical libraries
7. Industry

MEDICAL RESOURCE SITES

There are sites which cater specifically both to the gastroenterologist and to the generalist. Most of these sites have common aims and pattern, the main one being to educate the physician interested in gastroenterology with current medical information and practice guidelines. In addition, most sites have online continuous medical education (CME) with assigned credits, virtual patient simulated interactive cases, summaries of recent important conferences and important journal articles and access to a list of important journals in the specialty. Some sites like Medscape Gastroenterology are free (requiring free registration) but few others require paid subscription. Most of these sites also have a discussion group where one can interact with renowned global faculty in solving a difficult to manage situation or get a second opinion. Readers are requested to go through these sites to get more details.

Some of the important sites are the following:

Gastrohep.com-www.gastrohep.com: This is a paid site for accessing all the features. One of the best sites in gastroenterology backed by a renowned faculty with excellent features for both recent updates and patient management. The site offers a good database of endoscopic, radiological and pathological images of interesting cases to which any user of the site can contribute by uploading data.

Medscape Gastroenterology—www.medscape.com/gastroenterology: The specialty section of gastroenterology is an excellent site for information on gastrointestinal and liver diseases. There are other specialties as well as general medicine sections, which makes it a very comprehensive site for any physician. This is a free site requiring only a registration for most of the features except a few like access to online books in the library section.

emedicine—www.emedicine.com: Another good site offering not only gastroenterology, but lots of other specialty information as well. Most of the areas are accessible on free registration, but some features need payment like the section, which can be downloaded on to your PDA for use on the move and CME.

Gastrosource—www.gastrosource.com: A reasonably good site on topics in gastroenterology requiring only free registration. As the site is maintained by a pharmaceutical company with commercial interest in the specialty the drawback is that most of the topics covered are confined to a narrow area where the company has obvious commercial interest.

ORGANIZATIONS AND SOCIETIES

World Gastroenterology Organization – OMGE—www.omge.org: This is the official site of global gastroenterology organization first formed in 1964 under the leadership of Dr. Henry Bockus with an aim to promote education and training in gastroenterology, hepatology, endoscopy and GI Surgery. This site offers excellent resources on practice guidelines, conference information and training schemes. The section Gastropro offers excellent multimedia educational programmes on endoscopy, and various other GI diseases.

World Health Organization (WHO)—www.who.int/en: Official site of WHO with links to numerous other WHO sites. Provides global information on various diseases, country wise statistics, WHO publications and research tools.

Cochrane Foundation-www.cochrane.org: Good site for evidence based approach.

Indian Society of Gastroenterology—www.isg.org: Official website of Indian society of Gastroenterology. Contains information about organization, membership and access to Indian Journal of Gastroenterology and Pubmed.

American College of Gastroenterology—www.acg.gi.org: Some areas are unrestricted but others require ACG membership to access including the official journal American Journal of Gastroenterology.

Other Important Sites

- American Gastroenterology Association-AGA-www.gastro.org
- Canadian Gastroenterology Association-www.gi.ucalgary.ca
- British Society of Gastroenterology—www.bsg.org.uk

    In addition, most of the major endoscopic societies, liver associations, and major university gastroenterology departments have very good websites with updated GI information.

e-journals and e-books

Almost all of the major gastroenterology and general medical journals have online editions. Some like NEJM, BMJ have full free access but others have access to abstract only and the rest are fully paid either individually or by institution. More information about the journals can be obtained from www.omed.org/links.htm.

Imaging Sites

There are a large number of sites providing endoscopy, pathology and radiology images of interest to a gastroenterologist functioning as online atlas. These images can be downloaded for individual use and teaching. Some important sites are GastroLab (www.gastrolab.net), www.gastrointestinalatlas.com, http://medpics.findlaw.com, gastrosource.com, omge.org and gastrohep.com.

Medical Search Engines

Rather than using general search engines like Google, which throws up a lot of unreliable sites it may be better to use pre filtered medical search engines for specificity. "Garbage in Garbage out" holds true in computer search. The result of the search is directly related to how you frame your search question.

Specific pre-filtered search engines: The largest online medical database is medline. The specific search engines which retrieve information form medline are Pubmed maintained by National Library of Medicine (NLM) which is free, OVID which requires subscription, OMNI database of UK and Medscape's medline search facility. The advantage is that these sites throw up only relevant sites and give a grading of relevance in relation to search topic. For focused clinical queries it may be better to start with a "pre filtered" evidence based medicine resources such as best medicine, The Cochrane Library or Clinical Evidence.

The original MEDLINE database resides in a new access mechanism called **PubMed** (http://www.ncbi.nlm.nih.gov/PubMed), which was developed by the National Center for Biotechnology Information (NCBI). It is entirely free of charge and it is also one of the best search engines around.More details regarding how to effectively use pubmed search facility can be obtained from the excellent multimedia tutorial at http://www.ncbi.nlm.nih.gov/entrez/query.fcgi.

Tips for Effective Search

For effective search, the following principles may help:

1. Identify the database and search engine for the search
2. Proper framing of the search query. May need breaking up into simpler concepts and combining using Boolean terms. Use of inbuilt filters helps in improving specificity.
3. Knowledge about MeSH terminology (**MeSH** is NLM's controlled vocabulary used for indexing articles for MEDLINE/PubMed. MeSH terminology provides a consistent way to retrieve information that may use different terminology for the same concepts.
4. Use of Boolean terms like AND, OR and NOT

For details regarding e search strategies readers are requested to go through online tutorials by following the links like http://denison.uchsc.edu/tutorial/index.html for OVID tutorials or Pubmed tutorial at National Library of Medicine or online tutorial at http://www.tilburguniversity.nl/services/library/instruction/www/onlinecourse/ by Peter van Tilburg and Roger Schmitz, librarians at Tilburg University in the Netherlands.

Internet and Telemedicine

In most simple terms telemedicine is clinical care at a distance enabled by information technology (IT) and telecommunication. It is used for consultations, second opinion, diagnosis, clinical care, treatment, surgery, CME and research. Tele-gastroenterology is in a developing stage lagging behind other specialties like dermatology, radiology, pathology and psychiatry. With the availability of increasing bandwidth at cheaper rates internet based telemedicine is becoming more efficient, cost-effective and practical. This assumes great importance in India in bridging the divide between rural and urban population. The simplest internet tool for telemedicine is the email which can serve as an effective medium of information exchange between doctors and patients and between doctors themselves either directly or through online mailing groups or discussion groups with interest in a specific area. But this had thrown up new challenges like licensing of doctors between countries, malpractice litigation, liability and confidentiality of information exchanged.

CONCLUSION

Internet is aptly called an information super highway but it also has a lot of potholes and oil spills which one has to avoid carefully to reach the destination safely and efficiently. If used optimally it is a powerful and cost effective tool for improving health care and health related knowledge and gastroenterology is certainly no exception. In short, how effectively the power of Internet can be harnessed by a health professional for optimum use can be learned by an excellent online tutorial at http://www.vts.rdn.ac.uk/tutorial/medic.

SUGGESTED READING

1. Medical Informatics-A Primer—Dr. Mohan Bansal
2. GI Resources on the internet—Cohen. L. B—Am J Gastroenterology-March 2000
3. Gastroenterology on the Internet—1 to 5—Ramesh.H-Indian J of Gastroenterology-Jn 2000-Jan 2001
4. OMED—http://www.omed.org/links.htm-Medical Bookmarks for the Gastroenterologist
5. Hand book of medical informatics—J.H Van Bmmel, M.A. Muesen—http://www.mieur.nl/mihandbook/r_3_3/handbook/home.htm
6. A Students Guide to Medical Literature-http://denison.uchsc.edu/SG/main.html
7. Medical Literature retrieval on the internet-Renato M.E.Sabatini Phd-Intermedic-Sept-Oct 1997—http://www.epub.org.br/intermedic/n0102/sum0102_e.htm
8. E Europe 2002-quality criteria for medical web sites
9. All the websites given on OMED-http://www.omed.org/links.htm

46

Madhu S Menon

Normal Values in
Gastroenterology

INTRODUCTION

Laboratory values in the medical literature are referred to as 'normal reference values' or 'reference values'. Several variables are seen to affect the laboratory test results. Besides the obvious differences in the specific technique and methods of diagnosis, many other variables can influence the laboratory reference values. Age and sex are the chief physiological factors that change the 'norms'. Pregnancy as well as other physiologic factors such as diet, time of day, activity level and stress may alter what is 'normal' for a test.

The normal ranges are determined by testing a large sample of healthy people and then analyzing the results by statistical methods. From the wide variety of investigations and procedures that are currently available for the diagnosis of gastrointestinal and hepatobiliary disease, a list of normal reference values is made and appended below.

Liver Function Studies

Total bilirubin	0.1 – 1.0 mg/dl
Conjugated bilirubin	0 – 0.2 mg/dl
SGPT (ALT) Male	5 – 41 IU/L
SGPT (ALT) Female	5 – 31 IU/L
ALP Male	45 – 115 IU/L
ALP Female	30 – 100 IU/L
Serum Protein	5.5 – 8.0 gm%
Serum Albumin	3.5 – 5.5 gm%
Serum Globulin	1.8 – 3.5 gm%
A/G Ratio	> 1.5
GGT Male	11 – 50 U/L
GGT Female	7 – 32 U/L
Serum Ammonia	35 – 65 mg/dl

Pancreatic Function Studies

Serum Amylase	53 – 123 U/L
Urinary Amylase	4 – 400 U/L
Serum Lipase	3 – 19 U/dl
Fecal Elastase	> 190 µg/gm
Fecal Chymotrypsin	6 units/gm

Tumor Markers

AFP	< 12.8 IU/ml
CEA	0 – 3.4 ng/ml
CA19-9	0 – 37 U/ml
CA125	< 35 U/ml

Iron Studies

Serum Iron	30 – 160 µg/dL
Serum Ferritin	20 – 400 ng/mL
Total Iron binding capacity	250 – 410 µg/dL
Transferrin saturate	20 – 45%

Absorption Studies

24 hour stool fat	< 7gm/24 hour
D-Xylose test	> 20% ingested dose in 5 hours of urine
Schilling test [24 hour urinary excretion of Vit B$_{12}$]	10 – 40%

Gastric Function Studies

Serum Gastrin	50 – 100 pg/ml
Saline load test (750 ml saline infusion over 3-5 minutes)	Normally return of less than 300 ml is suggestive of and above 400 ml is diagnostic of gastric retention

Other Normal Values

Serum Ceruloplasmin	27 – 37 mg/dL
Serum Na$^+$	135 – 145 mEq/L
Serum K$^+$	3.5 – 5.0 mEq/L
Serum Cl$^•$	100 – 108 mEq/L
Serum HCO$_3$	24 – 30 mEq/L
Serum Calcium	8.5 – 10.5 mg/dL
Serum Creatinine Male	0.6 – 1.5 mg/dL
Serum Creatinine Female	0.6 – 1.1 mg/dL
BUN	8 – 25 mg/dL
Serum Phosphorus.	2.6 – 4.5 mg/dL
Serum Copper	114 ± 14 g/dL

Serum folic acid	3.1 – 17.5 ng/ml
Serum Vit B$_{12}$	200 – 600 pg/mL
Ascitic fluid WBC	< 250 cumm
Stool bulk Wet weight	60 – 250 g/day
Dry weight	20 – 60 g/day

Index